EDUCATIONAL PSYCHOLOGY

EDUCATIONAL PSYCHOLOGY

L.S. Vygotsky

Introduction by V.V. Davydov
Translated by Robert Silverman

S^{t}L

St. Lucie Press
Boca Raton, Florida

Library of Congress Cataloging-in-Publication Data

Catalog record is available from the Library of Congress

Visit the CRC Press Web site at www.crcpress.com

© 1997 by CRC Press LLC
St. Lucie Press is an imprint of CRC Press LLC

Published originally in 1926, in Russian
This volume is published as the result of an agreement originally made
with the Copyright Agency of the USSR (VAAP)
No claim to original U.S. Government works
International Standard Book Number 1-878205-15-3
Library of Congress Card Number 91-70614
Printed in the United States of America   2 3 4 5 6 7 8 9 0
Printed on acid-free paper

The development of our reactions is our life history...
If we were to seek an expression for the most important truth that modern
psychology can furnish the teacher, it would be simply this:
the pupil is a reaction apparatus.

Hugo Münsterberg

Table of Contents

EDITOR'S NOTE

The present volume consists of lectures delivered by Vygotsky at Gomel's teacher's college in the years between 1921 and 1923. It is thought that Vygotsky intended the book as an introductory psychology text for a new generation of Soviet teachers, who were to replace the pre-Revolutionary educational establishment. It is hoped that the publication of this book will reveal the unanswered questions posed by the book; at times it expresses views that are incompatible with other things he wrote and believed at the time.

It has been said that as a rule, the translation and publication of the works of a scholar such as Vygotsky who lived and worked over fifty years ago would be carried out because the ideas presented are seen in retrospect as being "ahead of their time." But in many ways, our publication of Vygotsky's work, as well as that of other publishers, is motivated by entirely different concerns. Our motivation follows the conviction of Vygotsky's students in the Soviet Union and in the West that his ideas and insights are in many respects considerably ahead of our time, and by the conviction that his influence on the development of psychology and the social sciences has not been nearly as considerable as it must be.

In translating the book we wished to leave the author's emphasis on certain words as Vygotsky wrote. Hence, the italicized words in the book were emphasized by the author in the original. Also, while we have "modernized" (or westernized) Russian spellings such as the ii-ending to y (such as Vygotsky rather than Vygotskii and Bernstein rather than Bernshtein in the front matter to this book, we have retained the original spellings used by the author in his text.

All notes at the end of the chapters are those of the translator, except for the notes at the end of Chapter 13, which are Vygotsky's own notes. Whenever possible, we have attempted to locate original sources such as book and year of publication for authors quoted by Vygotsky. There were instances where we were simply unable to locate such sources.

In these cases, we hope we have provided sufficient information in other parts of the book to guide the reader should a search for missing sources in this book be necessary.

LEV VYGOTSKY

Lev Vygotsky was born in 1896 to a middle-class Jewish family in Gomel, some four-hundred miles southwest of Moscow and of a predominantly Jewish population. Vygotsky was the second of eight children. His father held several managerial positions, and the family was well-respected, having been involved in public endeavors, such as the establishment of a library. The young Vygotsky must have been affected by the full-scale pogrom of Jewish businesses and dwellings in Gomel, in which his father was called as a witness.

Vygotsky is remembered as an intellectually precocious child. He had an unconventional education, studying with private tutors and entering the Jewish gymnasium only at high-school level. His interests lay primarily in the humanities and social sciences, and he graduated with honors and a gold medal. At this time, the beliefs and techniques of Hegel became the most important intellectual influences in his life and left a lasting imprint on his approach to formulating scientific problems and attempting their resolution. Other intellectual influences were the Ukrainian linguist, Alexander Potebnya and the works of the great German thinker, Wilhelm von Humboldt.

Besides the great authors, Vygotsky had a personal mentor in his cousin David, several years older and a promising philologist and critic, well-connected to the literary and academic circles of Moscow and St. Petersburg. David was probably the first to direct Vygotsky's attention to the world of the new literary theory of the so-called Formalists. Taking into account the range of Vygotsky's interests it seemed logical for him to enroll at the liberal arts program at one of the metropolitan universities. But because a liberal arts graduate at that time would most likely become a gymnasium teacher, a profession closed to Jews, it was better for Vygotsky to enroll as a law student. He enrolled at Shanyavsky Public University, where he majored in philosophy and history, as well as Moscow University, which was rife with political expulsions of large numbers of students, with the mass resignation of the faculty in protest. Shanyavsky was unable to award degrees, but it had a strong and progressive faculty and attracted gifted and independently-minded students.

Vygotsky's years as a student were marked not only by enthusiastic learning of all that was new in the sciences, humanities, and arts, but by his activities as an art critic. In the battle between the Formalists and the Symbolists, which was also a battle waged not only in Moscow and St. Petersburg, but also in Paris and Munich, Vienna and Rome, what was at stake was what made a given thing a work of art. It was at this time that Vygotsky wrote THE PSYCHOLOGY OF ART, which he later submitted as a Ph.D. thesis at the Moscow Institute of Psychology in 1925.

Vygotsky's legacy to modern psychologists revolves around how Vygotsky operated as a thinker: his whole psychological system appears to have been an attempt to build a new system through a careful analysis of the traditional problems of psychology. This quality of his scholarship becomes especially pronounced when viewed against the background of that of his contemporaries, reflexologists and "Marxist psychologists" and others who were ready to rearrange things in their mission to invent a new utopian science and society. What later distinguished Vygotsky was his ability to accept the task as it was posed by the turbulent Soviet social reality of the 1920s, but to approach it with methods informed by the Western intellectual tradition.

VASSILY V. DAVIDOV

Vassily Davidov (Introduction) is a Full Member of the organization formerly known as the U.S.S.R. Academy of Pedagogical Sciences, Honorary Member of the U.S. National Academy of Education, and has been a guest faculty member at several prominent U.S. universities.

ROBERT H. SILVERMAN

Robert Silverman (translator) has translated numerous scholarly works from Russian into English, for various organizations in the U.S.

PREFACE

The present book has as its goals chiefly those of a practical nature. It is offered as a contribution to the Soviet school of pedagogy and to assist the rank-and-file teacher, and to also promote the development of a rational understanding of the educational process in light of the most recent results of the science of psychology.

Psychology is now experiencing a crisis. The most fundamental and the most elemental claims of the field are being reconsidered, and utter confusion of thought rules in the laboratory and in the classroom. Faith in the old systems has been undermined, yet new systems are not yet so well developed that one might venture to extract from them an applied science.

The crisis in psychology inevitably means a crisis for all of educational psychology, and demands a reconstruction of the field from the very foundations. The new psychology is more fortunate than its predecessor, however, in the sense that it does not have to "arrive at conclusions" on the basis of its claims and does not have to go far afield when it wishes to apply its results in the realm of education.

The problem of education is at the very heart of the new psychology. The study of conditional reflexes constitutes a foundation on which the new psychology will have to be constructed. The term, *conditional reflex*, is the name given to that mechanism which carries us from biology to sociology and makes it possible to comprehend the very essence and nature of the educational process.

Quite frankly, there's no denying the fact that educational psychology, as a science, became possible only with this discovery. Until then, psychology lacked the essential basic principle that could have joined together into a unified whole all those fragmentary bits of factual information it made use of.

Now, the most important goal of the present monograph is to maintain such a fundamentally rational unity in the analysis of all the various aspects of education and in the description of the different elements of the instructional process. It is of extraordinary importance to demonstrate with exhaustive scientific rigor that, no matter what its subject matter and no matter what its methodology, at its very foundation education ultimately always rests upon the mechanism of the conditional reflex.

However, it would be wrong to see in this principle an all-encompassing and ultimately liberating tool, a kind of mystical "open sesame" of the new psychology. In fact, by the very nature of its goals, educational psychology deals with facts and with psychological categories of a more complex nature and of a higher order than the individual isolated reaction or reflex, and, in general, of a more complex nature and of a higher order than those areas which the modern science of man's higher nervous activity touched upon before actually studying them.

The teacher has to deal with more generalized forms of behavior, that is, with the unitary reactions of the organism. Naturally, therefore, the study of conditional reflexes can only form the basis and foundation for the present the course of studies. In the description and analysis of the more complex forms of behavior, it is necessary to make full use of all the scientifically reliable results that have been discovered by the old psychology, translating old concepts into the new language.

My objective has always been to disclose and demonstrate the motor, or reflexive aspect of every such form of behavior, and to thereby relate these more complex forms of behavior to the fundamental and initial standpoints taken toward the subject.

Together with Hugo Münsterberg, I am of the belief that the time is past when "the whole motor part appeared to be an unimportant appendix without which mental life might just as well take its course. Now everything is turned around. The attitude and action are now what give the real opportunity for the development of the central processes. We think because we are acting." (*Psychology and the Teacher*, page 116).

As regards terminology, I have nowhere hesitated over retaining the old terms, seeing in these terms the most understandable, convenient, and concise means of describing many phenomena. These terms will have to be retained for the time being, pending the development of a new scientific language. The creation of new words and terms would only be a pretense, or so it seems to me, since in the description of phenomena it is everywhere necessary to use not only the old names of these phenomena, but also the old results. It therefore seemed best each time to re-interpret the genuine content not only of these old terms, but also of the previously obtained results. The book, therefore, bears the clear imprint of the scientific epoch of that turning point, and of that crisis, in existence at the time it was written.

It seems appropriate in this regard to refer to some comments recently made by Pavlov. According to Pavlov, "The objective data we have obtained ... science will bring into our subjective world sooner or later and, thus, at a single stroke, and clearly, illuminate our concealed nature, clarify the mechanism and vital sense of what man is concerned with more than anything else — his consciousness, and the throes of his conscience. This is why in my presentation I have permitted myself a degree of inconsistency in my use of terms. In the title to my talk and throughout the entire presentation, I have used the term, mental [*psikhicheskii*], and in addition have always discussed only objective investigations, leaving entirely to the side all subjective studies. Those vital phenomena that are referred to as mental phenomena, though they seem to be observed objectively in animals as well, nevertheless differ, at least in terms of degree of complexity, from purely physiological phenomena. What could be the significance of calling them mental or complex nerve phenomena, as opposed to simple physiological phenomena, once it is acknowledged and recognized that the natural scientist may approach their study only from the objective side, without being at all concerned with the essential nature of these phenomena?"

In fact, in the present book, I have often had to present the views of other researchers, and to translate concepts developed by other writers into my own terminology, as in any systematic presentation. I have been able to express my own thoughts only in passing, and mixed in with those of other writers. Nevertheless, I am of the belief that the present volume represents not just a novel experiment in the construction of a course of educational psychology, but also an attempt at the construction of a new type of textbook. The very choice of system and the very arrangement of the material represents a novel, and as yet unrealized, experiment at a major synthesis of the most diverse scientific data and results.

In its present form, the book does not repeat any of the manuals on the subject I am familiar with, and for this reason I am well aware of being fully responsible for all the conclusions reached in the present volume.

How far this synthesis has succeeded, this I leave to the judgement of competent reviewers, inviting them to look upon the book as an interim work that will have to be replaced by other, more improved manuals in the very near future.

Besides my own personal mistakes, the inadequacies of a first attempt would appear to be entirely unavoidable whenever it is a matter of constructing something in entirely uncharted and uncleared territory. Rigorous and consistent application of a fundamental point of view on the educational process, understood as one involving the social re-orientation of biological forms of behavior, is the sole purpose of the present textbook. The construction of a course of educational psychology on a sociobiological foundation is, therefore, my principal intention.

I will consider my work to have attained its goal if, despite all the inadequacies of this first attempt, the path I have chosen will prove to have been the correct one, i.e., if the book will turn out to be the first step on the path toward the construction of an objective and rigorous scientific system of educational psychology.

Introduction

LEV VYGOTSKY AND EDUCATIONAL PSYCHOLOGY

V.V. Davydov

The name of the outstanding Soviet psychologist and scholar Lev Vygotsky (1896-1934) is well known throughout the world. Nearly all his scientific works (books, articles, etc.) have been published and reprinted many times in translation around the world. The six volumes of his *Collected Works* (*Sobraniva sochinenii*) (Moscow, Pedagogika, 1982-84) have been of especially great importance to the scientific community. There is also his remarkable book, *Educational Psychology. Abridged Course,* published in Moscow in 1926 but not reprinted for quite some time for purely ideological reasons, basically that it is not persuasive and even incongruous from a modern perspective. This book, in Vygotsky's words, was written with a practical purpose in mind and was "offered as a contribution to the Soviet school of pedagogy and to assist the rank-and-file teacher, and to also promote the development of a rational understanding of the educational process in light of the most recent results of the science of psychology".

The present edition of this book is, without a doubt, of considerable significance, since it will allow specialists to become acquainted with how a recognized leader of world psychology conceived of the "new data" of his science over 60 years ago. And, of course, in reading the book one cannot but get a sense of the author's skillful and vivid style in this popular presentation of the latest psychological results to an audience of public school teachers and university instructors, a style which is, moreover, highly distinctive and informative. The present edition of this work will, however, be of value to psychologists and educators engaged in scientific research who wish to transfer their results into the classroom. What is most important, though, is that the present-day teacher, and especially the rank-and-file teacher, who has read through the entire book cannot help but sense the resemblance and similarity of the topics covered in the book with all those conflicting and pressing problems in contemporary education which the teacher in the classroom and worker in the research laboratory have set their minds to solving. It is this which is the main purpose of the present edition; once this is understood, both the teacher and the researcher in education will be able to reach a deeper understanding of the psychological foundations of education.

In *Educational Psychology*, Vygotsky made the following fundamental theoretical assertions:

> The educational process must be based on the student's individual activity, and the art of education should involved nothing more than guiding and monitoring this activity ... From the psychological point of view, the teacher is the director of the social environment in the classroom, the governor and guide of the interaction between the educational process and the student ... The social environment is the true lever of the educational process, and the teacher's overall role reduces to adjusting this lever.

> And, further, "The psychological law simply says that before trying to get a child involved in some activity, get him interested in it, take care to discover whether he is ready for it, that all the forces necessary for the activity are tensed, and that the child is ready to act on his own, with the teacher left to simply guide and direct his activity" The principal psychological goal of education is the purposive and deliberate inculcation in the child of *new forms* of behavior and of activity, i.e., the deliberate organization of the child's development.

Thus, in the classroom the main figure, according to Vygotsky, is the child *himself* or *herself* as the *subject* of his or her own activity. By making use of the considerable opportunities afforded by the social environment in which the child dwells and functions, the teacher is able to direct and guide the child's individual activity with the purpose of achieving a further *development* of this activity. Throughout the entire abridged scientific and practical course in educational psychology which is set forth in the present volume, Vygotsky consistently imparts a coherent expression to, and gives a profound exposition of, these psychological purposes, which were in fact, quite new and almost radical at the time.

In fact, there is much in the present book which was new for its time. But what is it in the book which has retained its originality to the present day, and what is now out-dated? Let us try to consider both these questions.

Above all, our own experience shows us that there are any number of psychological observations in the volume touching on the special importance of the student's *independence* in processes of teaching and education which could sound like new ideas to many working teachers even today (see the quotations given earlier). These observations were hammered out early in the twentieth century by certain leading philosophers, educators, and psychologists who had fought to make the evolving system of public education effectively democratic. The remarkable American scholar John Dewey was one such educational philosopher. Vygotsky succeeded in comprehending many of the assumptions underlying these assertions and formulated them in explicit fashion in the form of a special psychological law.

Let us turn to various formulations of individual aspects of this law as given by Vygotsky.

Thus, he writes that

> ... the student's personal experience becomes the fundamental basis of pedagogical work. Strictly speaking, and from the scientific point of view, there is no other way of teaching ... Ultimately, the child teaches himself ... in the educational process, the student's individual experience is everything. Education should be structured so that it is not that the student is educated, but that the student educates himself ... The educational process must be based on the student's personal activity ... " (4:1, 4:2,)

But on the other hand, the student's experience

> is determined wholly and without exception by the social environment ... Though the teacher is powerless to produce immediate effects in the student, he is all-powerful when it comes to producing indirect, mediated effects in him through the social environment ... Education is realized through the student's own experience, which is wholly determined by the environment, and the role of the teacher then reduces to directing and guiding the environment.

And, finally, yet another decisive assertion from his overall review of the interrelation between student, environment, and teacher: "... and the child is ready to act on his own, with the teacher left to simply guiding and directing his actions".

In other words, according to Vygotsky, the teacher may educate students in deliberate fashion only by constantly *collaborating* with them, with their environment, with their desires and with their willingness to *themselves work* with their teacher. This fundamental idea was in contradiction to authoritarian pedagogy, which insisted that the teacher could supposedly influence the child effectively in direct fashion in accordance with his own instructional and educational goals without giving any thought to the child's motivations, interest, and willingness to undertake his own personal activity.

The reader of the present work book will, in all likelihood, notice that in his discussion of educational psychology, Vygotsky preferred to speak of *problems of education* [*problemy vospitaniya*] (in present-day educational psychology one speaks basically of *questions of teaching* [*voprosy obucheniya*]). This is no accident. As the outstanding psychologist he was, Vygotsky viewed educational processes as they occur in the child as an internal foundation of his *development*, and of the evolution of new forms of behavior in the child (the development of which in the appropriate period also constituted the principal goal of education). Moreover, within the context of the evolving system of public education, neither the classroom teacher nor researcher concerned with theoretical issues were inclined to discriminate between the two in any special way, and were even less inclined to oppose teaching and upbringing, and instead viewed both as components of a unified and integral formative process.

In looking through the present volume, which constantly draws the reader's attention to the child's independence in processes of teaching and education, the impression may arise that Vygotsky's argument is grist for the mill of those who advocate the notion of "permissive education." Such a conclusion would be utterly mistaken. Page after page of the book considers concrete forms of the genuine activity *all the participants* in the educational process — the child, the child's social environment, and the teacher — engage in, and expressly discusses the moral and pedagogical goals of education.

> Least of all should we think of the educational process as one-sided, and ascribe all activity without exception to the environment, making nothing of the activity of the student himself, of the activity of his teacher, and of everything that must come into contact with education ... Even lifeless objects, when they are brought into the educational arena, when they are assigned an educational role, acquire a sense of purpose and become effective participants in this process.

> And this thought is complemented with the following line of reasoning: ... the psychological theory of public education not only does not mean prostrating oneself before education, but, on the contrary, signifies the ultimate in our mastery of the flow of educational processes ... It must teach us how to grasp the very nature of education, guiding ourselves by its very own laws.

Note that Vygotsky did not recognize the existence of any kind of separate reality that would reduce to the pair "teacher-student," rather he was always identifying and investigating the dynamic *social environment* that *linked the two together*. The special complexity of the work of a teacher springs from the fact that, on the one hand, the teacher has to have a good idea of the laws governing the child's own activity, i.e., he has to know the child's psychology. On the other hand, however, he has to be oriented towards the dynamic features of the child's social environment in order if he is to guide the overall flow of the child's activity in a pedagogically proper course by skillfully altering this environment.

> This is also why an active role is the lot of the teacher in the course of education. The teacher fashions, cuts up, shreds, and carves up the elements of the environment and then combines them together in the most diverse way imaginable, in order to realize whatever goal he has need for. Thus is the educational process an active one on three levels: the student is active, the teacher is active, and the environment created between them is an active one.

These wise words, which are those of a remarkable thinker, both psychologist and educator, are far from out-of-date for those teachers who seek to organize the teaching of their charges and the overall educational process with an understanding of the psychological laws governing the child's activity and the pedagogical rules for altering his social environment. But such an understanding must be turned into creative striving and dexterity if the teacher is to succeed in his work with children of the most varied types in the highly multifaceted and unique social situation in which children live their lives. And it is forever necessary to reach unanticipated and *novel* pedagogical decisions, decisions that, moreover, have to be unerring, since the child's real fate and that of his *family* depends upon them. This is why the work of a true teacher always bears an especially creative character.

It is essential to particularly underscore the age-old truth, that the correct creative solution of a *an unusual* and complex pedagogical problem may be found only by the teacher who is already highly conversant with the essentials of his subject, who possesses a knowledge and understanding of the subtle turns of the child's soul and of the contradictory nature of the motivation and overall course of the child's activity, and who possesses an ability to "mold," "cut up," and "combine together" in the most diverse ways imaginable the different elements of the social environment in which the child is educated. This means that the teacher must master (of course, starting when he is still a student) the scientific foundations of child psychology, educational psychology, and social psychology, and the fundamentals of the theory and applications of pedagogics in order to subsequently fit them into the context of his own *practical* work.

A significant portion of the book is devoted to introducing the student and teacher to important aspects of the psychological elements of the skills that are part of the craft of education, on the one hand, and to an attempt at drawing both teacher and student into thinking about the vital pedagogical environments. Any effort at transcending these environments at once presupposes skillful use of the knowledge gained by educational psychology as regards the education of students in such realms as the emotions and attention, and thinking and memory, and in the realm of their moral, labor, and esthetic education. Vygotsky discusses the temperament and character of the child, the fundamental modes of investigation of the child's personality, as well as giftedness in children and individual goals in the education of children. A special chapter, the concluding one, is devoted to the psychology of the work of a teacher.

In the text where all these questions are considered, the reader will find the richest mine imaginable of wise thoughts and interesting aspirations, tied together internally by a common thread of psychological reasoning that underlies Vygotsky's approach to the education of children. In our view, it is not possible to agree with all these conclusions at the present time; educational psychology has, in fact, come a long way since the book was first written. Vygotsky's understanding of a "unified foundation" of the educational process, which he, with a nod to the prevailing wisdom, linked to the concept of "conditional reflex" (we will discuss this question somewhat later) requires a special review, and certain misunderstandings may arise due to his use of terminology that is no longer accepted in contemporary psychology.

Now it is a time for us to analyze in brief those general psychological standpoints which Vygotsky subscribed to at the time he wrote the present book and had it published. But before presenting this analysis, it would be a good idea to give a brief biographical sketch touching on the sources of Vygotsky's teaching and research. This task is even more significant if we bear in mind the fact that his book on educational psychology was written and published in the early period of his scientific career, a period that preceded the essential crisis in his creative destiny — the crisis and turning point which is the reason why the name of Lev Vygotsky is celebrated to the present day.

By formal university training, Vygotsky was an attorney (he had graduated from the School of Law of Moscow University in 1917). But at the same time he was at Moscow University, he was also a student in the School of History and Philosophy of the Shanyavskii People's University, an institution that existed in Moscow in the period just before the revolution. He received an excellent humanist education, had a serious interest in philosophy and psychology, esthetics and literature, and, of course, jurisprudence. Even in his student years, he had begun research on the psychology of art, research which he continued later on, writing his dissertation on just this topic, which he defended in 1925. (The dissertation was only published in 1965, and has since been published in translation in many countries, in English as *The Psychology of Art*). Upon completion of his studies at the two universities, he returned to Gomel', where he had lived for many years previously, and assumed a position in the field of education. He taught literature in high school, and lectured on esthetics, logic, and psychology at a number of educational institutions and gave courses in these subjects. In the early 1920s he organized a special psychological laboratory at the teacher training school where he was lecturing on psychology. The Gomel' period in his life defined his interests in the fields of pedagogics and psychology, and supplied him with all those resources which he then made active use of in his book on educational psychology. In

1924 Vygotsky moved to Moscow and began work at the Institute of Psychology of Moscow University.

While still living in Gomel', he had began serious study of the works of Ivan Pavlov, Vladimir Bekhterev, and other scientists who were at work on the investigation of the physiology of the nervous system, striving to relate the results of their investigations with outstanding questions in psychology. (The results of these studies served as the basis of his well-known paper, "The Technique of Reflexological and Psychological Investigations," which he presented at the All-Russian Conference on Psychoneurology held in January 1924; cf. *Collected Works*, Vol. 1, pages 43-62). Once he had settled in Moscow, Vygotsky began to work in the field of theoretical and applied "defectology" [the Russian term encompasses both rehabilitation and special education—trans.], and also undertook a critical analysis of the history of the contemporary state of psychology. In 1926, he prepared a major study, entitled "The Historical Meaning of the Psychological Crisis," making extensive use of the work of many non-Russian scientists (the study was only published in 1982; *Collected Works*, pages 291-436). It was during this period that he completed his abridged course in educational psychology. There is reason to believe that he had laid the foundation for the present volume while still working in Gomel'.

The essential shift in Vygotsky's creative life occurred following publication of the book. This, the most celebrated period of his scientific activity, began in 1927-8, when, working with a group of colleagues that included A. Leont'ev, Aleksandr Luria, A. Zaporozhets, and L. Bozhovich, he undertook a large-scale series of experimental investigations. From the results of these investigations, he was subsequently led to formulate the fundamental assertions of *cultural-historical theory,* the theory of the development of those mental functions which are not only specific to human beings, for example, attention, memory, and thinking, but which also possess a social, cultural, and life-history [*prizhiznennyi*] origin and are mediated by a special medium, called *signs,* that arises in the course of human *history.* A "sign," from Vygotsky's standpoint, is, above all, a social medium for man, a special kind of "psychological tool": "... a sign is located outside the organism, as is a tool, it is separated from the individual and is essentially a social organ or social medium" (*Collected Works.*, Vol. 3, page 146)

This theory was in contradiction with the *biologistic* (or vulgar natural scientific) approach to the study of man, which at the time was an intrinsic component of many psychological schools, particularly one of the most influential schools then in existence, that of American behaviorism, whose proponents often identified the distinctive features and mechanisms of human and animal behavior. For the behaviorist, the same laws of *adaptation* to the environment were supposedly characteristic of men and animals, in the form of the organism's reactions to appropriate stimuli, though it was acknowledged that in man these laws, of course, assumed more complex forms, inasmuch as man lives in a social environment and, moreover, unlike animals, possesses speech.

There is one important circumstance to keep in mind here, that at the early stages in his construction of cultural-historical theory, Vygotsky had suggested that the child's "elementary functions" possess an "innate" natural and hereditary character, that they were *not yet mediated* by the cultural medium). Later, though, working from a more extensive body of knowledge, he arrived at the following fundamental conclusion: "... the functions which are usually thought of as the most elementary, are subordinated in the child to laws that are entirely different than those which dominate the earlier stages of phylogenetic development, and are characterized by the same mediated psychological structure ... A detailed analysis of the structure of individual mental processes ... is enough to persuade us of the fact, and also demonstrates that even the science of the structure of the individual elementary processes of the child's behavior is in need of a radical review" (*Collected Works.*, page 38). The essential point is that in its very first hours the "infant acts in relation to its surroundings not directly, in unmediated fashion, but through another human being" (*Collected Works.*, page 29).

In other words, Vygotsky had reviewed his own previous ideas of the "biological" character of man's elementary (or lower) functions and had concluded that even the most elementary functions, even those that arise at the earliest stages of man's life, possess a mediative, i.e., specifically human, structure.

For cultural-historical theory, human behavior is radically different from animal behavior, since it is *social* in its very origin; it is linked to human intercourse internally and is inseparable from the various manifestations of the historically arising cultural medium which guides it (speech, mathematical signs in the form of the natural numbers, and so on). Within the overall course of this theory, Vygotsky formulated a *general genetic law* to describe the existence of any of man's mental functions, and of any of the psychological mechanisms of human behavior (or, better, *activity*): "... In the child's cultural development, every function appears on the scene twice, in two different contexts, first, as social, and then as psychological, first between people, ... and then within the child ... Functions first evolve in the group in the form of relations between children, and then become mental functions of personality" (*Collected Works.*, pages 145-7). "Man introduces artificial stimuli, he constructs a "signification" of behavior, and by means of signs he creates new relations in the brain through the influence he exerts from outside the brain... " (*Collected Works.*, page 80).

Thus, all of man's mental functions, all those functions which organize and steer human activity, possess, according to Vygotsky's cultural-historical theory, *their own deep-lying roots not within* each individual human being, not within each person's organism and personality, but *outside*, in the *intercourse* between individuals, in their relationships between each other and in their relationships to the objects created by people.

In the late 1920s and early 1930s, Vygotsky worked within the course set by the general assumptions of his cultural-historical theory, and, together with his colleagues, undertook broad and novel experimental investigations of child psychology and educational psychology. On the basis of the factual data which resulted, Vygotsky and his assistants wrote and published numerous scientific studies. After his early death, these investigations were enlarged upon and extended, which, naturally, led as well to definite changes in individual assumptions of the original theory. As a result, a powerful school of scientific psychology was forged in the Soviet Union, a school that we are now entirely justified in referring to as "Vygotsky's school." The basic assumptions of this school, together with Vygotsky's principal conceptions, are widely represented in the scientific literature of many countries around the world.

The adherents of this school, besides Vygotsky himself, Leont'ev, Luria, and others, arrived at an entirely clear-cut conception of the relationship between man's mental development and his education and teaching. That is, if *none* of man's mental functions are given to man at the time he is born, but are only *specified* in historically evolved, cultural forms, as in cultural-historical theory, then it is only in mastering, or, better, *appropriating,* these forms in the processes of teaching and education that man's mental development is realized. Vygotsky's well-known assertion, that "teaching must move development forward" (*Collected Works*, Vol.2, page 252) and not be a millstone on development, expresses this very notion. "Pedagogics," writes Vygotsky, "must be oriented not toward the point in the child's development from yesterday, but toward tomorrow's development. Only then will it be in a position to bring to life in the very process of teaching all those developmental processes that now lie in the zone of proximal development" (*Collected Works.*, page 251). It was Vygotsky, in fact, who introduced into scientific discourse the broad concept of the "zone of proximal development," which we should understand in the following sense. Everything which the child may initially do *together* with its peers or with grown-ups, and then all on its own, also lies fully within the "zone" of its proximal mental development.

It is entirely natural that the assertions of cultural-historical theory were not reflected in the present book of Vygotsky's. It is, moreover, remarkable that some of the preliminary reflections of this theory can nevertheless be sensed in the present "abridged course" of educational psychology. In fact, it was prepared during those years when Vygotsky was writing his book, *Psychology of Art*, and it is the belief of some specialists that the initial conceptions of the theory were already formulated in it (cf. D.B. El'konin. *Selected Psychological Studies*, pages 477-8).

In the first half of the twentieth century a theory of conditional and unconditional reflexes, which had been developed by the well-known Russian physiologist Ivan Pavlov, dominated the biological and psychological sciences. The concept of "reflex" (and the analogous concept of "reaction" or "response") was thought of by most materialistically minded psychologists as the foundation stone of objective, scientific psychology, and there was no way the young Vygotsky could avoid this powerful trend in science. "The study of conditional reflexes constitutes a foundation on which the new psychology will have to be constructed. The term, *conditional [conditioned] reflex*, is the name given to that mechanism which carries us from biology to sociology and makes it possible to comprehend the very essence and nature of the educational process". And, further, " ... ultimately, education always possesses in its very foundation the mechanism of the education of the conditional reflex".

Vygotsky was well aware that the concept of "reflex" refers to something which is biological and physiological in nature. But, from his point of view, the conditional reflexes in man may be educated through the medium of the *social environment*. In the preface to *Educational Psychology,* he therefore wrote that "Rigorous and consistent [realization] ... of the social re-orientation of biological forms of behavior, is the sole purpose of the present textbook. The construction of a course of educational psychology on a sociobiological foundation is, therefore, my principal intention".

Four chapters of the present book (Chapters 2-5) are given over to an attempt at realizing this intention. Vygotsky was fully devoted to a presentation of his theoretical understanding of the biological and physiological forms of behavior in man and in animals and the sociobiological foundations of man's education. (Note that the entire presentation is conducted on a high professional level, making use of all of the fundamental scientific results that had been achieved by that time.) And in many other chapters, he routinely resorts to such terms as "unconditional reflex," "conditional reflex," "reaction," "stimulus," and "instinct," and, of course, the description of the process of education in children and of new forms of behavior is conducted in conformity with what he supposes to be the structure of the fundamental mechanism of human behavior, that of man's reactions and reflexes (cf. the discussion in Chapter 2). Nevertheless, the reader should bear in mind that Vygotsky made an express effort to identify and to describe the distinctive features peculiar to human behavior as opposed to animal behavior [41-42].

We will not consider here the distinctive features of all those concepts which were commonly employed in biology, in the physiology of higher nervous activity, and in psychology in the early 1920s and which are made use of in this book; note, too, that a number of these concepts have been used in all these related disciplines, for example, the concepts of "adaptation," "reaction," "reflex," and "instinct". For our purposes, it is important to focus on and analyze the following questions: (1) Is it possible to concur with Vygotsky's claim of the necessity of educating "man's instincts"? (Chapter 2); (3) What is distinctive about his understanding of movement and does it coincide completely with its interpretation in contemporary stimulus-response theory?; and (3) How should we evaluate the overall approach of the young (or "early") Vygotsky as regards the sociobiological nature of man's education?

In many of the natural sciences that study man, particularly psychology, a long-standing assumption has been that, just as in the case of the animals, there are a number of instincts inherent to man. Though the various interpretations of their origin and mechanisms are quite varied, most scientists nevertheless are in agreement that any instinct constitutes an indissoluble unity of needs that have been passed down to the organism by heredity, and that the methods of satisfying these needs have likewise been inherited. (Proponents of the reflex theory, such as the young Vygotsky, suppose that the instincts are based on hereditary or unconditional reflexes.) But investigations carried out by a number of psychologists, physiologists, sociologists, ethnographers, and cultural historians over the past several decades have shown that though man, as a being in nature, is actually born with certain organic needs which he has inherited (for example, sexual and digestive needs), he does *not* possess any sort of vitally significant hereditary, or innate, methods of satisfying these needs. Consequently, man simply does not possess instincts as such, not even organic instincts, not to speak of "mental" [*dukhovnyi*] instincts. (This question was eventually treated in a sound and thorough fashion by Gal'perin, 1976.)

And, in fact, the studies conducted by Jean Piaget's co-workers on genetic epistemology, by George Meade, the child psychologist and ethnographer, by Mikhail Osipovich Gurevich, the specialist in cultural history, and others have confirmed this observation. Results of investigations carried out by the scientific school established by Vygotsky (Leont'ev, Zaporozhets, El'konin, and others) also lead to the same conclusion. Leont'ev, who had been a student and colleague of Vygotsky's, adopted a particularly strict approach to this question, and repeatedly declared that *all* of man's capacities (he is speaking of fully developed means of satisfying his needs) arise and develop in the course of his lifetime (cf. *Selected Psychological Works,* Vol. 1, page 79, etc.). And, as we showed earlier, Vygotsky himself in the latter period of his scientific activity came to the conclusion that even the most elementary mental functions, such as those of the child, possess a specifically human signifying mediation. In other words, the general meaning of Vygotsky's cultural-historical theory ran *counter* to any acknowledgement of the existence of instincts in man and, thereby, *counter* to any need to give pedagogical recommendations on ways and means of "educating" the instincts in children.

Several words are in order regarding the process by which man "lost" his instincts. There is reason to suppose that, in the course of human evolution, a process realized in the emergence of collective labor activity, instincts in the highly evolved apes, the phylogenetic precursors of man, simply collapsed, since their essential and obligatory component, that of specific methods of satisfying needs passed down by heredity, were "jettisoned." Now these methods of satisfying needs began to be created historically by early man, in culture, and were appropriated by each new generation of early man in the course of its existence.

And indeed, in Chapter 5, entitled "The Instincts as the Subject, Mechanism, and Means of Education," careful analysis of the educational psychology portion of the text, as opposed to the biological and physiological argument, reveals a rather interesting circumstance. Speaking in part of the child's instincts, Vygotsky, in fact, has in mind the child's *needs* and the intimately associated realm of the child's *interests*. "From the psychological point of view," writes Vygotsky, "the instincts appear to be powerful excitations which are associated with the most complex *organic needs* ... The instincts are the most powerful impulses and the most powerful stimuli to activity ... The instincts constitute a vast natural force, they are the expression and voice of the *organism's natural needs,* ... " [5a:19,20], and similarly, "In childhood the basic mode of appearance of the instincts is in the form of interest" [5b:12], and, "*Interests* are an expression of the child's organic needs" [5b:20] [emphasis added].

With such an interpretation of "instinct" in mind (note that out of the genuine content of the concept of instinct Vygotsky retains only its element of satisfaction, which, in and of itself, an instinct *is not*), neither psychologists nor educators could raise objections to the following line of reasoning: "It is not hard to show that, in the system formed by man's behavior and man's instincts, there is nothing permanent and inflexible, nothing that moves solely by the force of inertia. In a genuine behavioral system, the instincts are just as socially conditioned, just as adaptable and changeable, just as capable of assuming new forms, as are all the other reactions ... [5a:16]. Or, "All of man's culture as it relates to the individual himself and to the behavior of the individual constitutes nothing other than such an adaption of the instincts to the environment" [5:22]. But, it seems to us that biologists and physiologists who study genuine instincts in animals are scarcely in agreement with such reasoning, since real instincts are phylogenetically highly stable and emerge in conformity with the *innate methods* of satisfying needs and are not "changeable," do not "assume[e] new forms [like] all the other reactions."

Everything that Vygotsky, writing as an educational psychologist, actually understood by the term, "instinct," really constitutes man's needs and interests which, in the context of man's cohesive behavior, are, of course, changeable, dynamic, and, since they are socially conditioned phenomena, acquire new forms, especially when it is a matter of cultural methods of satisfying these needs. And Vygotsky was correct when he wrote (cf. above) that "all of human culture" represents an "adaptation" (better, *satisfaction*) of needs (in his terminology, of "instincts") to the social and historical conditions of people's lives.

In drawing upon the achievements of the biology and physiology of his time, the young Vygotsky was simply borrowing the popular term, "instinct," and conferring on it his own psychosocial content. The reader should be aware of this circumstance, but, in addition, should take note of Vygotsky's numerous valuable pedagogical aspirations expressed in the form of "pedagogical principles" having to do with conditions for the education of the child's interests and needs, and of methods of satisfying and developing these interests and needs. Vygotsky's line of reasoning on the sexual education of children, and of the role of games in the development of the child's interests are quite interesting in this regard.

Now let us consider Vygotsky's interpretation of the concept of "reaction" (Chapter 2). For Vygotsky, a reaction is a general biological concept inherent to all living matter. A "reflex" is a reaction of an organism that already possesses a nervous system; it is a physiological phenomenon [25]. But any reaction, like any reflex, possesses three components: a sensory component (perception of stimulus); a central component (processing of the stimulus); and a motor component (responding action). Human behavior represents a complex chain of reactions (conditional and unconditional reactions and super-reflexes).

All of this simply recapitulates the ABC's of behaviorism and the science of the higher nervous activity as it existed in the first quarter of the twentieth century. For the teacher and instructor in teaching methods of the time who wished to keep abreast of scientific approaches in educational psychology, these concepts were, in fact, novel. And an acquaintance with the content of the other chapters of Vygotsky's book assisted them in gaining the proper orientation to the corresponding terminology, which had also permeated studies in pedagogics, though the main thing was to understand and master the confluence of all those conditions in the work of their students that contributed to the formation in students of definite "reactions" or "conditional reflexes" (what in the ordinary language of pedagogics is referred to as "skills" and "habits."

Essentially, contemporary educational psychology no longer rests on the science of higher nervous activity, employing instead the age-old pedagogical concepts of "knowledge," "skills," and "habits." The fundamental conditions and laws governing the development of these elements in students have been studied in works published in recent decades, as, for example, in the study of problem-oriented teaching, the evolution of mental activity, the organization of educational activity, and so on. So there is not much that the teacher or university instructor of today can gain from a reading of Chapters 2-4 of the present volume, though from a practical and methodological standpoint there are any number of interesting points.

But for psychologists and educators there are certain views expressed in these chapters which are of definite interest, due not so much to the young Vygotsky's routine evaluation of the general state of the study of reactions. He was of the belief that the time had come when the main emphasis in the study of reaction had to be placed on the *motor component*. In the preface, Vygotsky quotes William James' colleague at Harvard, Hugo Münsterberg, as declaring that, "Now everything is turned around. The attitude and action are now what give the real opportunity for the development of the central processes. We think because we are acting" [P:5]. In fact, what is actually involved in the processing of stimuli is a subject which has been a special focus of studies carried out by physiologists. Their goal has been to explicate the physiological laws underlying the functioning of the basic centers of the nervous system, though investigations centered on the study of *movement* (actions) have made it possible to approach the study of the basic psychological functions of man, for example, thinking.

In Chapter 9, which is, in fact, devoted to thinking, there is a lengthy section entitled "The Motor Nature of Cognitive Processes" in which Vygotsky formulated an interesting theoretical assertion of direct relation to his general understanding of the psychological mechanisms governing human behavior. He writes that "[The] difference between thought and a complete reaction is that, since it manifests itself as internal movement exclusively, the reaction forfeits the meaning of reaction in general, i.e., as a given movement directed outwardly, and assumes an entirely new meaning, becoming an internal guide of our behavior ... Thought plays the part of an anticipatory guide of our behavior". Compare, in this regard, the corresponding assertion given earlier, in Chapter 3, "...thinking is always accompanied by various restrained movements, mostly by internal motor reactions of speech, i.e., by the rudimentary articulation of words".

In his characterization of the relationship between movements and the psyche, Vygotsky speaks of the fact that "that the subtlest forms of mental phenomena are always accompanied by particular motor reactions". Since behavior is a system of *externally* expressed movements, whereas mental functions constitute "*internal*" movements, Vygotsky was right to conclude that "...the psyche must be understood as consisting of especially complex forms of the structure of behavior". But the psyche (for example, thinking), which is based on "internal" movements, acts in the role of an "*anticipatory organizer*" of behavior. "... and if I think first and only then do something, this means nothing less than a duplication and complication of behavior in which the internal reactions of thought initially prepare and adapt the organism, and then the external reactions carry out *what had been established and prepared in thought ahead of time*" (emphasis added).

Such a conception on the part of the young Vygotsky of the basic functions of the psyche, in our opinion, carries his theory of movement beyond the limits of the views held at the time by proponents of the stimulus-response ("reactology") and reflex ("reflectology") theories, and, of course, behaviorism. But it also brought him to the threshold of certain conceptions that did not emerge until he was at work on the construction of cultural-historical theory. Only at that point did he write of the functions of the psyche (thinking) and of the role played by signs in thinking, thus, "... Man constructs new forms of action mentally and on paper, he manages battles from maps, he works on mental models, in other words, everything which in man's behavior is associated with the use of the artificial medium of thinking, with the social development of behavior, and, especially, with the use of signs" (*op. cit.*, Vol. 3, page 124).

El'konin is right in his assessment of the overall orientation of Vygotsky's *Educational Psychology* when he writes that in this book there is "still present the standpoint of a stimulus-response theorist, though one can already sense Vygotsky's dissatisfaction with an understanding of behavior based exclusively on stimuli and responses, and the necessity of considering behavior in a unity with the psyche and with consciousness as the regulator of the psyche (*Selected Psychological Studies.*, page 416).

Note that a similar sense of unease pervades Vygotsky's lengthy article, "Consciousness as a Problem of the Psychology of Behavior," which appeared around the same time as his book. In this article he writes that in the existing scientific environment, "biology devours sociology, and physiology devours psychology," and that so long as such a situation continues, psychology is "doomed to exist under the false impression that behavior seems to be a summing up of reflexes" (*ibid.*, Vol. 1, pages 80-1). Subsequently, Vygotsky and his followers did much to radically alter this situation, and to overcome more than just a single isolated false conception of human behavior whose roots were connected with the traditional teachings of reactions and reflexes.

Thus, as a psychologist Vygotsky had a profound sense of (one might even say guessed) the exceptional importance for man's psyche of the "inner movement" of living matter.

It so happened that N. Bernstein (1896-1966) worked at the same institute as did Vygotsky in the latter part of the 1920s. Bernstein had begun his investigations of human movement, the results of which led him some time later to the creation of a novel psychophysiological theory of the construction of movement. This theory was a distinctive *counterweight* to Pavlov's theory of reflexes. For Bernstein, human behavior was based not on reactions to external influences, but on *action*, which he interpreted as a process of overcoming internal and external obstacles in the course of solving a *problem* (in this case, human behavior does not constitute an *adaptation* to the environment, but its deliberate *transformation*). Afterwards Bernstein became a world-famous physiologist and psychophysiologist whose theories were attacked by many adherents of Pavlov's teachings. In 1990, a collection of his works, entitled *The Physiology of Movement and Activity,* was published in Moscow as part of the series, *Classics of Science.* The volume, *Human Motor Action: Bernstein Reassessed,* edited by H.T.A. Whiting and published in 1984 in the series, *Advances in Psychology,* is a good illustration of the value of Bernstein's works for contemporary science.

And it is hardly coincidental that Vygotsky's students, who, during the 1930s and subsequently, developed the theory of human activity brought into their scientific arsenal Bernstein's psychophysiological conceptions. Essentially, Bernstein's conceptions were (and remain) extremely close to the psychological understanding of the role of movement in genesis and in the functioning of the human psyche. We believe that this kinship between the two approaches is rooted in the views held by the young Vygotsky on the inner relation between movement and the psyche.

There remains for us to consider Vygotsky's intention to construct a course of educational psychology on the foundations of sociobiology. This he succeeded in accomplishing in a *formal* sense, inasmuch as throughout the entire volume his aim is to fit the concrete psychological and sociological data of man's education upon a matrix of biological and physiological terminology, meanwhile reaching specific conclusions within the context of educational psychology and proposing appropriate practical recommendations. But why have we referred to this accomplishment as a *formal* one?

As a true and exacting scholar and humanist, Vygotsky sensed the existence between the processes of education and the functioning of the nervous system of a complex and profound *psychological reality*. In order to reflect this reality in reasonable fashion, Vygotsky realized the need for a major transformation of the biological and physiological content of all those concepts which stood behind the terms used in these sciences. We have demonstrated this in our analysis of the biological term and concept of "instinct" which supposedly exists in people (cf. above). The point is that Vygotsky invested in this term his own psychological content; for him, "instinct" refers to "organic need" which, of course, exists in every person, though, in and of itself, in the exact biological sense, an instinct is not.

Moreover, by the time the book was published, he had begun to doubt the necessity of any direct connection between biology and sociology, or between physiology and psychology, thanks to the discovery of the sociobiological nature of man, inasmuch as he saw that any such connection would result in the humanist understanding of the vital activity of human beings being "devoured" by a simplified natural scientific interpretation of this understanding, i.e., by the utmost degree of reductionism (cf. above).

In his cultural-historical theory of the development of consciousness, Vygotsky demonstrated this circumstance *repeatedly* and numerous researchers by members of the school of psychology he established have substantiated the social nature of man on the basis of extensive factual data, though, of course, this does not preclude the presence in man of an *organic* nature (though not one which is *biological*!). Note that the very "organic nature" of man is, in its historical genesis and in its own genuine functioning, determined by *social* reality in an essential way.

Now, several words are in order regarding the obvious shortcomings of the present book. The first thing we have to note is connected with the fact that its author describes numerous important laws of the functioning of the nervous system which he has borrowed from general biology and from animal physiology, applying them to the case of man by analogic reasoning. Of course, this often keeps him from taking into account the distinctive nature of the physiology of the human nervous system and the distinctive nature of human behavior (though these distinctive features had received comparatively little study early in the century). This is a consequence of the formal realization in the book of Vygotsky's intention to place educational psychology on a sociobiological foundation, something we have already remarked on somewhat earlier. Vygotsky himself was well aware of this circumstance, and he wrote that "every theoretical border between animal behavior and human behavior has been effaced ... Human behavior may be studied to the extent that it is the behavior of a mammal ... " (*ibid.*, Vol. 1, page 80).

There is a further shortcoming on an internal level which is connected with the above. Within the pages of the book, there are, as we have already noted, many interesting pedagogical recommendations and reasonings that are still of practical value. In our view, many of these recommendations and reasonings are the result of much pedagogical experience, extensive fundamental observations (particularly, by Vygotsky himself) and their psychological analysis. But Vygotsky often seeks to place them on a biological and physiological basis, something which, in fact, is not always necessary, and, moreover, is often too broad a foundation, inasmuch as these observations are not specific to man.

From the point of view of the present-day reader who is interested in the topics that are part of educational psychology, the present book also suffers from the shortcoming that some of the terms used here are now out-of-date, and are no longer employed in the literature of contemporary psychology. At certain points of this introductory essay, we have already considered several conceptual and semantic misunderstandings of Vygotsky's book (of course, from the standpoint of our understanding of the scientific issues involved).

Our general analysis of the basic conceptions and assumptions of this interesting and instructive book is now complete, though we should also note that the book was, unfortunately, forgotten without reason. Bear in mind, too, the time the book was written, and the fact that its author was a young man who was just entering the field of psychological science. Vygotsky's true talent as an investigator developed only after the publication of the present book, though in our opinion it was an important stage in the preparation and evolution of cultural-historical theory for which the name of Vygotsky is celebrated throughout the world.

V.V. Davydov, 1990

References

Bernstein, N. The Physiology of Movement and Activity, Moscow, 1990 (translation in press).

El'konin, D.B. Izbrannye psikhologicheskie trudy (Selected Psychological Studies). Moscow, Pedagogika, 1989.

Gal'perin, P.Ya. "On the instincts in man." Voprosy psikhologiya, No. 1, 1976 (translated in Soviet Psychology).

Leont'ev, A.N. Izbrannye psikhologicheskie proizvedeniya (Selected Psychological Works), Vol. 1. Moscow, 1983.

Vygotsky, L.S. The Psychology of Art, translated by Scripta Technica. Introduction by A.N. Leont'iev. Commentary by V.V. Ivanov. Cambridge, MIT Press, 1971 (original publication Moscow, 1965, 1968, 1986, 1987).

Vygotsky, L.S. (edited by A.V. Zaporozhets) Sobr. soch. (Collected Works) Moscow, Pedagogika, 1982-84 (translation to be published by Plenum Press).

"Historical Meaning of the Psychological Crisis." In: Sobr. soch., Vol. 1, pp. 291-436.

"The Technique of Reflexological and Psychological Investigations." In: Sobr. soch., Vol. 1, pp. 43-62.

"Consciousness as a Problem of the Psychology of Behavior." In: Sobr. soch., Vol. 1, pp. 78-98.

Whiting, N.T.A. (ed). Human Motor Action: Bernstein Reassessed, New York, Elsevier North-Holland, 1984.

Chapter 1

PEDAGOGICS AND PSYCHOLOGY

Pedagogics

Pedagogics is the study of the education of the child. But what is education? It may be defined in any number of ways. We will use the definition given by Pavel Petrovich Blonskii, the Soviet psychologist and educational reformer, who wrote that education consists of a deliberate, organized, and prolonged effort to influence the development of an individual.

In pedagogics, as in the study of education, there is a need to establish clearly and precisely how this effort may be organized, what different forms it may take, what techniques it may utilize, and what direction it should assume. A further goal is to understand what the laws are that govern the very development of the individual we intend to influence. Accordingly, pedagogics encompasses, for all practical purposes, several entirely disparate domains of knowledge. On the one hand, since it has the responsibility of developing the child, it is a subfield of the biological (i.e., natural, sciences). On the other hand, since every form of education sets for itself particular ideals, goals, or norms, for that very reason it must deal with the philosophical or normative sciences.

Hence the never-ending controversy in pedagogics regarding the philosophical and biological aspects of the field. The methodology of the sciences establishes a fundamental distinction between sciences that study facts, and sciences that establish norms. Pedagogics, without question, is at the boundary between these two types of sciences.

However, facts, in and of themselves, cannot lead us to any sort of exact scientific conclusions regarding education, nor can norms give us any assurance that an ideal is truly realistic if it is not guided by facts. Blonskii wrote that

> philosophical pedagogics give rise to a spirit of educational utopianism. But scientific pedagogics will function not by establishing higher ideals, norms, and laws, but by studying the actual development of the individual who is being educated and the actual form of interaction between the individual and his or her educational environment. Scientific pedagogics is founded not on abstract speculation, but on data drawn from observation and experience, and is an entirely distinctive empirical science; it is not applied philosophy. [1]

1

However, even if it is an entirely original empirical science, pedagogics rests upon auxiliary sciences, for example, social ethics, which defines the overall goals and problems of education, and psychology together with physiology, which together define the tools for use in solving these problems.

Psychology

In the rigorous sense of the word, psychology denotes the science of the soul. This has been its definition from the very beginning.

In man's primitive outlook, there was a distinction made between body and soul, which were understood as individual *substances*. The assumption was that man possessed a dualistic nature. The emergence of this viewpoint goes back to primitive times, when man, having observed the phenomena of sleep, death, illness, and the like became convinced that a double or, a kind of soul, dwelled within him. In more developed forms of thought, this belief assumed the character of a conception of a soul that, in primitive man's thinking, recalled subtle physical substances like smoke or vapor. Even the Russian word for "soul," *dusha* is, in fact, related to the word *dyshat* which denotes the ability to breathe. [2]

Psychology, in fact, has been a science of the soul. Philosophers have studied the nature and properties of this soul and have raised any number of questions about it, for example, whether the soul is mortal or immortal, what might be the relation between the soul and the body, and what might be the essential nature and features of the substance of the soul, among others.

This trend dominated psychology for quite a long time, and, in all fairness, it may be referred to as *metaphysical psychology*, since it was always concerned with supra-sensible matter beyond our experience. With the appearance of a genuine science of psychology, the entire field of knowledge was divided up and branched out, subdividing into *metaphysical psychology* on the one hand, which was concerned with the subjects of truth and studied the world of the supra-sensible, and *positivist*, or *scientific psychology*, which, as far as it could ascertain, deliberately restricted itself to the domain of experience. (The Knowledge it gathered was nevertheless viewed as authentic).

In the 18th century, psychology split into two subfields, *rational psychology* and *empirical psychology*. Rational psychology continued to be referred to as metaphysical psychology, since its principal method of study was that of speculation. In opposition to rational psychology, empirical psychology defined itself outright as a science of facts based on experience, and attempted to place itself in the same kind of relationship with its object of study as did the natural sciences. Though it began with a severe critique of rational psychology, however, this form of empirical psychology likewise continued to occupy itself with the study of metaphysical problems for a long time.

Metaphysical psychology was subjected to severe criticism by John Locke, David Hume, and Immanuel Kant. These philosophers showed that the soul is nothing other than a product of our fantasy, and that, in our experience, in fact, only particular acts of perception confront us at every moment; in no way are we given any sensation of a soul in the form of a special substance.

Thus, in place of psychology as the science of the soul there arose a new science of mental data. This science was termed by N.N. Lange as a "psychology without a soul." Lange noted, however, that

> of course, isn't psychology called the science of the soul? How should we conceive
> of a science that leaves us in doubt as to whether there is, in general, a subject for it
> to study? We possess a traditional name for a large, but far from well-defined group
> of phenomena. This name has come down to us from a time when today's
> rigorously scientific constraints were unknown. Should we discard a name once the
> subject of the science has changed? This would be overly scrupulous and
> impractical. Thus, we will use without any hesitation the term 'psychology without
> any assumption of a soul'. The name is still appropriate as long as we are concerned
> with a subject that is not properly the subject of any other science. [3]

Empirical psychology also was transformed into a "psychology without any assumption of a soul," or "psychology without any metaphysics," or "psychology based on experience." It is necessary to note in this connection that this step was only a half-hearted one and only a compromise. Though a considerable proportion of metaphysics was discarded, psychology was still not entirely on the same footing as the natural sciences. It came to be thought of as a science of mental [*dushevnyi*] events or events of consciousness. Neither of these definitions could stand up to scientific criticism.

This form of psychology taught that mental events, by their very nature, differ absolutely from all other events in the world, that they are nonmaterial, without extent, and inaccessible to objective experience, and that they occur in conjunction with physical processes in our body without being related to them by means of causal connection. Though it assumed, therefore, the existence of nonmaterial, nonspatial events that were without causal connection, this form of psychology fully retained that dualistic viewpoint towards human nature, or "*dualism,*" which had been characteristic of primitive and religious thinking. It was no coincidence that it was closely related to idealistic philosophy, which taught that the soul is a special being unlike physical matter, and that consciousness possesses a special and primordial reality independent of being. Therefore, this form of psychology, which shut itself off, becoming estranged from the being of consciousness, was doomed to a lifeless existence, to isolation from reality, and to impotence when confronted with the most vital questions of human behavior.

First, consciousness constitutes only an insignificant portion of all of our mental [*psikhicheskii*] experience, since there is the entire vast world of the unconscious to consider. Second, consciousness either denotes only some single property of this experience, or constitutes, in disguised form, the very same entity as does the concept of soul, only under a different name. Blonskii noted that

> a psychology without any assumption of a soul, this form of psychology suddenly began to study phenomena of the ... soul. Of course, this was justified by the fact that the term, "mental [dushevnye] phenomena" simply denotes a group of distinctive phenomena that differ from material events or things by the fact that these distinctive, i.e., mental, events do not exist in space, do not take up any part of space, are not perceived by the eyes, ears, or any other sense organ, and are directly cognized only by being experienced. But could thoughts exist in the absence of that part of space called the brain? Can't you see, at least in part, my joy and hear my wishes? How can you claim after this that mental events are not associated with space, are not perceived directly by anyone other than myself and that they cannot be seen? [4]

Even empirical psychology, in the person of its strongest proponents, suggested the importance of the motor aspect in the study of mental processes. Empirical psychology showed that the development of the most complex central processes begins with movement and that movement is not a "minor appendix" of mental life. Indeed, all mental processes came to be understood as constitutent parts of an action, as the preliminary elements of a particular action. "We think because we engage in action," writes Hugo Münsterberg. Though Münsterberg cautions that the greatest caricature of this theory is expressed in that flagrantly mistaken understanding which claims the richness of inner life is a function of the quantity of one's movements and that, consequently, the athlete or circus acrobat possesses the richest inner life. In complex acts, the motor reaction consists not in a kind of muscular action, but in a novel expansion or closure of the motor pathways in the brain itself. However, with all due regard for the motor aspect, this form of psychology continued to distinguish particular mental events as being nonmaterial in nature, i.e., it continued to retain the dualism and spiritualism of empirical psychology.

Therefore, in place of a science of mental events, today psychology has begun to assume the form of a new science, one that American psychologists have referred to as the study of the behavior of living beings. By the term, "behavior," these psychologists understand the entire aggregate of movements, internal and external, which a living being has at its disposal. Psychology is guided by that long-established fact that every state of consciousness without exception is associated with particular movements. In other words, all mental events that occur in the organism may be studied from the standpoint of movement.

Psychology considers even the most complex forms of our consciousness as especially subtle and imperceptible forms of certain movements. Psychology, thus, becomes a biological science, since it studies behavior, which is interpreted as one of the most important forms of adaptation of a living organism to the environment. Therefore, it interprets behavior as the process of interaction between the organism and the environment, whose explanatory principle is that of the biological utility of the psyche.

However, man's behavior occurs within the complex framework of the social environment. Man engages in intercourse with nature in no other way than through this environment, and accordingly, the environment is the most important factor governing and establishing man's behavior. Psychology studies the behavior of *social* man and the laws of variation of this behavior.

Not only the subject, but also the methods of the science thus changed. Whereas in empirical psychology the principal method was that of introspection, i.e., the perception of one's own mental processes, the new psychology rejected this method, whether it was understood as the only method possible, or just a key method. In fact, the method of introspection is one that is marked by extreme subjectivism, since the person is, at one and the same time, the observer and the observed. It entails a division of attention, an act that can never be achieved in entirety; either the very feeling or some other phenomenon that is under observation vanishes under the influence of observation, or we run the risk of overlooking what is most important when in the grip of the intensity of immediate experience. "To observe one's own fear means not to be very afraid," writes Blonskii, "to observe one's own anger becomes a way of helping oneself begin to overlook things. But if we are consumed by a powerful fear or a powerful fear or a powerful rage, we do not have the time to observe ourselves."

Therefore, introspection must not be thought of as self-perception or as a passive state of consciousness in which mental events are, so to speak, themselves recorded in our consciousness, but rather as a special type of activity oriented towards the perception of our own experiences. This activity may influence other actions, may disturb them, and may itself be disturbed by other actions. Therefore, while rejecting the claim that introspection is the only source of psychological knowledge, the modern science of psychology nevertheless does not renounce the use of this method, for example, in the form of oral reports of a subject or the utterance of a subject which, naturally, itself has to be analyzed and interpreted, like all other aspects of a subject's behavior. These oral reports may lead us to take into account in our study of behavior inhibited or undisclosed internal movements and reactions that, in the absence of this method, would have remained outside the range of our observation.

However, the data accumulated by means of this method must be monitored and checked in the most rigorous way possible against objective results, inasmuch as we are always in danger of obtaining false and subjectively distorted results. Objective and experimental observation, therefore, remains the principal method of the science. By comparison with mere observation, experiment has the advantage of allowing us to produce whatever facts we require whenever we wish and as many times as we wish—to isolate them, to combine them together, to place them under different conditions, and to vary them in accordance with the conditions of the particular investigation.

The materialist basis of the new psychology is among its distinctive feature. That it is indeed a materialist psychology is clear from the fact that the new psychology considers all of man's behavior as consisting of a series of movements and reactions and possessing all the properties of material being. A second feature can be found in its objectivism, since it stipulates as the *sine qua non* of its investigations that these investigations be based on the objective verification of its material. Finally, its third feature consists in its dialectical method. According to the principle underlying this method, mental processes are understood to develop in indissoluble unity with all other processes in the organism and are subordinate to precisely the same laws of development as is everything else in nature. Finally, its last feature can be seen in its sociobiological basis, the meaning of which was defined earlier.

Scientific psychology is now experiencing a crisis of sorts, and the new discipline has only reached the initial stages of its construction. This, however, does not mean that it is constrained to rely only on its own results. On the contrary, it is often forced to rely on the entire body of scientifically reliable and accurate results of the old psychology. Once the original and fundamental view taken by the science of psychology towards its subject had changed, it found it necessary time and time again to re-interpret old results anew, to translate old concepts into a new language, and to elucidate and comprehend previously discovered facts and laws in the light of a new outlook. Hence, for quite some time to come there will unavoidably remain in psychology the impression of a duality at its very roots, beginning with the broadest generalizations and concluding with terminology. This situation is particularly unavoidable in our transitional and critical period, when the science of psychology is itself experiencing a serious crisis in its very foundations.

Educational Psychology

In the second half of the 19th century there occurred a turning point in psychology. Psychology entered into a period of experiment. In fact, it is precisely because of experiment that all the natural sciences have achieved their remarkable successes. Experimentation created physics, chemistry, and physiology. Physicians, physiologists, chemists, and astronomers were also the first to emphasize the potential for experimentation in psychology. Recourse to experimentation in psychology was accompanied by efforts aimed at the most exact study of phenomena, and psychology began to strive toward becoming an exact science. Hence, it was natural for psychology to attempt to make use of the theoretical laws of science in its practical applications, in the same way as had happened in all the applied disciplines.

"Educational psychology," writes Blonskii, "is that branch of applied psychology which studies the application of the conclusions of theoretical psychology to the process of education and teaching." Originally, when it first emerged, educational psychology aroused great hopes, and it seemed to everyone that, under the guidance of educational psychology, education would, in fact, become as exact a process as technology. These expectations proved to be illusory, however, and very shortly a general sense of disappointment set in in psychology. There were any number of reasons why this happened, some theoretical in nature and entailed by the very essence of the new discipline, and others of practical import, entailed by the historical development of psychology itself.

The first of these reasons lies in the fact that science can never serve directly as a handmaiden to practice. William James was quite correct in noting that it is a profound delusion to think that actual curricula, academic programs, or teaching methods could be taken right out of psychology for use in the school without further ado.

> Psychology is a science, and teaching is an art; and sciences never generate arts directly out of themselves ... The science of logic has never made a man reason rightly, and the science of ethics ... has never made a man behave rightly ... The pedagogics and the psychology ran side by side, and the former was not derived in any sense from the latter. The two were congruent, but neither was subordinate. And so everywhere the teaching must agree with the psychology, but need not necessarily be the only kind of teaching that would so agree; for many diverse methods of teaching may equally well agree with psychological laws. To know psychology, therefore, is absolutely no guarantee that we shall be good teachers. [5]

The inconsequentiality of educational psychology, which it assumed even in the studies of its greatest proponents, was yet another reason for this disappointment. Auguste Lay reproached Ernst Meumann for bringing it down to the level of a "mere craft." In fact, in the classical development, educational psychology stood far closer to a concept of mental health than to pedagogics proper.

Thus, psychology cannot directly produce any sort of pedagogical conclusions. But since the educational process is one of psychology, knowledge of the general foundations of psychology will, of course, help us in achieving a rigorous formulation of the discipline. Ultimately, education always denotes an alteration of inherited forms of behavior and a process of fostering new modes of reaction. Consequently, if we wish to view this process from a scientific point of view, we must, of necessity, have in mind the general laws of reactions and the conditions under which they are formed. Thus, the relationship between pedagogics and psychology recalls absolutely the relationship between all the other applied sciences and their theoretical disciplines. Psychology has begun to be applied to practical questions, to the study of crime, to the treatment of illness, and to labor and economic activity. According to Münsterberg,

...everything indicates that we shall soon have a real, substantial applied psychology. And then such an applied psychology would no longer be a mere heaping up of such bits of theoretical psychology as could possibly be utilized for practical purposes. Applied Psychology would thus stand in just the same relation to the ordinary psychology as that in which engineering stands to physics. It would deal exclusively with the question: How can psychology help us reach certain ends? ...Hence, educational psychology, a product of the last several years, is a new science which forms part of applied psychology together with legal and medical and economic and aesthetic and industrial psychology. ...Educational psychology is entirely at its beginning, and is unable to offer any complete system of prescriptions or advice... And yet it must rely on its own resources. Simply to take over the ready-made material of general psychology would be useless... A start has been made, however, and, no doubt, from humble beginnings a true educational psychology will soon arise. [6]

It is for this reason that we cannot agree with Blonskii when he claims that

Educational psychology, on the one hand, borrows from theoretical psychology chapters that are of interest to the teacher, for example, those on memory, attention, imagination, and the like, and on the other hand, discusses the pedagogical constraints imposed by everyday life viewed within the context of their correspondence with the laws of mental life, deciding, for example, how to teach writing skills in a way that would be most appropriate to the psychology of the child. [7]

Here Blonskii has it all wrong. First, any transference of fully worked-out chapters from general psychology will simply involve meaningless efforts at transferring fully worked-out, though foreign, results and fragmentary bits of knowledge, as Münsterberg has put it. Second, it is impossible to have any sort of life if there is no place for the sciences, nor is it possible to discuss the constraints of pedagogy; here it is a matter of theoretical pedagogics. Finally, it also does not make sense for psychology to serve only in the role of expert.

The correct relationship between strengths and scientific goals can be established only if the different subfields of psychology were distributed among the individual pedagogical disciplines in the following way: (1) history of pedagogical systems; (2) history of educational concepts; (3) theoretical pedagogy; (4) experimental pedagogy. (This latter was identified too hastily, and wrongly, with educational psychology, as in experiments, though any investigator may have to deal with experimental investigations of this or that educational technique which are in no way psychological in nature); and, finally, (5) educational psychology, which must exist as a separate science; those authors who speak of the "transformation of pedagogics into educational psychology" are, therefore, entirely mistaken. This notion, in fact, appeared only because of a misunderstanding of what constitutes the problems of each science and an inadequately clear distinction between these problems.

Blonskii also declares that pedagogics must be based on educational psychology, in the same way as animal husbandry is based on experimental biology.

That's one thing; but to claim that pedagogics is experimental vocational psychology is something altogether different. By the same token, it's one thing to say that animal husbandry depends on experimental biology, but it's quite another matter to take it into one's head to merge animal husbandry with experimental biology. The former is correct, but not the latter.

Pedagogics must discuss the goals and problems of education, while educational psychology can do no more than designate the means of implementing the process of education.

> The florist loves his tulip and hates the weed; the botanist who describes and explains does not and, from his standpoint, cannot hate or love anything; the weed is to him as real and, therefore, as important as the most beautiful flower ... As the botanist cares no less for the weed than for the flower, the science of mankind cares for human foolishness no less than for human wisdom; all is material which must be analyzed and explained without passion and without partisanship. The most noble deed is, from this point of view, no better than the most hideous crime, the most beautiful sentiment no more valuable than disgusting vulgarity, the deepest thought of the genius not to be preferred to the inane babble of the insane; all is neutral material, which has only the one claim, that it exists as a link in a chain of causal events. [8]

In precisely the same way, educational psychology can be oriented towards any system of education equally. It may tell us how to educate the serf and the free man, the career-minded just like the revolutionary. We see this quite eloquently in the example of European science, which is equally creative in the invention of tools of creation as of tools of destruction. Chemistry and physics serve equally in war and in culture. Every educational system, therefore, must possess its own system of educational psychology.

The absence of such a science may be explained by purely historical causes and aspects of the development of psychology. Blonskii is right when he says that the present-day shortcomings of educational psychology may be explained by vestiges of spiritualism and an individualistic point of view, and that only that form of psychology will be of use in pedagogy which constitutes a bio-social science discipline.

The old psychology, which had considered the psyche in isolation from behavior, was, in fact, unable to find a genuine soil for an applied science. On the contrary, because it was concerned with constructions out of thin air, and abstractions, it was always out of touch with genuine experience and, therefore, too insubstantial a discipline to become a source from which an educational psychology could be created. Every science arises out of practical demands and is, ultimately, directed also towards practical application. Marx has said that it was enough for philosophers to have interpreted the world, now it's time to change it. Such a time comes for every science. But philosophers have interpreted the soul and mental phenomena until they were no longer able to figure out how to recast these phenomena simply because these phenomena fell outside the realm of experience. Now, however, when psychology has begun to study behavior, it is natural to wonder how to alter behavior. Educational psychology is also a science of the laws of variation of human behavior and of the means of mastering these laws.

Thus, educational psychology should be thought of as an independent discipline, as a special branch of applied psychology. It is wrong, as most writers on the subject have done (e.g., Meumann, Blonskii, and others) to identify educational psychology with experimental pedagogics. That this is indeed the wrong approach is demonstrated quite convincingly by Münsterberg, in whose view experimental pedagogics is a subfield of vocational psychology. "If this is so," writes Gessen,

> are we then justified in referring to this branch of psychotechnics as pedagogics only because it is concerned with the search for technical means that could be applied under practical conditions in pedagogics? In fact, when it is applied in the field of justice vocational psychology does not, therefore, turn into jurisprudence. In precisely the same way, when applied in economic life, vocational psychology does not, therefore, become part of political economy. Just as obviously, there is no basis for claiming that, when applied in education, vocational psychology will, in time, become all of pedagogics, nor that it can be considered a subfield of pedagogics. Experimental pedagogics, under the best of interpretations, could be called educational vocational psychology. [9]

It would be correct to distinguish between (1) experimental pedagogics, as involved in the solution of purely pedagogical and instructional problems by means of experiment (e.g., as in a pilot school); and (2) pedagogical vocational psychology, analogous to the other branches of vocational psychology and concerned with *psychological* investigations applied in the field of education.

But the latter constitutes only one *part* of the discipline of educational psychology, since according to Münsterberg, "psychotechnics is hardly the same thing as applied psychology, but rather constitutes only one half of it." Its other half consists in the "psychology of culture." Together they form a "genuine educational psychology," the actual construction of which will be a task for the very near future.

"Isn't it because experimental pedagogics still has so little to boast of in the way of precision in its conclusions," writes Gessen, "that it is the concern mostly of teachers and philosophers instead of physicians and specialists in psychology?" [10]

[1]Original source not known.

[2] *Dusha* also can refer to the mind and to mental phenomena (trans) deliberately restricted itself to the domain of experience, though the knowledge it gathered was nevertheless viewed as authentic.

[3]Original source not known.

[4]Original source not known.

[5] *Talks to Teachers on Psychology and to Students on Some of Life's Ideals,* now available from Harvard University Press, 1983, pp. 15-16.

[6] *Psychology and the Teacher*, Münsterberg, *ibid.*, 1909, pages 25, 30.

[7]Original source not known.

[8]Original source not known.

[9]Original source not known.

[10]Original source not known.

Chapter 2

THE CONCEPT OF BEHAVIOR AND REACTION

Behavior and Reaction

Reactions are the fundamental elements out of which all human and animal behavior is composed, both in the simplest and in its most complex forms. In psychology, a *reaction* is understood to refer to the responding action of an organism which has been induced by some stimulus. If we look at man's behavior, we may easily note that, under ordinary conditions, all movements and actions arise in response to some impulse, impetus, or stimulation, which we usually call the cause of the particular action.

Every one of our actions is, without fail, preceded by some inducing cause, either in the form of an external datum or event, or in the form of an inner desire, excitation, or thought. All the motivations of our actions will also be stimuli of one of our reactions. Thus, a reaction should be understood as a special relationship between an organism and its environment. A reaction is always a response of an organism to various changes in its environment, and constitutes an extraordinarily valuable and biologically useful mechanism of adaptation.

The reactions arise at the lowest stages of development of organic life. Bacteria, for example, respond to such minute stimuli as one-billionth of a milligram of potassium chloride. Other protozoa, for example, amoeba, infusoria, etc., also possess a quite pronounced capacity to enter into reactions. Plants are no exception. Darwin established that sundew glands are stimulated by a speck of iron dust weighing as little as 1/250,000 of a milligram.

A reaction constitutes the primitive and fundamental form of every behavioral act. *Movement away from something* and *movement toward something*, the simplest forms of a reaction, express the striving of an animal to avoid undesirable stimuli, to contract its mass, or turn away from danger, or, conversely, approach a desirable stimulus, extend its body, or grasp hold of something. A vast collection of the most diverse forms of behavior has developed in man over the course of a lengthy evolution starting from these, the simplest forms of behavior.

The Three Components of a Reaction

Every reaction, whether we consider it in its most primitive form, as in the simplest organisms, or in the highly complex forms of man's conscious activity, will inevitably consist of three basic components. The first component is the organism's perception of particular stimuli that are transmitted by the environment. This component is, by convention, usually termed the *sensory component*. The next, or second component, involves the transformation of this stimulus into those internal processes of the organism that have been excited by this impetus into undertaking some activity. Finally, the third component consists in the organism's responding act, mostly in the form of movements that are the result of internal processes. The third component is called the *motor component*, and, in the case of the higher animals and man, in which it is associated with the functioning of the central nervous system, may be termed the *central component*. These three components—the sensory, the central, and the motor—or the perception of a stimulus, its transformation, and the responding act, must be present in every act of reaction.

An example, consider some of the simplest types of reaction, for example, when the stems of a plant stretch toward the sun (heliotropism), when a moth flies toward the light of a candle, when a dog produces saliva in response to a piece of meat placed in its mouth, when a person who has heard the bell ring at the front door goes to open it, and so forth. In all these instances, it is a simple matter to discover the presence of all these three components. The effect of the sun's rays on a plant, of the light of a candle on a moth, of a piece of meat on a dog, of the ringing of a bell on a person all serve as the stimulus of a corresponding reaction. Internal chemical processes that arise in a plant or in the body of a moth under the effect of the sun's rays, the nerve excitation transmitted from a dog's tongue and from a person's ear to the central nervous system—each is the second component of a corresponding reaction. Finally, the very bending of the stem of a plant, the flight of a moth, the secretion of saliva in a dog, the steps a person takes together with the unbolting of the lock—these all constitute the third, concluding component of a reaction.

These three components are not always so obvious as in the examples just presented, however. Sometimes, the stimulus will be in the form of certain internal, invisible processes of the organism, such as a change in the circulatory system, respiration of internal organs, glandular secretions, and so on. In these cases, the first component of the reaction will remain hidden from our eyes.

In other cases, internal processes, which are the most difficult to observe and are the least studied of all processes, either are of such complexity that they cannot be taken into account because of the contemporary state of psychological science, or, on the other hand, assume such accelerated forms as to appear to be entirely absent. The third component of a reaction may then seem to follow immediately after the first, i.e., the organism's movement seems to occur immediately following the perceived stimulus, as in the case of a cough, a reflexive shout, and so on.

The third component of a reaction, i.e., the actual responding action of the organism, occurs even more often in concealed form. It may be expressed in slight and visually imperceptible movements as, for example, in the rudimentary speech movements we make when we pronounce some word in our minds. It may be expressed in a series of movements of the internal organs, and then it also remains concealed from our eyes.

Finally, reactions may occur in such complex interdependence as to make it virtually impossible to divide behavior up into individual reactions for the sake of simple observation, or to distinguish all three components of a reaction. This also occurs whenever the responding action is slowed down or delayed by comparison with the action of the stimulus. In this case, it is not always possible to easily or fully establish the three-component process of a reaction.

We should, in general, note that these three components manifest themselves with absolute clarity in the simplest reactions. In the more complex forms of human behavior, they assume increasingly more concealed, implicit forms, and highly complex analysis is needed in order to discover the nature of the reaction. However, even in its most complex forms, human behavior is constructed, in terms of type and model, in precisely the same way as in the simplest forms in plants and one-celled organisms.

Reaction and Reflex

In animals that possess a nervous system, reactions tend to assume the form of what is known as a *reflex*. By a reflex we generally understand in physiology any act of the organism that is induced by some external stimulation of the nervous system, which is transmitted along an afferent nerve to the brain, and from there along an efferent nerve, automatically inducing a movement or a secretion of a working organ. The actual pathway of an ordinary reflex is composed of (a) an afferent nerve, (b) the afferent and efferent neurons of the spinal cord, and (c) an efferent nerve, which are collectively referred to as the reflex arc. This is also the most general scheme of any nerve act. Certain scientists have recently begun to insist on referring to human reactions as reflexes, and have begun to call the science of human and animal reactions, *reflexology*.

However, such a substitution of terms is unwarranted. As can be easily seen from its description, a reflex is only a special case of a reaction, that is, it is a reaction of the nervous system. Thus, a reflex is a concept which is narrowly physiological in nature, while a reaction is one which is broadly biological in nature. Reflexes are present neither in plants nor in animals without a nervous system, though we are entirely justified in speaking of reactions in these cases. Thus, the concept of a reaction helps us to include human behavior in the lengthy chain of biological adaptive movements all organisms engage in, from the lowest to the highest, to locate it relative to the basis of organic life on earth, and to discover the unlimited horizon for studying its evolution and for considering it from the broadest biological perspective. In contrast, the concept of a reflex restricts us to the comparatively narrow circle of the physiology of the nervous system and places a limit on the range of phenomena that may be observed.

To this we must add that whether there exist reactions that cannot be associated with a reflex arc, but arise directly from chemical stimulation of the central nervous system is a question that is far from solved and one that is still under discussion. Thus, Lazarev, in his theory of the ionic excitation of nerves, established the full theoretical feasibility and possibility of such autochthonous, arbitrary excitation of the nervous system, which occur as a consequence of the dissocation of potassium chloride in cerebral matter. The movements which arise thereby constitute a fully developed type of reaction, since all three essential constituent components are present: a stimulus in the form of the dissociation of potassium chloride, central processing, and a responding act. However, it is only by a stretch of the imagination that such action can be considered a reflex. What is missing here is the first component of the reflex arc and the participation of an afferent nerve to conduct a peripheral stimulation to the brain.

For all these reasons, everywhere in the presentation below we will retain the term, "reaction," to denote the basic forms of human behavior. Moreover, this term possesses a genuine scientific tradition, chiefly in experimental psychology, the most exact part of the discipline, where it has been used to denote the elementary acts of human behavior.

The Inherited Reactions and the Acquired Reactions

For the simplest observation of human or animal behavior, it suffices to note that behavior itself consists in reactions that originate in different ways. Some reactions are *inherited* or *innate*, and seem to be conferred on the child at the very moment of birth, or arise as the child grows up without any training or outside action. Such reactions include, for example, the reflexes of crying, deglutition, and sucking, which may be observed in the infant in the very first hours after birth and which, in general, remain unchanged throughout the individual's life. These inherited forms of behavior are easily broken down into two classes, the reflexes and the instincts.

Other reactions, in contrast, arise in the course of individual experience at different points in a person's life and are indebted for their origin not to inherited constitution, but to individual elements of one's own experience. The principal difference between *innate* and *acquired reactions* becomes clear once we note that the former constitutes an inherited reserve of useful, adaptable movements which are absolutely the same for all the individuals of an entire species. The latter, in contrast, present an extraordinary variety and are distinguished by extreme diversity and variability. Australian aborigines and Eskimos, Frenchmen and Negroes, workers and millionaires, children and the elderly, ancient man and modern man all experience fear in nearly identical ways. In the inherited forms of behavior there is much that is common to animals and man. In contrast, the acquired reactions are highly diverse, and depend on the circumstances of history, geography, sex, and social class, and on the particular individual.

Inherited or Unconditional Reflexes

The group of inherited or unconditional reflexes should be thought of as the principal group of reactions of the newborn infant. The infant cries, moves its hands and feet, coughs, and takes food—and this it does all thanks to a well-regulated reflex-nerve mechanism that begins to function in the very first minutes of life.

Among the distinctive features of the reflexes, we should note, first, the fact that each is a responding action to some stimulus, second, that each is mechanical, involuntary, and unconscious, so that even if the individual wishes to inhibit some reflex, he is often unable to do so; third, they are, for the most part, biologically useful. For example, if a human infant were unable to cough reflexively, he could easily choke when ingesting food; through the existing reflex, expulsive, ejecting movements are forced as a means of dislodging food particles that have fallen into the cavity of the windpipe and present a danger. The reflex of closing one's eyelids in response to some unpleasant mechanical stimulation of the eyes is just as useful a reflex, serving to protect this extraordinarily important and essential organ from mechanical injury.

From the foregoing, we may already see that the newborn infant exists principally by virtue of inherited forms of behavior. While he can eat, breathe, and move his organs, for all this he is indebted to reflexes. A reflex is nothing other than the simplest connection between particular elements of the environment and corresponding adaptive movements of the organism.

Instincts

The most complex forms of inherited behavior are referred to as *instincts*. One point of view recently proposed insists that the instincts should be considered as compound or chain reflexes. By this we should understand a linkage of several reflexes in which the responding part of one reflex serves as the stimulus for a succeeding reflex. As a consequence of a slight impetus or some isolated external stimulus, therefore, a complex sequence of actions may arise, associated with each other in such a way that each action automatically induces the succeeding action.

As an example, consider the digestive instinct as it manifests itself in the infant. In this approach we have to proceed by thinking of those internal processes that induce the infant to reflexively perform a series of searching and positioning movements with his mouth, eyes, and head as constituting the initial stimulus. When, in response to these movements, the infant's mother brings her breast near the infant's lips, there arises a new stimulus along with a new reflex in which the infant grasps its mother's teat with its lips. This movement induces, in turn, a new reflex of suction movements, as a result of which milk is drawn into the infant's mouth. This new stimulus induces a deglutition reflex, and so on.

With this understanding, an instinct is nothing other than a series of successive reflexes connected together like links in a chain. Provisionally, and schematically, an instinct may be represented by means of a formula. If an ordinary reflex is denoted ab, where a denotes a stimulus and b a reflex, then we may express an instinct in the following way: $ab—bc—cd—de$, and so on.

However, such an interpretation of the concept of instinct brings up a host of objections. First, there is the fact that an instinct exists in far less limited and far less rigorous connection with the elements of the environment than a reflex. A reflex is an connection that is elementary, strictly defined, and deterministic. In contrast, in an instinct, this connection is far less well-defined and for more arbitrary in nature.

Observers have declared that even young squirrels who have been separated at the moment of birth from their parents and who were raised as house pets, never having seen open spaces or forests and who had always gotten their food out of human hands, begin to exhibit the instinct of gathering together food stores for the winter when autumn comes round. They begin to bury nuts in a carpet or sofa, or pile them up in a corner of the room. Under these conditions, it is utterly impossible for training to have had any effect, and any possibility for those elements of the environment which usually accompany the manifestation of this instinct is excluded. It is, therefore, necessary to suppose here a far more extendable and flexible connection between the instinctive reaction and the environment than is observed in the case of the reflexes.

Further, the system of movements that compose a reflex is strictly defined and given in advance in a precisely stipulated form. In contrast, instinctive movements can never be guessed at or taken into account from start to finish, there is never an exact and stereotypical pattern to work from, and instead these movements vary from one moment to the next.

Finally, the third feature of an instinct can be seen in the greater complexity of the movements that compose it. Whereas usually only a single organ is involved in a reflex, in any instinct there occurs a sequence of coordinated movements involving different organs.

To this we should further note the anatomical and physiological differences between the instincts and the reflexes. In the development of the instincts, an extraordinarily important role is played by the vegetative nervous system, as well as the hormonal or endocrine system.

For all these reasons, the instincts have to be thought of as constituting a special form of inherited behavior. That a reflex constitutes a reaction that is transmitted from one particular organ, whereas an instinct constitutes a behavioral reaction that involves the entire organism is the feature which underlies this distinction. (This feature was suggested by Vagner.)

It is simplest to understand this distinction using Vagner's example of the mating of flies that have been decapitated. Decapitated flies are capable of mating, but only if mating occurs between a single decapitated fly and a normal specimen. Moreover, the normal specimen engages in all those movements that are performed prior to mating, movements that cannot be precisely taken into account in advance or predicted and which involve a number of different organs. The decapitated fly is capable of engaging in the actual act of mating. In this case, we are dealing with an experimentally performed subdivision of behavior into instinctual and reflex forms. All the reactions in the behavior of the entire organism that precede the sex act must be ascribed to instinctual behavior associated with the functioning of the cerebral centers. The actual act of sexual union proves to be a simple reflex that does not require the participation of the cerebral centers and is localized at lower centers.

Origin of Inherited Reactions

The question of origins is one of the most difficult of all scientific questions. Here it is necessary to deal with conditions that have existed for many thousands of years, with conditions that are long gone, and to make judgements about the past on the basis of the present. Questions as to the origin of the inherited forms of behavior are no different. Given the present state of scientific knowledge, it is entirely impossible to determine the origin of a particular instinct or reflex even approximately.

The general principle underlying the origin of the instincts was established and elucidated by Charles Darwin in his study of natural selection. In this sense, there is no essential difference between the origin of the useful inherited forms of animal organization and the behavior of animals.

During the epoch of religious thinking, a conception of miraculous purposefulness, by means of which animal and plant organisms were supposed to have been constructed, was everywhere dominant. It was also assumed that there was a correspondence between the organism and its conditions of existence. Prescientific thinking saw in this a direct proof of an intelligent and well-meaning providence that equipped the bird with wings, the fish with fins, and man with reason. It was only by conceiving of a deity that man was able to understand himself, understand how the unreasonable adaptability of all living matter to life could have come about and, reasoning about all of living matter the way he reasoned about himself, anthropomorphised nature, ascribing to it an intelligent and deliberate origin and turning the concept of purpose into a foundation of his understanding of the world.

The rejection of this world view, a rejection that reached its most fully developed form in Darwin's study of the origin of the species, was the greatest conquest of scientific thought. Darwin always advanced the conception of an intelligent creator from the domain of science, and he was the first to set forth the principle of natural development, or evolution, of living organisms and the principle of a natural explanation of the origin of the world and of man.

It is well known that Darwin viewed the harmonious coordination of the organism and the environment not from the naive point of view of expediency, but instead from the standpoint of scientifically comprehensible causality. His focus was to set forth as the fundamental motive mechanism of evolution the struggle for existence in the animal and plant kingdom. It is precisely this principle which confronts every living being in the form of a dilemma: either be capable of adapting to life or perish. And in this struggle those who do not adapt perish and vanish. In this struggle only those organisms survive that, for one reason or another, prove more adaptable than others to existence.

The same process of struggle occurs time and time again between the surviving organisms, a struggle that leads to the creation of a selection of the most adaptable, most viable specimens of a species every time. And just as this process of struggle does not cease even for a single moment, neither does the process of perfecting the species and the survival of the fittest. Furthermore, those organisms that do survive retain the right to life only through the unceasing straining of all their strengths and the active participation of all their adaptive capacities. It is for this very reason that they practice, develop, and bring to as perfect a state as possible all their essential and useful organs, while unnecessary and idle organs gradually atrophy as a consequence of lack of use.

There is also the effect of sexual selection to consider in this connection, for it is directed to the very same ends. It is because of sexual selection, in fact, that only the most viable, or fittest, specimens leave descendents, and, because of inheritance, these descendents receive and reinforce the biological features of their ancestors.

It is only because of the tragic law of struggle, the basic law of life, that the evolution of organisms can extend from the one-cell infusoria right up through man. The science established by Darwin has recently received a major corrective in the development of the so-called "theory of mutations." Its most essential import is that new species arise in the course of development not only by means of evolution, i.e., slow and gradual accumulation of slight variations, but also by means of sudden jumps, by means of the revolutionary path of sudden and abrupt transitions to features surfacing anew.

The origin of the instincts and of the simple reflexes are also explained wholly by these fundamental principles of evolution and the theory of mutation. They must be understood not as the wise and expedient workings of some sort of intelligent will, but rather as a fearful and useful experiment developed in the course of the struggle for existence whose costs have been borne by the deaths of countless individuals. And since the instincts and reflexes, i.e., the inherited forms of behavior, must be considered a type of biological adaptation, there can be no doubt that, in its fundamental and principal aspects, the instincts and the reflexes have precisely the same origin as does the structure of the body and the organs of animals. It is entirely understandable that, in the struggle for existence, those species have survived which produce protective reflexes when confronted by danger, and jump back from fatal bites and stings more rapidly and more dexterously.

It is just as obvious that the remarkable adaptability of all the instincts can only be explained by the fact that those species that were unable to develop such complex and highly perfected forms of adaptation have perished. There is a story told of a Greek who was taken to a temple. He took a look at the votive plaques erected as offerings to the deity, next to which was a painting depicting those who had perished in shipwrecks and those who had been saved by prayer. Said the sceptic, "Show me a painting of those who, despite their prayers, nevertheless perished. Otherwise I will not believe in an all-powerful God." Thus it is with life. Those who have adapted are simply those who have been saved, but adaptation does not constitute the fundamental law of organic life. The species that do not adapt are far more common, but we don't take notice of them, since they perish.

It should be clear to the reader why it is that, because of the general law of natural selection, such biologically useful adaptive work has occurred in the behavior of animals, and in the structure of their body. The fact that there has developed in man a coughing reflex, or in the rabbit the instinct of fear, or in the bird the instinct of flight, may be ultimately explained by the fact that those organisms have perished who were unable to cough or prick up their ears when in fright or take to flight once cold weather set in.

Conditional Reflexes

Until quite recently, the origin of the non-inherited reactions remained unclear and only dimly understood by science. Teachers had long been inclined to assume that the newborn infant constitutes a blank screen, like a clean sheet of paper on which the teacher may write anything that might seem appropriate. It is not too hard to see how wrong such a view is from just a brief description of the manifold and complex types of inherited forms of behavior.

The child is not a clean sheet of paper, but a sheet covered everywhere with the imprints left by the biologically useful experience of his or her ancestors. However, it is very difficult to find out what precisely is the mechanism responsible for the appearance of newly acquired reactions. Only in the past several decades, thanks to advances principally due to Russian physiological thought, has it been possible to catch a glimpse of this mechanism. The study of the conditional reflexes, developed mainly by Ivan Pavlov, has revealed the laws governing this mechanism with the indisputable precision of experimental natural science.

The essence of this science may be easily understood if we consider the example of a classical conditional reflex experiment. In this experiment, a piece of meat or biscuit powder is placed in a dog's mouth, or hydrochloric acid is instilled into its mouth, etc. In response to these stimuli, the dog begins to produce saliva, in strictly determined quantities and of an entirely determined quality, depending on the nature of the stimulus. For example, in response to hydrochloric acid the dog reacts by producing abundant salivation, though the composition of the saliva is extraordinarily watery and thin, since in this case the function of the reflex is to wash down an unpleasant stimulus. In response to dry and pungent food, an extremely viscous, thick, and slippery liquid is secreted, in far lesser quantities. By acting as a protective cushion around the membranes or bone, saliva serves to protect delicate internal membranes from damage. Thus, we have a complete reflex with all three fundamental components and with all the typical features of a reflex: adaptability, automaticity, etc.

If we flash a blue light in a room, ring a bell, stroke, scratch, or prick a dog at the same time we place a piece of meat or drops of hydrochloric acid in its mouth or, more precisely, several seconds later, after a given number of trials a new connection will have been captured, or "locked in," in the dog between the alien and indifferent stimulus (blue light, bell, etc.) and its salivary reflex. It is now sufficient to turn on a blue light without giving the dog any meat in order to cause it to produce saliva in the same quantity, and of the same quality, as when it is presented with a piece of meat. This new salivary reflex should be termed a *conditional reflex*, since it arises only under particular conditions, that is, when a new alien stimulus coincides with, or is *combined with*, a previous basic stimulus (e.g., blue light + meat). This reflex has, therefore, elsewhere been called a compound reflex.

The inherited or unconditional reflexes must be distinguished from the conditional reflexes, and the previous or unconditional stimulus must be distinguished from the new, conditional stimulus. How should we distinguish a conditional reflex from an unconditional reflex? First, in terms of origin; a conditional reflex is not present in inherited experience but arises in the course of an individual's own experience. Second, it is individualized and entirely different in different members of the same species. Third, it possesses far more transient and far less stable forms, and tends to vanish and break down if not reinforced again and again by unconditional stimuli.

Even from this brief description, it is clear that a conditional reflex possesses all the features of the acquired reactions and constitutes the property of the individual, forms the aggregate of his individual experience, i.e., experience that had not been imparted to him by inheritance. This remarkably simple discovery explains extraordinarily important aspects of animal behavior. It reveals the mechanism that makes animal behavior especially flexible, manifold, and quick to adapt. In its most general form, the law of formation of the conditional reflexes may be expressed in the following way. In addition to the inherited connections that exist between the environment and the organism, throughout its life the organism develops and establishes new connections between individual elements of the environment and its own reactions, and the diversity of these reactions is quite inexhaustible. This law asserts that a new connection may settle in under particular conditions between any element of the environment and any of the animal's reactions. Thus, any event, datum, or phenomenon of the environment may become a stimulus of any of the animal's reactions. For this to hold, it is only necessary that the effect of this phenomenon occur while the original stimulus is in effect.

It is not hard to see how extraordinarily critical are such reflexes in terms of biological importance, and the degree to which they can cause the animal's behavior to adapt and render it appropriate to the demands of the environment. It is precisely these reflexes which make it possible for the animal to produce adaptive reactions to stimuli that have just appeared, to respond to remote signals, and to guide its behavior not only under the influence of genuine stimuli, but also in expectation of future stimuli.

This same law shows us that the acquired reactions do not constitute something essentially novel by comparison with the innate reactions and, in theory, are in no way different from the innate reactions. On the contrary, it establishes that individual experience arises in no other way than on the basis of inherited experience, and that every acquired reaction is really an inherited reaction, except for having been altered in accordance with various conditions of existence. The process of development of the conditional reflexes is nothing other than a process of adaptation of the inherited experience of the species to individual conditions.

It is also extraordinarily significant that the environment is the decisive factor in every event in individual experience. It is precisely the structure of the environment that creates and defines those conditions which ultimately govern the development of all of individual behavior.

It is conceivable that the environment plays for each of us the very same role that Pavlov's laboratory plays for the dogs in his laboratory. In fact, what is it that ultimately defines the development of a particular reaction in a dog? Why does one dog learn to respond to blue light by salivating, while another to the beating of a metronome, and a third to being combed with a brush?

It should be clear to the reader that, in this case, the real cause is the way that the environment in the laboratory has been organized. If the infusion of an acid is accompanied by a flash of blue light, a reflex in response to blue light is formed, and so on. The same thing happens in the everyday environment, where, because of particular features of the structure of this environment, particular groups of stimuli occur at the same time, a feature which is also responsible for the nature and forms of the acquired reactions. Thus, the science of conditional reflexes establishes that acquired reactions are developed and arise on the foundation of innate reactions under the decisive influence of the environment.

If we bear in mind the fact that the innate reactions are developed and form ultimately under the influence of the environment, we can then define the conditional reflexes as an "environment that is itself a product of an environment." It is highly unlikely that there is any reaction in man that is not already present in latent form in the infant in its cradle. The infant possesses the elements of all those highly complex forms of behavior that lead to the discovery of spectral analysis, to Napoleon's campaigns, and to the discovery of America. No genuinely novel reaction arises in the course of individual experience, though, note, these elements are present in the infant as formless, uncoordinated, unorganized agglomerations. The entire process of growth, which distinguishes the behavior of the adult from that of the child, reduces to the construction of new connections between the environment and the reactions of the organism, and to the organization of mutual coordination between the two.

The psychologist of today might even say, "Give me absolutely every one of the newborn infant's reactions and absolutely every single intersection of influences in the structure of its environment, and I will predict with mathematical precision the behavior of the adult at any given moment."

Thus do we see the unusual plasticity and variability of behavior in the sense of an infinitely complex and infinitely subtle adaptation of behavior to the environment.

Super-reflexes

Using the same experimental techniques, it has been possible to establish that new conditional connections may settle in not only on the foundation of the innate or unconditional reflexes, but also on the foundation of the conditional reflexes. For example, if we develop in a dog a conditional salivary reflex in response to blue light, the dog will salivate every time we turn on a blue light in the room. If we now accompany the blue light with a new foreign stimulus, for example, the beating of a metronome, after a certain number of trials a new conditional reflex will have been formed in the dog, and it will begin to produce saliva only in response to a single beat of the metronome without any blue light.

We would be justified in calling this new reflex a *second-order conditional reflex*, since it itself arises and is formed on the foundation of a conditional reflex. The mechanism responsible for the formation of higher-order conditional reflexes, or *super-reflexes*, does not differ in essential respects from the formation of first-order reflexes. In order to arise, they likewise require a pre-established connection, moreover the old and new stimulus must occur at the same time.

In experiments on dogs, it has been possible to develop conditional reflexes of order no higher than the third, though this is only because investigations were only begun quite recently, and involved working with the primitive nervous system of the dog. Furthermore, the experiments have been performed on a reflex which, by virtue of its very biological function, cannot be considered a favorable medium for the development of super-reflexes, i.e., higher-order reflexes.

It is, however, easy to imagine that in the more highly developed nervous system of man, and even, in certain instances, in the animals as well, it is possible for conditional reflexes of extraordinarily high order that happen to be quite remote from the initial conditional reflex that engendered them, to manifest themselves. There is every reason to believe that, in the vast majority of all its forms, man's behavior is constructed out of such super-reflexes of extraordinarily high order.

It is extremely important to note in this connection that every conditional reflex that arises in individual experience is capable of serving as the basis for a new connection, and that, in principle, the process by which the conditional reflexes form is one that is infinite and without limit. This once more underscores the enormous biological value assumed by human behavior, thanks to the super-reflexes and the conditional reflexes.

Complex Forms of Conditional Reflexes

As studies have shown, highly complex forms of conditional reflexes are possible. If some unconditional stimulus, for example, offering a dog a piece of meat, is not initiated right after the onset of a conditional stimulus (turning on a blue light), but in each instance only after some given length of time, for example, after a three-second pause, a *delayed conditional reflex* will develop in the dog. The dog will produce saliva not immediately after the light has been turned on, but only three seconds afterwards. This type of reflex helps us to understand those reactions in which the responding action is separated from the stimulation by a more or less lengthy interval of time.

Another type of conditional reflex is the *vestigial reflex*. It arises whenever an unconditional stimulus begins to act before a conditional reflex has terminated. For example, if a blue light has been turned on in a room, but a piece of meat is given to the dog only after the light has been turned off, after a series of trials the dog will produce saliva once a blue light is turned off. This reflex would seem to be in response to the imprint of the stimulus, after, that is, the stimulation has itself ceased functioning. This type of reflex helps to explain how complex forms of conditional reactions arise where the structure of the environment assumes complex forms.

In all forms of human and animal behavior, from the most elementary to the most advanced, Pavlov sees the links of a common chain, as a boundless adaptation in all its variety, which constitutes life on earth. The movement of plants toward the light and the search for truth by means of mathematical analysis, aren't they, in essence, phenomena of the same type? And aren't these the final links of a nearly infinite chain of adaptations that manifests itself throughout the living world?

Chapter 3

THE MOST IMPORTANT LAWS OF HIGHER NERVOUS ACTIVITY IN MAN

The Laws of Inhibition and Disinhibition

The diversity of animal behavior and the complex forms of conditional reflexes become understandable only by taking into account the law of inhibition of the reflexes. It is not hard to see that abstention from a reaction or its suppression may otherwise constitute the essential conditions of behavior. From the standpoint of behavior, it is often just as necessary to abstain from a reaction as it is to execute a reaction.

Let us suppose that an animal had decided to attack or rush upon an enemy. It then becomes extraordinarily important that the defense reactions of fear and flight be suppressed or inhibited, and that the ordinary course of the aggressive reaction not be disturbed. In certain cases, it is just as necessary, biologically speaking, to suppress a reflexive shout as it is to produce it. Thus, the inhibition and suppression of certain reactions become an essential condition for other reactions to proceed correctly.

Simple external inhibition is the simplest form of inhibition. If an external stimulus acts on a dog at the same time as a conditional reflex, and is strong enough, the effect of the reflex either ceases or is inhibited. The effect of the new stimulus acts as a kind of brake. For example, if a dog produces saliva in response to blue light, and if at the same time, a loud knock is produced, the dog's salivary reflex will be inhibited. In precisely the same way, in man all reactions are either inhibited or cease entirely when a gunshot, shout, and so on are heard all of a sudden.

A second form of inhibition consists in the *conditional inhibitions*. If an external inhibitor acts repeatedly, *seriatum*, it will lose its power to delay the reflex. For example, if a salivary reflex produced in response to blue light is accompanied each time by the beat of a metronome, the beat will eventually forestall the reflex, and salivation will occur in a perfectly normal manner. Consider as an example a stimulus that has lost the power of inhibition in this way, or simply a stimulus that is not powerful enough. Let us carry out the same experiment in such a way that a blue light acting alone is accompanied by a piece of meat (i.e., we reinforce a conditional reflex with an unconditional reflex). At the same time, a blue light, now accompanied by some new stimulus, for example, the beat of a metronome, is present without being accompanied by a piece of meat. After a certain period of time, the beat will become a conditional inhibitor of the salivary reflex; that is, once it has been associated each time with the effect of blue light, it will halt the reflex. It differs from a simple external inhibitor, in that it also appears through the action of the complex structure of the environment along the same pathway as the conditional reflex, and is formed under the influence of the same conditions.

Alongside external inhibition, there also exists *internal inhibition*, related not to the effect of a particular external stimulus, but rather to internal processes in the nervous system. The simplest type of internal inhibition consists in the extinction of a conditional reflex. If a strongly developed conditional reflex is excited in a dog for a prolonged period of time without being reinforced by an unconditional stimulus, it will begin to gradually weaken and diminish, as if extinguishing and growing feeble, and will finally cease entirely. In fact, in this case we are dealing with the inhibition of a reflex, and not its utter disappearance, and it is not too hard to see that if the dog were allowed to rest, or if the experiment were conducted some other day, the reflex would be re-established.

The extraordinary biological utility of this form of internal inhibition becomes perfectly obvious once we note that it protects the animal against fruitless and useless waste of energy, and helps him consume his energy in a careful and economical manner. It safeguards the animal against the reinforcement of false and random *conditional connections*. There is every reason for believing that sleep is nothing other than a highly evolved form of such a universal, internal inhibition of reactions.

The inhibition of reactions, or *differentiation*, is of no lesser importance. If a conditional reflex in response to an arbitrary stimulus is fostered in an animal, the animal will respond to all analogous stimuli as well. For example, if an animal already produces a conditional reflex to a metronome beating at a rate of 100 beats per minute, it will also respond to both 50 and 100 beats per minute. But if the stimulus consisting of 100 beats per minute of a metronome is accompanied each time by an unconditional stimulus, and if everything else remains unreinforced, a process of differentiation will be established in the animal. It will begin to distinguish the stimulus with increasing accuracy and respond only to the desired stimulus, while everything else will be inhibited by internal inhibitors. Because of such a mechanism of differentiation, the organism is able to achieve an extraordinarily high degree of specificity and subtlety of relationships, a capacity to make highly refined distinctions between different elements of the environment and, by means of this capacity, to correlate its reactions to desired actions.

The same mechanism of internal inhibition underlies the vestigial and delayed reflexes. We may be convinced of this in the following way. It is known that inhibitors possess a reverse capacity, i.e., if they have been applied to an inhibitor, they inhibit the inhibitor or disinhibit the reflex. If we have created a delayed or vestigial conditional reflex to blue light in a dog, it will not produce saliva immediately after the blue light has been turned on; instead, the reflex will be inhibited for a period of time. But if during this time an external stimulus of sufficient strength, for example, the beat of a metronome, acts upon the dog, the reflex will quickly manifest itself. The beating of a metronome, which is invariably the inhibitor of every conditional reflex, inhibits the inhibitor once it is applied to the inhibited reflex and, thus, *disinhibits the reflex.* What sort of complex forms may be assumed by behavior depending on different combinations of inhibitors and reflexes may be seen from just one of Pavlov's experiments. A conditional reflex to light was created in a dog, and the dog produced 10 drops of saliva. If some musical tone was produced on a piano during the action of this reflex, the reflex was inhibited absolutely. If the metronome was then allowed to start beating, the effect of the reflex was restored, though the dog produced only 4 drops. To explain this phenomenon, these three stimuli were tested, in all possible combinations, first one at a time, then two at a time, and finally all three together. The results of the experiment may be written out most conveniently in the form of a table in which the initial letters in each row denote the particular stimulus (L, blue light; P, musical tone produced on piano; M, beat of the metronome), and the plus sign indicated concerted action:

$$L = 10 \text{ drops}$$
$$P = 0 \text{ drops}$$
$$M = 0 \text{ drops}$$
$$L + P = 0 \text{ drops}$$
$$L + P + M = 4 \text{ drops}$$
$$L + M = 6 \text{ drops}$$
$$P + M = 0 \text{ drops}$$

This table demonstrates that light by itself induces the production of 10 drops. The sound of the piano and beating of the metronome are inhibitors and do not produce any effect either when operating on their own or together. The tone inhibits the reflex completely and reduces it down to zero. The metronome, understood as a stimulus of the same acoustic order, i.e., a secondary and weaker stimulus, inhibits the reflex only partially, reducing it down to 6 drops. In combination, all three stimuli produce 4 drops, and this result is composed of the complex interaction of all three stimuli; i.e., the light induces the production of 10 drops, the tone inhibits all 10 drops, and the metronome inhibits the inhibitor and disinhibits 4 of these drops, as it did when acting in combination with the light.

From this example, it is not hard to see that even when we are dealing with only three elements all told, i.e., light, musical tone, and metronome, an animal's behavior may assume extraordinarily complex and manifold forms, depending on the combinations and structure of these elements. It is easy to imagine how highly complex an animal's behavior may become under the influence of the collection of elements forming the complex structure of a genuine environment and influencing the organism for many years.

Psyche and Reaction

The study of the conditional reflexes makes it possible to consider all of man's behavior as a system of acquired reactions built up upon the foundation of the inherited reactions. With a careful analysis, the most complex and the most subtle forms of mental activity disclose their reflexive nature, and show us that the psyche should also be considered as consisting in particularly complex forms of behavior.

Formerly, psychologists claimed that mental phenomena constituted something isolated and unique in nature, having nothing in common with, indeed differing radically from, the physical world. Psychologists would usually point out that mental phenomena do not have physical extent, that they are inaccessible to the observation of another person and are closely connected with personality—in all these features seeing an essential difference between the mental and the physical.

It was not too hard for scientific analysis to discover that the most subtle forms of mental phenomena are always accompanied by particular motor reactions. All we have to do is to consider the perception of objects, and at once it becomes clear that no one single act of perception occurs without some movement of the appropriate organs. To see means to perform highly complex reactions with our eyes. Even thinking is always accompanied by various restrained movements, mostly by internal motor reactions of speech, i.e., by the rudimentary articulation of words. Pronouncing a sentence out loud or saying it mentally to oneself—the whole difference between the two phenomena is that in the latter case, all movement is suppressed, attenuated, and imperceptible to the eyes of another person, but only to this other person. In essential respects, both thinking and audible speech represent the same motor speech reactions, except for being of differing degrees and strengths.

It was just this result that led Ivan Sechenov, the physiologist who laid the foundations of the science of mental reflexes, to declare that thought is a reflex broken down into two thirds, or the first two thirds of a mental reflex.

It is even easier to demonstrate the reflexive motor nature of every sensation. It is well known that nearly every sensation a person may feel may be "read" in his face or in the movements of his body. Both fear and anger are accompanied by such palpable body movements that, from a single glance at a person, we can correctly tell whether he is afraid or angry. These body movements all involve motor reactions of the muscles (mimicry or pantomime), secretory reactions (production of tears, foaming at the mouth), and reactions of respiration and circulation (paleness, gasping for breath).

Finally, the third realm of the psyche, called the <u>will</u>, is always concerned with particular deeds, and even traditional psychology recognized its motor aspect. The study of drives and motivation, the motive source of the will, must be understood as the study of systems of internal stimuli.

In all other cases, we are presented with nothing other than the most perfected of organic phenomena, and the very same reactions, but only in infinitely complex forms. This is why the psyche must be understood as consisting of especially complex forms of the structure of behavior.

Animal Behavior and Human Behavior

For modern natural science the common origin and common nature of man and animal is no longer open to question. For science, man is only a higher and far from the ultimate species of animal. Similarly, there is much in common in the behavior of man and animals. One might say that man's behavior grows out of the roots of animal behavior and, quite often, is only the "behavior of an animal that has assumed an upright position."

In particular, the instincts and the emotions, i.e., the inherited forms of behavior, are so similar in man and the animals that they doubtless share a common origin. Certain naturalists are not inclined to make any essential distinction between human and animal behavior, and tend to reduce all the differences between the two to different degrees of complexity and subtlety of the nervous system. The proponents of this viewpoint believe it is possible to explain human behavior exclusively from the standpoint of biology.

However, it is not hard to see that this is not so. There is a fundamental distinction between human and animal behavior, as is apparent from the following argument. From the standpoint of the study of conditional reflexes, all of an animal's experience, his entire store of behavior, may be reduced to inherited reactions and conditional reflexes. All of an animal's behavior may be expressed by means of the following formula: (1) inherited reactions + (2) inherited reactions x by individual experience (conditional reflexes). That is, the behavior of an animal is composed of these inherited reactions plus the inherited reactions multiplied by the quantity of new relations that are present in the individual animal's experience. It is obvious that this formula does not cover human behavior even in the slightest degree, however.

By comparison with animal behavior, human behavior displays, above all, an expanded use of the experience gained by prior generations. Man makes use of the experience of prior generations not only to the extent it is reinforced and transmitted by physical inheritance. Everything we use in science, in culture, and in everyday life is enriched by the vast quantity of experience accumulated by prior generations but not transmitted by means of physical inheritance. In other words, unlike the animals, man possesses a history, and this historical experience, i.e., not physical inheritance, but social inheritance, distinguishes him from the animals.

The second new term in our formula is that of collective social experience, which is also a new phenomenon in man. Each person makes use not only of those conditional reactions that have formed in his or her individual experience, as happens also with animals, but also by means of conditional relations that have formed in the social experience of other peoples. In order to establish a conditional reflex to light in a dog, it is necessary that the two effects, of light and of a piece of meat, "intersect," i.e., occur simultaneously, in the individual dog's personal experience. Man, in contrast, uses in his everyday experience reactions which evolved in, and became part of, someone else's experience. I may know about the Sahara without ever having left my native city, or I may know quite a bit about Mars without ever having looked through a telescope. Those conditional reactions of thought or of speech in which these pieces of knowledge are expressed are part not of my own experience, but of the experience of people who have lived in Africa or have, in fact, looked through a telescope. Those new forms of adaptation, which we encounter for the first time in man, are the most essential feature which distinguishes human behavior from the behavior of animals.

The animal adapts passively, responding to changes in the environment by varying his own organs and the structure of his body. He changes himself in order to adapt to the conditions of existence. Man, on the other hand, adapts nature to himself deliberately. Instead of his own organs undergoing changes, bodies in nature are altered by man, becoming tools for him. He responds to cold not by growing a protective coat of wool, but by making deliberate adaptations to the environment, through the production of dwellings or of clothing, i.e, by adapting nature to himself.

According to one researcher, the whole difference between man and the animals may be summed up by saying that man is an animal that makes tools. From the moment labor, in the human sense of the term, i.e., the deliberate and intentional intervention in the workings of nature on the part of man, for the purpose of regulating and controlling vital processes between nature and himself, became possible—from this very moment mankind ascended a novel biological stage, and something novel that was foreign to his animal ancestors and to his fellow creatures became part of his experience.

It is true that we encounter in animals purposive adaption in rudimentary form, for example, nest building in birds, the construction of dwellings in beavers, and so on. These examples all recall labor activity in man, but nevertheless occupy such a small place in the experience of the animal that, on the whole, it alters the basic character of passive adaption only slightly. The main point is that, despite all apparent similarity, the labor of an animal differs from human labor in the most decisive and categorical respects. This difference was expressed by Marx with consummate force, in *Das Capital.*

> The spider carries out operations reminiscent of a weaver, though the cells of wax which bees build in the sky would be the disgrace of any architect. However, there is something that distinguishes the labor of the worst architect from the labor of the most skillful bee, in that before an architect builds a box out of boards he first builds it in his mind. By the end of a process of labor, he has obtained something which already existed in his mind ideally before he began to build.

The fact is that the spider's weaving of a web or the bee's construction of the cells in its hive constitutes the same passive, instinctive, inherited forms of behavior as do all its other passive reactions. The labor of the least experienced human weaver or architect constitutes deliberate forms of adaptation simply because the weaver or architect is conscious.

What constitutes the conscious aspect of human behavior and what is the psychological nature of consciousness—these questions are very nearly the most difficult questions in all of psychology, about which we will speak later. But even now it is clear that consciousness must be considered as consisting in the most complex forms of organization of our behavior, in particular, as Marx has shown, as a kind of doubling of experience, that makes it possible to predict in advance the results of labor and to direct one's own reactions to this end. This doubled experience also constitutes the third and final distinctive feature of human behavior.

Thus, the entire formula of human behavior, which is based on the formula of animal behavior, complemented with new terms, assumes the following form: (1) inherited reactions + (2) inherited reactions x individual experience (conditional reactions) + (3) historical experience + (4) social experience + (5) doubled experience (consciousness).

Thus, the decisive factor of human behavior is not only the biological factor, but also the social factor, which brings with it entirely novel elements behavior. Man's experience is not just that of an animal that has assumed an upright position, but is rather a complex function of the entire social experience of mankind and of his individual groups.

The Build-up of Reactions into Behavior

The concept of a reflex or reaction is, essentially speaking, an abstract and provisional one. In fact, we almost never encounter a reflex in pure form. In actuality, we encounter more or less complex groups of reflexes. In the real world there exist only complex groups of reflexes, not individual reactions.

An isolated reaction or reflex may be obtained in the laboratory with a frog specimen, but in no way in a living person. In a living person, the reflexes exist in permanent and indissoluble unity, and, depending on the nature and structure of each group of reflexes, the nature of any one reflex occurring in this group proves to vary as well. Thus, a reflex turns out to be, not a constant entity given once and for all, but a variable entity that changes from one moment to the next. Moreover, it is not an independent entity, but rather is governed by the overall character of behavior at the particular moment. A reflex is defined, therefore, not as a constant property of a given organ, but as a function of the state of the organism.

The simplest example of the interrelation between reflexes may be observed in the inhibition and disinhibition of reactions. From these phenomena, it is clear that reflexes may weaken or reinforce each other, or one reflex may inhibit or excite another.

In his studies, Pavlov found it necessary to also work with more complex examples in which there was conflict between two reflexes. In certain experimental dogs, a *sentry reaction* towards one of the investigators developed in the course of the experiments, in the form of a violent, menacing reaction on the part of the dog, expressed in aggressive barking at every strange person passing through the room. Every time it appeared, the reaction checked the salivary reaction that had already formed, and was of such significance that the investigators made it the subject of a special study.

While a sentry reaction developed in the dog in relation to one of the investigators, a conditional reflex type of feeding reaction developed in response to the appearance of the other investigator, to his utterance of the word *kolbaski* [sausages], and to the appearance of the dish from which the dog was fed the sausages. When both reactions occurred simultaneously, i.e., when the second investigator entered the room while the first was working with the dog, a clear pattern of struggle between the two reactions could be observed. It was apparent that the sentry reaction gradually attenuated and faded away as one stimulus after another was added to the feeding reaction. The moment someone appeared in the room, the dog ran at him barking furiously, but once he uttered the conditional word, the barking toned down, and the two reactions seemed to balance each other out. The dog did not run at the new arrival, but neither did he reach out towards him. Finally, when shown a small glass, he produced a vigorous and unequivocal food reaction. "Two reflexes," notes Pavlov, "constitute virtually two scales of weights." One could say of a pair of reflexes, all you have to do is reinforce one and the scales turn in its favor, but reinforce the other, and it will prevail. The overall complexity of human behavior becomes understandable if we bear in mind the fact that every reflex, as Pavlov puts it, is limited and controlled not only by another, simultaneously acting external reflex, but also by the weight of internal stimuli, whether chemical, thermal, etc., and that these reflexes are all in constant interaction.

To understand this mechanism, this means of coordinating the reflexes, it is necessary to familiarize ourselves with the principle of the *struggle for the total motor field*, a principle established by the English physiologist Charles Scott Sherrington. Sherrington's idea is that purposive behavior may be carried out only where there is a relative adjustment of the individual reflexes, otherwise the individual would not be an integral organism possessing a unified system of behavior, but would rather constitute a haphazard collection of individual organs with utterly uncoordinated individual reflexes. Physiologists have long assumed the existence of special centers in the nervous system that inhibit and control reflexes. However, subsequent investigation has not confirmed this supposition, and it has been found that an entirely different mechanism is responsible for the unification of the reflexes into the integral behavior of the organism.

In fact, in the human nervous system the number of perceiving (afferent) fibers, called *receptors*, is not equal to the number of motor (efferent) fibers. Calculations have shown that there are five times as many receptors as there are efferent fibers. Thus, every motor neuron is connected not to one, but to several receptors, possibly with even every receptor. This relation is of varying duration and strength, though it has been found that in strychnine poisoning in man, *any nerve will enter into a reflex with any muscle.* This underscores the fact that every motor system exists in relation to different groups of receptors, possibly with all these groups, and, consequently, there cannot exist any isolated and independent reflex in the organism. It is, therefore, understandable that an extremely complex struggle for the general motor field may arise between different groups of receptors, and that the outcome of this struggle would depend on innumerable conditions of extraordinary complexity.

The mechanism of the struggle for the general motor field is also the mechanism involved in the coordination of the reflexes; it underlies the unity of personality and the extremely important act of attention, it is the "marksman" that steers the behavior of any one of our own reactions, and the behavior of an animal, Sherrington remarks, constitutes a series of sequential transitions of the motor field from one group of receptors to another.

Pavlov has compared the workings of our central nervous system with that of a telephone system, where more and more connections between the individual and the elements of the world are being created all the time. It would also be correct to compare the nervous system to a narrow doorway leading into some large building or outdoor theater towards which a crowd of many thousands of people has rushed in a panic. Those who have passed through the doorway and were thus able to save themselves represent only a small fraction of the many thousands who have perished, and the very struggle at the doorway bears a close resemblance to the struggle for the total motor field that is incessantly going on in the human organism, giving human behavior the tragic and dialectic character of an incessant struggle between man and nature, and between the different elements of nature within man himself.

The relationship between the different forces in this struggle, and consequently, the entire pattern of man's behavior is changing from one moment to the next. Everything is uncertain and up in the air, what happens one minute is overturned the very next minute, every reaction turns into its opposite, and all of behavior recalls, on the whole, a struggle of forces, a struggle that never ceases, even for one minute.

The Principle of the Dominant in Behavior

In this struggle between the reactions the deciding factor is not only the skirmish over the total motor field, but more complex connections between individual centers in the nervous system as well. Experimental investigation has demonstrated that if some powerful center of excitation is dominant in the nervous system, it will possess the property of attracting to itself other excitations arising in the nervous system during this time, and will therefore become amplified.

For example, if a frog is taken while the clasp reflex is in effect, i.e., during the period of heightened sexual excitation, and if some external stimulus (e.g., acid, electric current, injection) is applied to its skin, the clasp reflex not only is not weakened, but is even reinforced. The ordinary defense reaction in response to a new stimulus vanishes. In precisely the same way, external stimuli amplify the ordinary acts of swallowing and elimination in a horse. In a female cat which has been separated from male cats while in heat, the basic reflex is reinforced, depending on the most exotic external stimuli, for example, the noise produced by forks and dishes being beaten together, which usually reminds the cat of feeding.

In experiments on frogs, it has been possible to ascertain that a dominant excitation in the central nervous system is capable of inhibiting all other excitations or of deflecting a reflex, steering it in an entirely novel direction. Because of the overriding role of a strong excitation, which subordinates all other excitations to itself, it makes sense to refer to it as a *dominant excitation*, and to refer to all the other excitations as *subdominant excitations*.

Experiments have even shown that if a sensory dominant is artificially induced in a frog, it will respond to the most diverse stimuli by rubbing an outstretched leg, i.e., all reflexes will be directed towards the area of the skin associated with the center of the sensory dominant. Thus, if the sensory centers of a frog's rear right leg are stimulated by means of strychnine, then by stimulating each of the other legs, a defense reflex may be observed. This reflex will be directed each time towards the rear right leg, however, no matter what area of the skin the strychnine is applied to. Thus, a sensory dominant does not check the other reflexes, but rather steers them in an entirely new direction.

If a dominant is induced in the same frog at the motor centers of the same leg, an entirely different effect is obtained. Now, if different areas of the skin are stimulated by means of acid, a licking reflex will always be directed towards the genuine site of the stimulus, but the first leg to respond will always be the one whose motor centers were stimulated. Thus, a motor dominant presupposes the selection of a responding organ and consigns all other reflexes to some delay.

The principle of the dominant introduced by Ukhtomskii thus proves to be a fundamental operational principle of the nervous system, in the sense that it places all other reflexes of the different organs under the authority of an overriding or dominant reflex, and coordinates their activity in a unified direction.

Above we saw that man's behavior constitutes only one of the several forms of behavior that are possible. Now we can define behavior as consisting of a triumphant dominant and of subdominant reflexes that have acceded to it. This principle also explains the source of the unity and purposefulness of human behavior.

Human Constitution and Human Behavior

The composition of the human organism, together with the inherited laws of man's behavior, constitutes the primary biological factor of human behavior. Corresponding to the three components of a reaction, we may distinguish from the standpoint of human behavior (1) a perceiving system, (2) a central processing system, and (3) a responding system.

In the human organism, the perceiving system consists of the entire system of special organs of sense, including the eyes, ears, mouth, nose, and skin (*exterio-receptive field*), i.e., specially designed systems for the perception of external stimuli, the analysis of these stimuli, and the transmission of these stimuli to the center. These systems possess afferent nerves whose function it is to transmit stimuli to the center. By means of special terminal systems, these nerves terminate in the brain, which has the identical purpose of further analysis. Pavlov was quite right to refer to the entire system, beginning with a peripheral organ and ending in the terminal system of a sense nerve, as an analyzer, since it has essentially no function other than that of analyzing and distinguishing the most minute and subtlest elements of the world, and of adjusting the individual's reaction to the subtlest and slightest variations of the environment.

This effort of analysis, which makes it possible for the organism to establish the most complex and subtlest relations with the world, constitutes one of the principal functions of the cortex of the large hemispheres of the brain. Irradiation and concentration of nervous excitation are the basic laws governing its activity. Initially, upon the development of a conditional reflex, the organism will respond to every analogous stimulation. The excitation spreads, spilling over into adjacent sectors, i.e., it *irradiates*. Gradually there occurs a *concentration* of the excitation, i.e., the excitation is focused in an increasingly narrow and constricted region, and is, moreover confined to a single region. By virtue of the concept of irradiation, we are able to understand the various ways in which we respond to analogous stimuli by means of various movements, and the various ways in which we are able to generalize upon our experience. Similarly, the concept of concentration serves to explain the different ways in which we refine and focus our understanding of our experience, and seem to adapt it to familiar stimuli in an entirely rigorous fashion.

The internal-perceiving system, or *interio-receptive* field, possesses the same construction. It is adapted for the perception of internal stimuli and is localized in internal integuments that seem to be turned inward and cover the interior cavities of our organs. It is also adapted for the perception of chemical, thermal, and other internal stimuli of the interior surfaces of the body.

It is by virtue of the exterio-perceptive system that we are able to perceive the external world. Similarly, the interio-perceptive system is adapted to the perception of the most important organic processes occurring within the organism, in the stomach, intestines, the heart, blood vessels, and other organs associated with the most important internal functions of the organism.

Finally, the third perceiving system is that of the *proprio-ceptive* field. This system serves for the perception of the organism's own reactions in precisely the same way, in response to peripheral stimuli that arise in the functioning organs, for example, in the muscles, joints, tendons, etc.

The organism can also learn about its own reactions by means of the first two systems, whenever, that is, the result of its reaction affects it anew through the exterio- or interio-receptive field. For example, the salivary reflex acts through the perceiving system just like any external stimulation. Likewise, it is possible for a reflex to act through the interio-receptive field if it results in particular changes in internal organs. In this case, the reaction is perceived in the same way as is the environment or ordinary organic processes. But there also exists a special system which is entirely analogous to the first two in terms of mechanism and which pervades all the regulating organs of the body, whose sole function it is to perceive all the different peripheral changes that accompany a particular reaction.

A person who places his hands and fingers together in some special way with his eyes closed can always report the position in which he has placed them, thanks to the internal motor or kinaesthetic sensations of the proprio-receptive field. For all further understanding of the psyche, in fact, there are three points which are extraordinarily important to take note of and keep in mind. First, the proprio-ceptive field is organized in the same general way as are the other fields. In other words, man recognizes his own movements by virtue of the same mechanism with which he perceives the external world.

Secondly, the proprio-ceptive field may be excited by effects that come from outside only secondarily, i.e., through the individual's own reaction. In other words, a feedback [*krugovji*] reaction is possible which consists in the reversion of its own reaction back to the organism. Such a feedback reaction consists of six components, unlike the ordinary three-component reactions: (a) external stimulation; (b) central processing; (c) reaction; (d) proprio-ceptive stimulation; (e) processing of proprio-ceptive stimulation; and (f) amplification or delay of the initial reaction. Because each reaction produces a "report" about itself, it becomes possible for the organism to regulate and adjust the course of these reactions.

Thirdly, reflexes from the proprio-ceptive field may enter into precisely the same types of connections with all the other reflexes as with everything else. They may exert extinction and reinforcing, or deviating and steering effects.

The processing system in man's constitution consists of the central regions of the nervous system, i.e., the bulk of the spinal cord and brain. In terms of genetics, the spinal cord is the oldest component, and the most primitive and lowest functions in the life of the organism are, therefore, associated with it. In particular, all the inherited reflexes are localized in the spinal cord and the subcortical centers, which is also where all the motor centers are found. The cerebral cortex constitutes a kind of superstructure over the central nervous system, and essentially possesses no independent connection with the periphery of the body, other than through the subcortical centers. It is a kind of hearth and receptacle of all the conditional reflexes.

If we were to consider the spinal cord as the region where inherited experience and inherited reactions are localized, i.e., those connections that were settled in, or became embedded in, the experience of the species, then the cerebral cortex would have to be thought of as the organ of the individual's personal experience, the domain of the conditional reactions. Thus, the cerebral cortex, which, in and of itself, lacks motor functions, executes only delaying and other, increasingly complex functions, constructs new pathways, and establishes new conditional relations.

Accordingly, it is associated in most intimate fashion with the entire perceiving system, and seems to constitute an exceedingly subtle extension of the entire system by means of which it becomes excited when the appropriate points on the periphery of the body are stimulated. This primary function is best referred to as the *analyzer* function, since it has the task of decomposing the environment as finely as possible into constituent elements so that the most subtle connections may be established between the organism and the environment.

Another, but no less important function of this system consists in the synthesizing or securing activity of the cerebral cortex. In this function, new connections are created and "secured" in the form of conditional reflexes. The activity of the processing system consists largely of these two types of activity. Following Pavlov, it is, in fact, best likened to a telephone switchboard through which every possible new connection is temporarily "secured," i.e., connected, and "opened," i.e., disconnected, from one minute to the next in a versatile and flexible fashion, and which therefore presents an inexhaustible wealth and diversity of forms of behavior—the infinite and inexhaustible variety of all possible combinations of a set of distinct elements. It is precisely for this reason that human behavior can never be reduced to a mere collection of stereotypical patterns given once and for all, rather it constitutes an entirely unpredictable mass of possibilities that can in no way be foreseen in advance.

It is important to note that the same struggle for the total motor field occurs in this processing system, which, as we saw above, is the fundamental regulator of all of behavior. The excitations that occur here merge into a single general system of behavior. Thus, this system is also responsible for the coordination of the reflexes into a behavioral system. The very process of securing a conditional reflex is in direct dependence on all these processes.

It is curious that such a process of connection constitutes only a special case of a dominant process. In fact, if we take a close look at the mechanism of the conditional reflexes, it is not hard to see that it constitutes a conflict between two stimuli, for example, a piece of meat and a blue light in our example. It should not be overlooked that conditional stimuli (here: light and sound) also induce a reaction of their own, for example, the steering and adjusting reaction of the eyes and the head, the pupillary reflex of the eyes, and so on. The question arises, why is it that a conditional reflex to light is secured by the piece of meat, and not the other way round, i.e., why is it that as a result of the concerted action of a piece of meat and blue light, the dog begins to produce saliva in response to light, but does not produce the pupillary reflex or reflex of the eyes in response to the sight of meat. Obviously, here there is a conflict between two reflexes, where the stronger one, that of the feeding and salivary reflexes, possesses the capacity of a dominant reflex, i.e., to attract and delay a weaker stimulus.

It remains for us to consider the responding system in man's constitution. This system consists of absolutely all the functioning organs of the organism, the muscles and tendons for the motor reactions; the heart and blood vessels for the somatic reactions; and the endocrine and exocrine glands for the secretory reactions. Taken together, these systems constitute nothing other than the governing, "effector" working system of the organism. The same may be said as regards each part of this reflector system as regards each muscle. Just as every muscle is associated with an entire group of receptors, so can any group of perceiving cells capture any effector, motor, or secretory organ or blood vessel. In other words, every organ may respond to any stimulus and constitutes, like the muscles, a "check payable to the bearer on demand," as Sherrington has put it.

Of special importance in this system is the activity of the endocrine glands. It has long been acknowledged that there are special glandular bodies in the organism of man and the animals. In terms of their overall structure, these bodies are highly reminiscent of the ordinary glands, for example, the salivary gland and others, and differ from the latter only in their lack of an external outlet duct. It is for this reason that, until recently, it had not been possible to study their discharges, or secretions.

For a long time, the purpose of these glands could not be understood, and could only be conjectured about. Only in the past several decades has scientific knowledge begun to get a clue as to the nature of this extremely complex system in the make-up of man. There have been studies of pathological cases which showed that the absence or hypertrophy of a particular gland produced particular changes or disturbances in certain functions. Other studies have focused on the medicinal action of certain extracts of these glands, which happen to restore these functions. Together with results learned from the experimental removal and grafting of these glands in man and in animals, these studies have made it possible to establish beyond all reasonable doubt that these glands discharge their secretions directly into the blood, and therefore have been termed the hemodynamic, incretorial, or *endocrine glands.*

Alongside these glands, there also exist glands with a dual purpose, i.e., those which produce external and internal secretions simultaneously. These include the sexual glands, the pancreas, and others. It has not been possible so far to establish with any degree of precision what are the actual secretions produced by these glands, and the products they discharge into the blood have been provisionally termed *hormones* (from the Greek word, *hormao*, or "I move" or "I excite").

Even the very name shows that internal secretion is extremely important for the activity of the entire organism. Thus, it has been established that people who have been born without a thyroid gland but who are entirely normal in all other respects suffer from congenital cretinism; however, it is only necessary to graft a thyroid gland into such a person and he begins to regain his health; the same thing occurs in animals if their thyroid gland is removed immediately after birth. But if an animal is fed thyroid extract taken from the gland of another animal, their illness subsides gradually. Conversely, the over-development of the thyroid gland encountered in certain illnesses produces highly accelerated metabolism and leads to a high rate of consumption and exhaustion of the organism. The removal of the parathyroid gland leads to the appearance of fatal convulsions. Abnormality in other glands, in cerebral processes, or in the pituitary gland all have a pronounced influence on the growth, size, and formation of the bones; thus, an increase in the size of the parathyroid gland produces gigantism, or abnormally huge growth and the abnormal enlargement of one gland in particular. Conversely, the removal of the parathyroid gland is associated with diminutive growth.

It has been further established that castration, i.e., the removal of the sex organs, rapidly affects the entire structure of the body. In men the voice becomes high-pitched and begins to resemble a woman's voice, facial hair vanishes, and the entire body begins to take on a feminine appearance. In studies carried out by Steinach, Voronov, Zavadovskii, and others, two remarkable facts relating to internal secretion were experimentally established. It was shown, first, that absolutely every element of the sexual character of the human body depends on the internal secretions of the sex organs. Experiments were performed in which the sex organs of the hen were grafted onto a castrated rooster, and conversely, and as a result a change in sex was obtained experimentally. Such a rooster lacked all its own (secondary) sexual features, for example, voice, comb, tail, spur, and even disposition, and behaved exactly like a hen. It has been possible to transform a hen into a rooster in the same way. Thus, it was possible to establish a direct correlation between virtually the entire structure of the animal's body and its character, on the one hand, and the internal secretions of the sex organs, on the other; thus, everything that we refer to as masculine and feminine, whether in the structure of the body, in the personality, or in the psyche, prove to be ultimately conditional by nothing other than the internal secretions of the sex organs.

Secondly, it is no less remarkable that a direct dependence con be shown to exist between the secretions of the sex organs and all those manifold changes in the organism—whether in the body or in the psyche—that are usually referred to as ageing. It had long been noted that the age and sex of a person seem to represent parallel streams in their development, but only recently has it been possible to show that ageing is ultimately dependent upon a cessation of the secretion of the sex hormones into the blood. In Steinach's well-known experiments, sex organs taken from a young animal were grafted to an arbitrary spot of the body of an aged and senile animal. Once the glands had begun to discharge their secretions into the blood, rapid and clear-cut rejuvenating effects set in every time. The animal regained its strength, senile characteristics vanished, wool again began to grow, sparkle returned to eyes that had become lackluster, and the animal began to experience a kind of second childhood. Rejuvenating effects have been produced in man in precisely the same way, though here it was a matter of adjusting the functioning of the sex organs by increasing its internal secretion.

From this survey, it is clear that such phenomena as the growth and structure of the body, the size and shape of the organs, the sexual features of the body and the psyche, imbecility and consciousness, all the developmental features of man, which are expressed equally in both the organic and mental aspects, ultimately prove to be dependent upon internal secretion. The nature and substance of this dependence have yet to be conclusively unraveled, though even with the present-day state of scientific knowledge there can be no doubt that the chemistry of the blood plays a decisive role. Because of the secretion of various hormones, the chemical composition of the blood undergoes changes, and accordingly, absolutely all processes in the organism, including nervous processes, vary in the most essential respects. Consequently, absolutely all the organism's vital processes are directly dependent upon the chemical composition of the blood, which, moreover are regulated principally and primarily by the endocrine glands.

This may be explained quite simply and persuasively. Everyone knows the miraculous effects of intoxicating substances on the body; only a small amount of alcohol is sufficient to entirely change our consciousness, heart beat, respiration, perception of the world, mood, sensitivity, and will. In every epoch, the widespread use of intoxicants as a method of inducing particular changes in the body artificially has always been based on this circumstance. Morphine and opium, cocaine and ether—all change our consciousness in different ways, and though their effect on the organism is a disruptive one, nevertheless they plunge man into such a fantastic and magical world and possess such an improbable capacity to change our senses, mood, and perception, all our experience in the world, as to appear to be the source of every imaginable fable the world over. But what actually happens in all these cases of intoxication of the organism? As can be easily seen, all that occurs is the introduction into the blood of certain new intoxicating substances that radically alter, first, the chemical composition of the blood, and then the nature of all those processes, principally the nervous processes upon which our behavior depends.

Something like that happens in the endocrine glands. By virtue of their effect on the chemical composition of the blood, the endocrine glands also regulate nervous processes and contribute to substantial changes in our psyche. In the secretory system, man possesses a kind of perennial apothecary within himself capable of exciting and intoxicating his organism with all different kinds of hormones. The endocrine glands, thus, are not an uncoordinated collection of organs existing independently of one another. On the contrary, they are joined together into a harmonious system whose existence has been established with indisputable certainty, though its nature has still not been completely unraveled. Undoubtedly, the glands influence each other through the blood, which carries the hormones throughout the entire body and which is, therefore, the best source of "news" about the organism. The hormones produced by one gland excite or inhibit another gland, and in the organism as a whole, a specialized system of internal secretary equilibrium and interaction that depends on the presence of the different hormones is established at every given moment following prolonged and complex struggle.

In turn, the hormonal or secretary system is in intimate dependence upon, and exists in relation to, all the other unified systems of the organism, i.e., the circulatory system and the nervous system. Its relation to the circulatory system is entirely obvious, since it is by virtue of this mechanism that the hormones are transported throughout the entire body and exert an influence at remote sites in the body. In other words, the hormonal system exerts its influence through the circulatory system, and thus do we return to the ancient view of the blood as the true seat of the soul and of life. Ancient man believed that the blood is the soul, and present-day science has begun to believe that, in fact, it is the chemistry of the blood which is responsible for our behavior. It is appropriate at this point to note yet another relation that exists between the hormonal and the nervous system. "The nervous system," writes Weyl, "governs all the other organs of the body, as well as the endocrine glands, and conversely, internal secretions may, in turn, influence the peripheral termini of the nerves and the nerve centers." These glands are just as capable of transmitting an excitation to the center as of receiving directive impulses from it, just like any muscle; in this regard, they exist as part of the responding mechanism of the nervous system and are governed by all the laws involved in the establishment and education of conditional reflexes. Experience has shown that if an action occurs in response to intra-chemical stimulation, it nevertheless serves to secure a conditional reflex. For example, if we put a mouse in a glass box partitioned into three parts, and place the mouse and a piece of food at opposite ends, the mouse will run for the food each time because of what is known as "hungry blood," i.e., by a change in the chemical composition of its blood. If the experiment is accompanied every time by a bell, after a series of experiments the mouse will learn to run in response to the bell alone, even if stimulation of hungry blood cannot be said to have occurred, for example, if the mouse had eaten several minutes before. Thus, intra-chemical stimulation is not something isolated from the environment, but occurs as a constituent element of the overall functioning of the nervous system.

But if the nervous system affects the hormonal system, the inverse influence of the hormones on the brain is no less obvious. Above it was noted what sort of changes occur in the nervous system and in behavior when a particular gland is surgically removed. The brain influences the hormonal system, and through the hormonal system, again influences itself. With this in mind, it is clear that an American scholar was speaking a profound truth in remarking that, "Man thinks not only by means of his brain, but also by virtue of the coordinated and strictly defined activity of the contents of his cranium in conjunction with all the endocrine glands."

Finally, the last corollary of the study of the endocrine system, one that is, moreover, extraordinarily suggestive from the standpoint of psychology, is that the physical and the mental, the mind and the body, the structure of the body and the nature of essence, are all processes that are profoundly identical, and closely intertwined, and that any separation of the one from the other cannot be justified by any kind of real consideration. On the contrary, a fundamental premise in psychology asserts the unity of all the processes that occur in the organism, the identity of the mental and the organic, and the falsity and impossibility of any division between the two. It is by studying the endocrine system that we will be able to get an idea of the nature of one of the psychophysical mechanisms that underlie this unity. The endocrine system constitutes one part of the responding mechanism of our behavior and, consequently, depends on it. But by the same token, such functions of the organism as growth, sexual activity, and the shape and size of the different parts of the body all depend on the nervous system, i.e., on the psyche, and conversely, the psyche depends on the activity of the endocrine system. The unity of the mental and the physical nowhere shows through so clearly as in the study of the endocrine system.

Chapter 4

BIOLOGICAL AND SOCIAL FACTORS IN EDUCATION

There are extraordinarily important psychological conclusions regarding the nature and essence of the educational process which we draw from the foregoing remarks. We have seen that man's behavior is composed of biological and social features of man's own developmental conditions. The biological factor defines the foundation, the basis or groundwork, of the innate reactions without which the organism could not exist and upon which the system of acquired reactions is constructed.

That this new system of reactions is wholly determined by the structure of the environment in which the individual grows and develops is entirely obvious. Every form of education, therefore, unavoidably bears a social character, whatever else it might be.

We have seen that the individual's own experience is the only teacher capable of forming new reactions in the individual. Only those relations are real for an individual that are given to him in his personal experience. This is why the student's personal experience becomes the fundamental basis of pedagogical work. Strictly speaking, and from the scientific point of view, there is no other way of teaching. It is impossible to exert a direct influence on, to produce changes in, another individual, one can only teach oneself, i.e., alter one's own innate reactions, through one's own experience.

"Our movements—they are our teacher." Ultimately, the child teaches himself. It is in his organism as nowhere else that there occurs the decisive engagement between all those different factors that determine his behavior for many years to come. In this sense, education, in every country and in every epoch, has always been social in nature, indeed, by its very ideology it could hardly exist as antisocial in any way. Both in the seminary and in the old *gymnasium*, in the military school and in the schools for the daughters of the nobility, just as in the schools of ancient Greece and those of the Middle Ages and in the East, it was never the teacher and the tutor who did the teaching, but the particular social environment in the school which was created for each individual instance.

From the scientific point of view, therefore, the assumption that the student is simply passive, just like the underestimation of his personal experience, is the greatest of sins, since it takes as its foundation the false rule that the teacher is everything and the student nothing. On the contrary, the psychological point of view forces us to acknowledge that, in the educational process, the student's individual experience is everything. Education should be structured so that it is not that the student is educated, but that the student educates himself.

The traditional European school system, which always reduced the process of education and instruction to a passive apprehension by the student of a teacher's lessons and outlines, was the ultimate of psychological nonsense. The educational process must be based on the student's individual activity, and the art of education should involve nothing more than guiding and monitoring this activity. In the educational process, the teacher must be like the rails on which trains travel freely and independently, receiving from the rails only the direction in which they are to travel. The school which is run on scientific grounds is inevitably a school of action.

The effect of education on the students themselves must be based on a total process of reaction which combines all three components of any reaction—the perception of a stimulation, the processing of the stimulation, and the responding action. The old pedagogics placed extraordinary emphasis on, and greatly exaggerated, the first component of perception, and treated the student like a sponge which absorbs new knowledge the more eagerly and the more thoroughly, the better it fulfills its function. Meanwhile, knowledge that is not gained through personal experience is not knowledge at all. Psychology requires that students learn not only to perceive, but also to respond. To educate means, above all, to establish new reactions and develop new forms of behavior.

In attaching such exceptional importance to the student's individual experience, should we reduce the role of the teacher down to nothing? Should we replace the old formula, "the teacher is everything, and the student nothing," with its opposite: "the student is everything, and the teacher nothing"? By no means. If, speaking from a scientific standpoint, we have to reject the thesis that the teacher has the power to produce an immediate educational influence, that he possesses a mystical ability to directly "mould another person's soul," this is precisely because we are assigning to the role of teacher something incomparably more important.

From the foregoing, we see that the student's experience, the formation of conditional reflexes, is determined wholly and without exception by the social environment. It is only necessary to change the social environment, and human behavior likewise changes at once. We have already mentioned earlier that, for each of us, the environment plays the same role as did Pavlov's laboratory for his experimental dogs. There, the conditions in the laboratory determined the dog's conditional reflexes, while here it is the social environment that determines how behavior evolves. From the psychological point of view, the teacher is the director of the social environment in the classroom, the governor and guide of the interaction between the educational process and the student.

Though the teacher is powerless to produce immediate effects in the student, he is all-powerful when it comes to producing direct effects in him through the social environment. The social environment is the true lever of the educational process, and the teacher's overall role reduces to adjusting this lever. Just as a gardener would be acting foolishly if he were to try to affect the growth of a plant by directly tugging at its roots with his hands from underneath the plant, so is the teacher in contradiction with the essential nature of education if he bends all his efforts at directly influencing the student. But the gardener affects the germination of his flowers by increasing the temperature, regulating the moisture, varying the relative position of neighboring plants, and selecting and mixing soils and fertilizer, i.e., once again, indirectly, by making appropriate changes in the environment. Thus it is that the teacher educates the student by varying the environment.

It should be kept in mind that the teacher has a dual role to perform in the classroom, and in this regard the job of the teacher does not constitute an exception in any sense of the word from the general run of human labor. Every form of human labor is dual in nature. In the most primitive and in the most complex forms of human labor, the worker has a dual role to perform, on the one hand, as the director and foreman of the production process, and on the other, as a part of his own machine. Consider, for example, the labor of the Japanese rickshaw driver who transports passengers through a city, and compare it with the labor of a streetcar conductor. It is clear that the rickshaw driver is a simple source of physical force, or thrust, substituting for the power of a horse, or steam or electrical power, simply by virtue of his muscular and nervous energy. But at the same time, the rickshaw driver performs another role, a role in which he could not be replaced by horse, steam, or electricity: He is not only a part of his machine, but also its lord and master, the foreman and director of his very own simple workshop. He lifts the shaft, starts to move the carriage and brings it to a halt at the right time, avoids obstacles, swings around turns, and selects a desired direction.

The same two components are also found in the work of a streetcar conductor. He likewise moves the braking handle or power lever from one point to another by the force of his muscles, and transmits signals through the mechanical impact of his foot. Thus, he is also a simple part of his own machine, a part that, moreover, alters the relative position of all the other parts. What is far more noticeable is the streetcar conductor's other role, in which he is the director and foreman of a whole complex system of engines, brakes, and signals.

From this comparison, it is evident that though both components of labor are equally present in the streetcar conductor and in the rickshaw driver, they have, however, changed places. In the rickshaw driver, the job of director and foreman plays a negligible and unremarkable role by comparison with physical labor. If the rickshaw driver happens to get tired by the end of the day, this exhaustion will, of course, come not from directing the machine, but rather from running in harness with the shafts. On the contrary, in the case of the streetcar conductor physical labor is nearly nonexistent, and the importance of mental labor has grown enormously. It is because of improvements in technology that the development of labor points in the direction from the rickshaw driver to the streetcar conductor. The worker in modern industry is increasingly becoming the director of the production process and foreman to the machine.

In precisely the same way, the teacher is, on the one hand, the director and foreman of the social environment in the classroom, and on the other, a part of this very same environment. Whenever he takes the place of a book, of a map, of a dictionary, or of a colleague, there he is acting like a rickshaw driver who has replaced a horse. Wherever he plays the role of a part of the educational mechanism, like a rickshaw driver, there, from the scientific point of view, he is not acting like an educator. He is acting like an educator only where, in self-effacing fashion, he calls upon the services of powerful forces of the environment, directs them, and places them in the service of education.

Thus, we arrive at the following formula of the educational process: Education is realized through the student's own experience, which is wholly determined by the environment, and the role of the teacher then reduces to directing and guiding the environment.

To be perfectly clear as to the nature of this role, it is necessary to discuss in somewhat greater detail the concept of an educational environment. At first glance, it may be easily seen that no special educational environment is needed, that education may be accomplished in any environment whatsoever, and that, in particular, the best educator is that environment which also happens to be the place of the student's future activity. Every artificially constructed social environment will always encompass relationships that distinguish it from genuine reality, and, consequently, will always retain a degree of divergence from real life. Hence, it is not very hard to conclude that no sort of artificial educational environment has to be created, that life educates better than any school, just plunge the child up to his neck in the noisy flow of life, and you can be sure ahead of time that a spirited and resolute adult will come out of this education.

This view is wrong, however. There are two points that have to be kept in mind here. First, education has always had as its goal not adaptation to an already existing environment, which may, in fact, happen anyway in the natural course of events, but the creation of an adult who will look beyond his own environment. In the first year of the revolution, there were many people who saw the goal of education as a matter of demolishing the school. The path of revolution, the revolutionary avenue, is the best teacher, our children must become children of this avenue, the school must be demolished in the name of life— such were the slogans of the day. There was much healthy enthusiasm expressed in this view, a genuine reaction against the school fenced off from life as if by a kind of Great Wall of China, and it may very well be true that the abolition of education is the most correct of all educational methods in the turbulent times of a revolution. However, this is not quite the way things work in more peaceable, times nor in the light of sober scientific reflection. It is true that we educate for life, that life is the highest judge, that our ultimate purpose is not to inculcate any sort of special academic virtues, but to teach vital habits and skills, and that acculturation to life is our ultimate purpose. But the most varied habits may be met up with in life, and acculturation may assume the most diverse properties. We cannot relate equally and with indifference to all aspects of life, we cannot say "yes" to absolutely everything, just because it exists in real life. Consequently, we cannot agree to leaving the educational process in the control of life's elements. We are never able to judge ahead of time which of life's elements will triumph in our student without ending up with a parody of life, i.e., a medley of all its negative and worthless aspects. There is so much muck and mire along our way together with the beautiful and the sublime that, were we to leave the outcome of the struggle for the child's motor field up to the free play of stimulation, we would be acting just as foolishly as a person who jumps into the ocean and yields to the free play of the waves out of a desire to get to America.

Second, it must be kept in mind that the elements of the environment may sometimes include effects that are quite harmful and destructive to a young child. Bear in mind that we are dealing not with a well-established member of the environment, but with a growing, changing, fragile organism, and much that would be entirely acceptable for an adult can be destructive to a child.

Thus, both these considerations, on the one hand, the fact that the adult environment is not suitable for a child, and on the other, the extraordinary complexity and diversity of environmental influences, compel us to reject a spontaneous foundation for the educational process, and to oppose to it a program of judicious resistance to, and guidance of, this process, attained through rational organization of the environment.

Such is the nature of every form of scientific knowledge. Every theoretical claim is verified or tested under practical conditions, and its truth established only when praxis that has evolved on the basis of such claims demonstrates its value. Man discovers the laws of nature not in order to be resigned to, and helpless before, its omnipotence, nor in order to deny his own free will —nor, incidentally, in order to act foolishly and blindly in spite of his own will. Rather, by wisely subordinating himself to the laws of nature, and working in conjunction with these laws, he subordinates them to his will. Man forces nature to serve him through the agency of nature's very own laws. The very same thing may be said as regards public education. If we learn which laws governing the nature of public education happen to be true independently of the teacher's will, this does not in the least mean acknowledging our impotence to affect the educational process, nor does it mean rejecting all intervention in it and leaving all of education to the mercy of the elemental forces of the environment.

On the contrary, just like any increase in our knowledge, by learning these laws we will find ourselves more in control of this process, and have greater opportunity for actively intervening in it. Knowledge of the true nature of education will lead us to the various ways in which we can become master of it in its entirety. Thus, the psychological theory of public education not only does not mean prostrating oneself before education, but, on the contrary, signifies the ultimate in our mastery of the flow of educational processes.

Thus does educational psychology become an extraordinarily effective applied science. It is not restricted to the purely theoretical goals of comprehending and describing the nature of education, and of discovering and formulating its laws. It must teach us how to grasp the very nature of education, guiding ourselves by its very own laws. Now we can understand the thought expressed above, that in the process of education the teacher is, in this new understanding, not only of no lesser importance than before, but, indeed, is of incomparably greater importance. And although his role seems to diminish in terms of apparent activity, since he teaches and educates less, he nevertheless gains with regard to inner activity. The control such a teacher exerts over the educational process exceeds that of the teacher of old just as much as does the power of the streetcar conductor exceed that of the rickshaw driver.

Activity of the Educational Process and its Participants

Least of all should we think of the educational process as one-sided, and ascribe all activity without exception to the environment, making nothing of the activity of the student himself, of the activity of his teacher, and of everything that must come into contact with education. On the contrary, in education there is nothing passive or inactive. Even lifeless objects, when they are brought into the educational arena, when they are assigned an educational role, acquire a sense of purpose and become effective participants in this process.

From a superficial approach, it is very easy to conclude from the study of the conditional reflexes that human behavior and education should be understood as exclusively mechanical, and to think of the individual as a robot that responds to stimulations from the environment with machine-like regularity. We have already pointed out how wrong is such a view. From the above, it is clear that the very process in which a conditional reflex is formed arises out of a struggle and a conflict between two elements that are inherently entirely independent of each other and which come into conflict, cutting across each other and interlacing in the organism in accordance with the laws of this very organism.

Man confronts nature as if a force of nature; the individual confronts the world as a deliberate contending quantity. The individual brings to bear all his inherited experience in his encounter with all the influences of the environment. Like a hammer, the environment pounds and forges this experience, and reshapes it, and meanwhile the individual struggles for self-affirmation. Behavior is a dialectical and complex process of struggle between man and the world, and within man. And the conditions of the individual's inherited construction play no lesser a role in the outcome of this struggle of forces within the individual himself than do all the impinging influences of the environment.

Thus, to recognize that our experience is "socially impregnated" through and through by no means represents an acknowledgement of man as a robot and the rejection of any significance for man. The formula we have presented above, therefore, which is meant to predict each individual's behavior with mathematical rigor and to abstract it from his or her inherited reactions and all environmental influence—this formula is in error in one essential respect: It does not take into account the infinite complexity of the intra-organic struggle, as a result of which it is never possible to predict a person's behavior or say what it will be ahead of time, in that this behavior is always nothing but the outcome of this struggle. The environment is not something located absolutely outside man. It is not even impossible to determine where the influence of the environment ends and the influence of one's own body begins.

Thus, man's body itself is, for itself, an element of the social environment in the same way as are the interio- and proprio-ceptive fields. The process by which the acquired reactions and conditional reflexes are formed is a two-way, active process in which the individual is not only subjected to the influence of the environment, but in which he influences the environment in particular ways through each of his reactions, and also influences his own being through the environment. In this two-way process, the reflex, understood as a pre-set reaction, is the possession of the individual, while to the environment belong the conditions under which new reactions may arise. The formation of the reactions is thus forever dependent upon the outcome of a struggle between the individual and the environment.

But the environment is not something absolutely hardened, inflexible, and unchanging. On the contrary, in real life there is no indivisible environment. The environment is composed of a series of more or less independent and disjointed fragments, and these fragments can just as easily become the subject of man's rational action, as anything else. Ultimately, for man the environment is a social environment, because even where it appears to be a natural environment, nevertheless, in relation to man, there are always definite social elements present. In his interaction with the environment, man always makes use of his social experience. If, in looking at a forest, at a river, at a tree, we are conscious that here there is a forest, here there is a river, here there is a tree, we will refer to them, and we will understand what they themselves constitute, and consequently, we will relate to them by means of complex operations of social experience which we tend not to notice simply on the basis of a law which declares that we don't notice that we breathe, that we grow, that we revolve together with the earth, i.e., that we don't notice all those sorts of changes that occur continuously and constantly.

Therefore, it makes sense to oppose the social environment to the natural environment only in a very narrow, limited, and provisional sense. But if the social environment is understood provisionally as a collection of human relationships, the extraordinary plasticity of the social environment, which makes of it very nearly the most flexible of all tools of education, becomes entirely understandable. The elements of the environment are not in a forced and rigid state, but rather exist in a state that is variable and readily changes its shape and form. By putting these elements together in a certain way, man creates ever newer forms of the social environment.

This is also why an active role is the lot of the teacher in the course of education. The teacher fashions, takes apart and puts together, shreds, and carves out elements of the environment, and combines them together in the most diverse ways in order to reach whatever goal he has to reach. Thus is the educational process an active one on three levels: the student is active, the teacher is active, and the environment created between them is an active one. The educational process, therefore, may least of all be considered a benignly indifferent and straightforward process. On the contrary, the psychological nature of the educational process discloses itself as a complicated struggle in which thousands of highly developed and heterogenous forces join battle, as a dynamic, deliberate, and dialectical process that recalls not the slow, evolutionary process of growth, but a wavering and revolutionary process of unceasing combat between man and the world.

On the Goals of Education from the Psychological Standpoint

What might be the goals of education is a question that, in its totality, is not truly part of educational psychology. The function of educational psychology is to expose the formal side of every educational process, independently of its goals, and to elucidate the laws governing it independently of the direction of their effects. It is the responsibility of general pedagogics, and of social ethics, to pinpoint and map out the goals of education.

The psychological nature of the educational process is entirely the same, whether we wish to educate a goon [fascist] or a worker, whether we are training an acrobat or an efficient office worker. Our concerns must be focused only on the very mechanism involved in the formation of new reactions, whatever the ultimate benefits we hope to achieve by means of these reactions.

However, there is a certain formal aspect to this question, an aspect that may be considered only from a psychological standpoint. In psychology, the question is not a matter of this or that particular goal of education, rather the sorts of goals which may, in general, be given to the educational process from a scientific viewpoint. What are the conditions which, when present, push our goals counter to the educational process is a question which may be properly answered by the psychological theory of education, and only by this theory.

From the foregoing, it is clear that the educational process is thoroughly original. It consists in nothing less than the formation of new relations, each of which is always fully realized and fully specific. Even from this one remark, it is quite understandable that only specific goals may be assigned to the educational process. From the scientific point of view, one may speak equally of the education of a goon or of a revolutionary, of an acrobat or of an office worker, since in all these instances we are always dealing with the fully defined character of those reactions, the entirely explicit system of the form of behavior, the exact ideal of that form of activity we wish to realize.

But, from the scientific point of view, it is meaningless to speak of abstract ideals for education, for example, the development of an indivisible and harmonious personality, or of an educated and civilized person, since this says absolutely nothing about all those relationships we have to make use of in the educational process. Thus, to formulate the goals of education in a scientific fashion means to have in mind, in an entirely specific and exact form, the particular system of behavior we wish to realize in our student.

We only have to glance over the various educational systems in their historical development in order to discover that the goals of education have, in fact, always been entirely specific and fundamental, and have always corresponded to the ideals of the epoch and of those particular economic and social structures of society that defined the whole history of the epoch. And if these ideals have been formulated in new ways each time, this has always been because of the scientific helplessness of the particular philosopher, or because of the class-based pretense of the epoch.

Feudalism, which was concerned only with the education of obedient and uncomplaining serfs, could not, of course, speak of this openly, and had to hide behind the theological theme of the saving of souls. Such has been the case in all those epochs when the ruling class of exploiters, who were also in control of the educational system, concealed the true goal of education behind abstract words. Now that class contradictions have been exposed, the demand for such concealment is past, and the man of our epoch is inclined to formulate the vital goals of education exactly and specifically.

It must be kept in mind that education has, at all times and in all places, borne a class-based character, whether or not its adherents or apostles were aware of it. In fact, in human society education is an entirely well-defined social function whose direction is defined always by the interests of the dominant class, and the freedom and independence of the lesser artificial educational environment from the greater social environment is essentially a matter of very relative and very conditional freedoms, and to an independence that exists within certain narrow limits and boundaries.

There always exists a certain interaction of influences and relationships between the greater and lesser social environment, and the full complexity of the psychological problem of education involves nothing other than establishing the true limits of this independence. It is not difficult to discover and demonstrate the class-based character and content of every educational system. One need only recall the educational system of the tsarist school, which created lyceums and institutes for the nobility, secondary schools for the urban middle classes which did not involve a classical education, and orphanages and trade schools for the poor.

From the psychological point of view, therefore, it does not make sense to speak of different abstract and general goals of all of education in general. Each form of education has its own goals, indeed, one might say that every epoch has its own form of education, and however these goals are expressed, they will always develop certain aspects and a form of behavior which this education would like to bring to life. It is only these educational goals which can be of genuine value in selecting and guiding the educational process, since only they give us rules by means of which we are able to discern what educational effects are needed and to learn how to combine these effects together correctly into a rigorous pedagogical system.

Education as Social Selection

We have now come close to finally formulating the psychological nature of the educational process on the basis of all the results we have reviewed. It would, however, be extremely difficult to do this in a single sentence, since every definition is, as a French saying goes, a restriction, i.e., a partial, one-sided illumination of an object. Therefore, let us try to take a look at the subject of education from several important aspects.

As a first, rough definition of education, note that the educational process reduces essentially to the formation and accumulation of conditional reactions on the basis of innate reactions, and the development of forms of behavior that are useful in terms of adaptation to the social environment. In other words, education may be defined as the adaptation of inherited experience to the given social environment.

But it is not difficult to see that such a definition is too broad, because in this case under the concept of education would be subsumed every new conditional reaction, and we would lose all criteria for making distinctions between education and the formation of all the new conditional reactions we routinely form, for example, when we decide to greet a new acquaintance, to learn a new foreign word, or to respond to a new event. From this point of view, it is necessary to distinguish education from everyday life.

There can be no doubt that every time such new types of reactions are formed in the course of everyday life, there is, basically, a psychological effect produced on oneself, what may be thought of as a self-teaching process. This fact is particularly striking wherever we encounter, not isolated and random formations of reactions, but a rational, purposeful, and prolonged process of development of whole systems of behavior in adults that are entirely novel. For example, when we are concerned with teaching soldiers, or with teaching a new game, with this or that course of stenography or typing, we are most certainly dealing with psychological processes that are educational in nature, since in all these instances it is a matter of developing and forming whole new systems of reactions, and forms of behavior, that are entirely novel.

For the sake of clarity and precision of discussion, however, it would be more correct to speak of re-education in the broad sense of this term rather than of education. The distinction we wish to make between the two words differs somewhat from the ordinary meaning given to them in common usage. In everyday language, by re-education is usually understood a thorough remaking, or re-orientation, of already existing systems of reactions. Thus do we commonly speak of the re-education of the criminal, of the mentally ill, and so on. No one would begin to speak of re-education in typing or stenography courses in everyday terms. From the popular point of view, we are not involved in any sort of re-education here, but are instead inculcating and developing what would seem to be new habits. But from a scientific viewpoint, in all these cases it would be correct to speak re-education proper, since, from the standpoint of psychology, here we are dealing everywhere with the formation of certain new relations in an already existing system of behavior.

The element of uncertainty, of fluidity of growth, and of original changes in the individual should be considered the essential feature of education. Thus, in pure form the concept of education is applicable only to the child, i.e., to the growing and self-changing individual. It is entirely analogous to all the other physical processes which occur in the individual. Changes occur in the individual without stop throughout his or her lifetime. Those changes which are usually referred to as growth, however, possess an entirely different biological meaning. Their ultimate purpose and goal consist in the preparation of the young for the complex and multi-faceted activity of life. The term, "education," is applicable only to growth.

Thus, education may be defined as a systematic, purposeful, intentional, and conscious effort at intervening in and influencing all those processes that are part of the individual's natural growth. Consequently, only that formation of new reactions will be educational in nature which, actually intervenes in growth processes to one degree or another, and steers these processes. Not all those new reactions which are formed in the child, consequently, will constitute educational events.

If, upon leaving home, I arrange with my child where I'm going to leave the key for him, there can be no doubt that I am thereby forming a new relation with my child. But if this reaction does not have any purpose other than help him find the key, from the psychological point of view it cannot be termed educational. Consequently, not everything we do with children is education, in the scientific understanding of this term.

Hence, it is evident that education may form the subject and problem of child psychology. What might be the meaning of this process? It would be most correct to define it as a process of social selection. Recall that a reaction is a complex process of interaction that exists between man and the world and is determined by adaptation. Behavior is a higher form of adaptation to the environment. But the child possesses a collection of social abilities, and from this set the most highly diverse personalities may develop. "The child," says Frank, "who 'imagines' he is a pirate, a soldier, or a horse, and who 'acts out' these characters is actually more correct than his parents or learned psychologists who see in him only a small, helpless being, living in a nursery. For beneath this exterior, there is *actually* concealed a potential reserve of forces and potentialities that are not part of the outwardly objective reality of the child's life. In this little being, there *actually lives* the forces and yearnings of a pirate, of a soldier, and even of a horse; this being is, *in fact*, one that is infinitely greater than what he appears to be to an outside observer." The child harbors as potentiality a collection of all those future personalities he may become, and not just those of a pirate, of a soldier, or of a horse, but of others as well. Education creates a social selection of the outward personality. Out of the individual, as biological type, it forms, through selection, man as social type.

Chapter 5

THE INSTINCTS AS THE SUBJECT, MECHANISM, AND MEANS OF EDUCATION

Instinctive activity in man and in animals has always appeared to observers as something clandestine and mysterious. Until recently, it had remained the most obscure and unexplained of all features in the psychology of man and the animals. Why this question has remained obscure and unexplained is due, above all, to the very obscurity of instinctive activity.

We encounter the instincts at the lowest levels of life as well as at the highest, and, strange as it may seem, not only do we not notice their evolution and progressive development, but, quite the contrary, are able to establish beyond all reasonable doubt that purely instinctive behavior is incomparably more perfected among the lower animals than among the higher. In man, the instincts are virtually never expressed in pure form, but always manifest themselves as constituent elements of a more complex unity, and therefore function always in highly discrete fashion, as if a concealed well spring at the base of all the explicit mechanisms of behavior.

As to the nature of the instincts and their classification, science still has no answer. From earliest times, there have been researchers who have insistently held to the view that the instincts as such, as special forms of behavior, do not exist at all. Others, on the contrary, have seen in the instincts something special, something not fully reducible to anything else, a kind of special class of reactions in man and in animals.

One researcher has remarked quite correctly that we call instinct everything we do not understand. And, truly, in common word usage, the term, "instinct," is applied to all those cases when we cannot discern the most immediate and genuine cause of our deeds.

It is easiest to explain the nature of the instincts by comparing them with an ordinary reflex. There is the belief that the instincts constitute only complex or serial reflexes. However, as we saw above, there exists a whole series of distinctions between instincts and reflexes. Bekhterev suggested that the instincts could be thought of as complex organic reflexes, and that they could be placed in a class of their own consisting of the simple and unconditional reflexes.

This also means essentially acknowledging the instincts as constituting a special class of reactions that exist independently.

Before placing the instincts in a special class of reactions, we have to consider how they are related to physiology and anatomy. Modern-day science divides the entire nervous system into two fundamental systems, the animal or mammalian nervous system, and the vegetative nervous system. The former supervises all the animal functions of the organism, primarily the motor reactions, and maintains the relationship between the organism and the external world. The latter governs the vegetative functions of the organism, operating in the internal organs, cavities, tissues, and so on. According to all our data, unlike all the other reactions, the instincts are connected most closely with this, the interior, vegetative part of the nervous system. It is precisely the nerves of the vegetative nervous system, which radiate throughout the glands and internal cavities of the body, which permeate absolutely every tissue, and which line the blood vessels, that are the primary pathways by means of which intra-organic excitations associated with the instincts reach the central nervous system.

Instinctive activity is rooted in the anxious urges of the body for organic satisfaction, in the complex vegetative and chemical processes of the organism. It would appear to be the result of the innermost needs the organism addresses to the world.

Further, from the physiological point of view, it is not at all hard to see that the internal, innermost processes of internal secretion also serve as stimuli of the instincts. It may be considered established beyond all reasonable doubt that the sex instinct is excited principally in two ways, either in a pathway through the ganglia of the vegetative system, or directly, by means of hormonal excitation of the nerve centers of the brain. In this latter case, the instinctive reaction will differ so substantially from a reflex as to lack anything comparable to the reflex arc, and instead appears to be due to stimulation applied directly to the cerebral centers. This imparts to the reaction a seemingly independent, autonomous character, so unlike the responsive character of a reflex.

Consider, next, the biological difference between reflexes and instincts. On the whole, this difference may be reduced to the claim that, like the reflexes, the instincts constitute inherited reactions associated, however, with such palpable features as age, recurrence, and so forth. In other words, a reflex is a reaction that is constant, remaining unchanged throughout one's lifetime, whereas instinctive reactions may change, appear and disappear, depending on age, physiological and physical time, and so forth.

Finally, from the psychological point of view, the instincts constitute deviations, and as such cannot be reduced to a simple summation or series of reflexes. There is, above all, not so strict a dependence between a stimulus and a reaction as is characteristic of an instinct. Scientists have long spoken of the blindness of the instincts. To say the instincts are blind is to say, incidentally, that an instinct does not notice the absence of a stimulus and is able to function even when it finds itself in an entirely novel situation. Note, too, the irregular arrangement of the actual collection of reflexes that occur in an instinctive reaction. It is never possible to enumerate and determine ahead of time these movements—nor the order of these movements—which go to make up an instinctive reaction. In contrast, a reflex functions with machine-like regularity. And although it constitutes a complex and composite whole, nevertheless this whole is so well-formed that, in a compound reflex, in which any number of individual muscles may participate, one can predict precisely in what sequence they will appear one after the other.

Earlier we noted the distinction between the instincts and the reflexes which Vagner had discovered in his experimental observations of the mating of decapitated flies. This experiment showed, above all, that an instinct may be encountered in particularly complex interactions with reflexes, but nevertheless constitutes something entirely different from a reflex, since the very nature of the relation and association of the reactions present in it is altogether different.

Taken together, the foregoing results give the psychologist sufficient grounds for placing instinctive behavior in a class of its own, and, following Vagner, we recognize that the instincts constitute a behavioral reaction of the entire organism, in contrast, viewing the reflexes as reactions in which individual organs perform a function.

In contrast to the reflexes, in an instinct we may easily discern an integration of the reflexes that is pre-defined by heredity, a predestined dominance of the process, a pre-determined outcome of the struggle for the total motor field, and the integral nature of behavior.

Origin of the Instincts

Just as scientists disagree as to the nature of the instincts, so do they disagree as to the origin of the instincts. Some scientists believe the instinctive reactions to be primordial and once conscious, rational types of reactions which the animal, whether for fortuitous reasons or through trial and error, had selected and reinforced because of their usefulness and handed down to future generations. Proponents of this view find confirmation in the involuntary character assumed by man's rational and conscious actions if repeated often and in the same way and in the same order.

In fact, virtually all of our behavior occurs entirely automatically, i.e., mechanically, independent of consciousness. The nerve centers that supervise these movements seem to function autonomously. We breathe, walk, write, and speak, play our parts, read, and get dressed entirely automatically, i.e., without our having to think each time what it is we have to do. Our feet seem to carry us on their own, without requiring any volitional impulse on our part each time, the decision, to lift up and put down one foot after the other; in precisely the same way, the fingers of an experienced pianist perform their work independently, as do the vocal cords of an ordinary person.

It is only necessary to compare the effect, the degree of straining, the expenditure of attention, that man makes when learning a foreign language for the first time, or when learning how to play a piano, with that facility and freedom he brings to these same actions later on, in order to understand how great is the force of mental automatism. Just look at a child who is only beginning to walk. His entire face expresses a strained state, as if he were engaged in the most difficult of mental effort. Every time he lifts up one of his little feet and looks about for a solid point of support, and then pulls up his other foot, it's as if he's solving the most difficult of all problems. One need only compare him to the child freely running about two years later to get a vivid idea of the substantial difference that automatism contributes to human reactions.

One might easily imagine that automatism depreciates the character of human reaction, reduces it to a lower type, mechanizes it, and, in general, is a step backwards and a step down by comparison with the conscious, rational type of reaction. This is not quite the case, however. It is not at all hard to demonstrate that the automatism characteristic of our movements is a necessary psychological condition for the appearance of the higher forms of activity proper. This is clear from the fact that, first, only certain automatic or involuntary acts constitute fully perfected types of reactions. The playing of a pianist, the manner of speaking of an orator, the dancing of a ballerina, everything that requires the utmost subtlety and exactitude of movement reaches the height of perfection and its full measure once the nerve centers that direct the necessary movements seem to function autonomously, in isolation from all extraneous influence of the nervous system, performing their work with the utmost elegance and harmony, and, by its very nature, is accessible to only one of man's nerves.

Moreover, the automatism of man's movements is essential for relieving the central nervous system of a whole series of extraneous labors. It would appear to constitute a unique division of labor between nerve centers, a freeing of the higher centers from a veritable host of forms of lower and habitual tasks. If walking were not performed mechanically, but instead required the conscious awareness of one's movements at every moment, it would consume such an enormous quantity of nervous energy as to leave virtually no space for other acts. It is precisely for this reason that a public speaker can impart to his speech the meaning of his own speech, that the very process of articulation of sounds is performed as if all on its own, requiring on the part of the speaker neither attention nor thought. This is also why it is so difficult to speak a language we are little accustomed to, in which our very pronunciation has yet to become mechanical.

Thus, the automatism assumed by our movements constitutes a universal law of our activity, and is of an extraordinarily great psychological importance. The foundation of this law is rooted in the distinctive plasticity of our nerve matter, in which the nerve pathways seem to travel along well-worn tracks, in which the imprint of previously experienced excitations seems to have been preserved and in which a predisposition to the replication of these excitation has evolved.

To create a sheet of writing paper, i.e., to fold a piece of paper in half, means bending the paper in order to create a fold, which becomes the imprint of the movement just completed, a kind of deformation and rearrangement of the molecules in the paper. Now the sheet is ready to be folded just at this spot. All that's needed is the slightest puff and it's done. Something similar occurs in the nervous system, though one should scarcely understand this comparison in the literal sense and imagine that the imprints of nerve excitations are like the fold in a sheet of paper.

Understanding the process of automatism leads us to an understanding of the process whereby the instinctive reactions are supposed to originate from the conscious reactions. Proponents of this view suppose that the instinctive reactions arise in roughly the same way that the conscious movements involved in learning how to play a piano subsequently become mechanical, and that the instinctive reactions arise through a selection of conscious and spontaneous actions. Thus, the instincts are understood by these psychologists as mechanical, rational acts, which leads us to affirm that everything which today is instinctive and mechanical was once creative and rational. "The instinct is our fallen reason," thus declares this standpoint in an exact formula. From this standpoint, in fact, the schema of the development of the reactions may be represented thus: reason—instinct—reflex.

Even though it is confirmed by striking analogy with the involuntary aspect of man's movements, this view cannot be considered very likely, however. Automatism only illustrates how random acts become exact and mechanical after a series of repetitions, but this does not in the least mean that these acts are initially rational. It only says that rational acts may also become mechanical, but this likewise does not at all mean that this capacity is inherent only to such acts. On the contrary, as is evident from what was presented earlier, all our observations show that the rational type of activity that arises with the direct participation of the cerebral cortex is built up upon the foundation of the inherited reactions and occupies a later stage in the evolutionary process than the instincts.

Another view, according to which the instincts should be considered earlier in terms of origin than the rational actions, is a far more likely one, however. From this point of view, reason is conscious, i.e., built up through the individual experience of the instincts. The schema for the development of the reactions, according to this view, may be represented thus: reflex—instinct—reason.

Thus, the reflexes, understood as the most primitive form of behavior, become the elemental foundation, the basis of all forms of human activity.

This does not mean, however, that the instincts may be reduced to the reflexes. An instinct may arise on the basis of a reflex in the course of evolution, as a form of behavior that is entirely different from it, even if it is genetically associated with it. "From the foundation of a house," writes Vagner, "one cannot say what will be built up upon it, whether a grocery store, a chemical laboratory, or the office of a notary public. The class of reptiles forms the foundation of both the class of birds and the class of mammals; however, it would be foolish to see the teeth of lizards in the beak of pigeons, or the webbed feet of birds in the claws of crocodiles."

But neither is this second schema entirely satisfactory, since we know that "rational" forms of behavior arise directly from the reflexes, and that there is really no need for an intermediate link in the form of the instincts. We could just as well say that, in a multitude of organisms, even the development of the most highly advanced instincts does not in the least reduce to the formation and development of rational reactions. For all these reasons, it is more proper and more correct to adopt the schema proposed by Vagner for the origin of the instincts. According to this schema, reason and the instincts, though they share the reflexes as their common foundation, nevertheless developed in parallel and on its own into independent and distinctive forms of behavior. The schema assumes the following form:

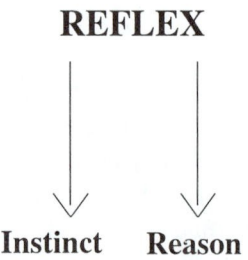

REFLEX

Instinct   Reason

Relationship Between the Instincts, Reflexes, and Reason

The relationship that exists between the instincts, the reflexes, and reason, a relationship that was first found in animal psychology and has clearly been confirmed in man, is of extraordinary interest for the educator.

In this relationship, the instincts are understood to exert a delaying effect upon the reflexes. This is clear from the following experiment. If a decapitated insect crawling in a straight line in a given direction is struck by a pair of tweezers, it will engage in reflexive, rotating movement to the left and the right, basically a defense reaction intended to evade danger; the oscillations will continue until simple fatigue and exhaustion of the nervous system puts an end to it. Such is the purely reflexive nature of behavior. The normal insect that has not lost its instinctive reaction will react quite differently to this very same stimulation. It will reflexively turn aside, but further reflexive movements will halt and be suppressed after awhile, by virtue of the instinct of self-preservation, which forces the insect to resort to more complex movements in order to avoid danger.

Consciousness exerts precisely the same delaying action on the reflexes. There is a well-known story of Darwin making a bet with 20 young people that the strongest snuff would not cause them to sneeze and, in fact, none of them did sneeze during the experiment, though before, as well as afterwards, the very same snuff had had a strong effect on them. The powerful desire to win the bet arising here, due to the large sum involved, the concentration of attention on the event, the fear of losing, and other conscious processes paralyzed and inhibited the reflex.

Incidentally, there is an interesting pedagogical conclusion that should be drawn from this law. If a powerful emotion associated with desire and fear so affects behavior as to undermine it and upsets even the normal run of the lowest reactions, it is easy to understand how counter to psychological wisdom are all those pedagogical techniques such as tests and the like which deliberately place students in the same position Darwin placed his colleagues and which, as a rule, distort the course and replication of reactions in the strongest way possible.

As a general and unquestionable psychological rule, it should be declared that tests and all such techniques always produce an entirely false and distorted picture of behavior and, for the most part, tend to have a diminishing and distorting effect on the system in which the reactions are reproduced. The reverse case, when test anxiety serves as a stimulus for extraordinarily sharp recall and quickness of response should, naturally, be well known to the reader, though, from the psychological point of view, this, too, is unnatural.

Just as well, there is every reason for supposing that, in the same way that the instincts exert a delaying effect on the reflexes and tend to suppress them, so are the instincts themselves subject to the same effect from the direction of the rational reactions.

Instincts and the Biogenetic Law

Scientists have long noticed the somewhat odd relationship that exists between the ontogenesis and phylogenesis of organisms, i.e., between the development of the species and the development of the individual. In the human embryo, for example, gills, tail, scalp may be observed at a certain stage, a stage that is, moreover, analogous to those long-gone stages of evolution when man's ancestors dwelled in the water and possessed tails.

There is a multitude of facts that point to a correspondence between the history of the development of the organism from an embryonic cell and the development of the species as a whole. These circumstances led Haeckel to formulate the *biogenetic law* in roughly the following form: The history of the individual constitutes an abbreviated and compressed history of the species. Thus, the evolution of the organism repeats the evolution of the species, and in the course of their own development, the embryo and young of any species pass through all those stages through which the development of the species passed. Thus, the embryo accomplishes a kind of truncated and accelerated passage through the entire path of evolution. [1]

Many thinkers have translated this law into the realm of psychology. By now, it has been introduced into numerous systems as a fundamental principle of the child's psyche and the fundamental normative principle of the development of educational psychology. It has been suggested, for example, that the child repeats in its development, though in abbreviated and altered form, all those critical stages that mankind has experienced from the moment man first appeared on the earth right up through the present day. From the very first moment of life, the infant is a simple grasper of objects. He drags everything over to himself, everything he puts into his mouth, and this corresponds to that epoch in which primitive man, like an animal who knows nothing of work, would feed himself by reaching out to edible substances. The migratory instinct appeared somewhat later on in man, involving running, climbing, the investigation of everything around him, and this corresponds to the second stage of historical development, when mankind assumed a nomadic way of life. The child's interest in domestic animals at a certain stage thus corresponds to primitive cattle-breeding. His combativeness and fighting instincts are considered echoes of mankind's bloody strifes in ancient times. Finally, the child's tendency to endow all objects with life, his love for everything imaginary, his attachment to fables, the primitive forms of his drawings and his language, all find their analogy in the animism of savages, in primitive religious beliefs, and in myths.

Taken together the foregoing remarks lead to the claim that the child, in fact, experiences in his few short years the many thousands of years mankind has existed. Hence, the pedagogical conclusion regarding the legitimacy of all these primitive events in childhood, the recognition of the child as a little savage, and the rule that insists we not fight all these phenomena, but instead let the child get over its primitive instincts and its wild tendencies all on its own. Thus, the extraordinary emphasis placed on fantasies, and similarly the child's routine animistic explanation of events in the world, his belief in imaginary beings, in the "aliveness" of inanimate objects, and so on, all of which became a general pedagogical technique, a theme which even the most progressive and the most rational educator finds it difficult to guard against.

This principle should not be taken in such a definitive form, however, since we do not know enough about mankind's historical development to make judgements about analogies. What we do know constitutes no more than isolated, fragmentary, often highly strained analogies that scarcely permit us to declare that, in its general course, the child's whole development repeats the entire historical development of mankind. The only thing we can be absolutely certain of is that individual points in the child's development may be associated together in a relation that, at times, is closer to, at times more distant from, individual points in mankind's history. Following Marshall, we have to admit that if the history of the individual does repeat the history of the species, in this repetition there are whole chapters, moreover rather lengthy chapters, that are missing entirely, others are so distorted as to be unrecognizable, while a third group are in such disarray that, on the whole, this repetition is in no way recognizable as a true reproduction, it is more of a distortion, and not only is it not an explanatory principle for the child's development, but, on the contrary, itself requires explanation.

With such a limited meaning, the law loses all force of attraction, and from a universal explanation it becomes a problem. "To explain the child's development by the development of mankind," writes Kornilov, "is to explain one unknown by another."

As regards the psychology of the instincts, this means that here we have to limit ourselves to drawing comparisons between certain instincts observed in children and analogous forms of the behavior of primitive man, though this does not in any way mean conceding that in the development of the instincts, there is a straightforward and passive mechanism present which consists in the simple repetition of already experienced history. Such a recognition would be in utter contradiction with the dynamic social conditionality of the psyche, a result we established earlier as a fundamental principle. It is not hard to show that, in the system formed by man's behavior and man's instincts, there is nothing permanent and inflexible, nothing that moves solely by the force of inertia. In a genuine behavioral system, the instincts are just as socially conditioned, just as adaptable and changeable, just as capable of assuming new forms, as are all the other reactions. Hence it is not the principle of parallelism in the development of the instincts which holds such great importance for pedagogics, but rather the mechanism responsible for the social adaptation of the instincts and their inclusion in the general scheme of behavior.

Two Extreme Views of the Instincts

There were two extreme views in the psychological and pedagogical interpretation of the older, traditional point of view of the instincts. Some saw in the instincts the legacy of the animal in man, the voice of the wildest and the most unbridled passions, a residue of the burden of all those primitive and savage epochs that had been experienced by mankind and since left far behind. To these scientists, the instincts appeared to be of the nature of rudimentary organs, i.e., organs that had once possessed particular biological meanings and functions corresponding to the lowest stage of evolution of the organism. With the transition to a higher stage, however, these "organs" had become unnecessary and were doomed to gradual atrophy and condemned to disappear. Hence the extraordinarily poor evaluation of the instinctive capacities from the standpoint of psychology, and the pedagogical slogan that repudiates as mere instinct all educational values, the utter absence of any concern for the development of the instincts, and, at times, the pressure to struggle against, and suppress and curb, the child's instincts. There was a whole system of pedagogics that guided education under the banner of such a struggle against the instincts.

Another view, one that was in utter contradiction with the latter, preached admiration for the instincts, and viewed the instincts as being of paramount importance in the educational system. Those psychologists who held to this view saw in the instincts the wise voice of nature itself, the most advanced of all the mechanisms of faultless and exact behavior, and considered instinctive behavior to be the ideal and prototype of the most advanced forms of behavior. Hence, they arrived at a pedagogical conclusion that took the instincts to be wise guides in matters of education. And where the former systems called for a struggle against the instincts, these latter systems saw the full meaning of education to lie in the most painless of pursuits after all those natural processes that confound the instincts.

It is not hard to see that none of these points of view can be taken as correct, that each possesses a degree of truth and a degree of error. In a scientific view of the instincts, there has to be the recognition that the instincts possess both positive and negative aspects, and there is the inclination to agree with that general point of view on the educational process which views it as a matter of taking control of the child's spontaneous growth, and that the instincts constitute a vast educational force that can be just as useful as harmful. The electricity in lightning can kill, but under the control of man it moves trains, illuminates cities, and transmits human speech from one end of the earth to the other. Thus the psychologist approaches the instincts as if a vast natural, elemental force that, in and of itself, produces a result capable of being equally useful and harmful. The instincts must be forced to serve one's own purposes; "they are terrible when they are the masters, and beautiful when they are the servants," says one American psychologist. Therefore, the question has to be not of a struggle or pursuit of the instincts, but only of the genuine psychological nature of the instincts, knowledge of which will give us the opportunity to take control of this educational force.

Instinct as a Mechanism of Education

From the psychological point of view, the instincts appear to be powerful excitations which are associated with the most complex organic needs, sometimes turning into an entirely insurmountable force. The instincts are the most powerful impulses and the most powerful stimuli to activity. It is quite clear from the above, therefore, that this enormous natural motive force must be used to the fullest extent possible in education. It is precisely because instinctive behavior does not constitute a kind of stiff, ingrained pattern given once and for all, as we noted earlier, that it may instead be cast, as in a mould, in the most varied forms of activity, and the instincts themselves may initiate, as if a kind of engine, the most diverse types of reactions imaginable.

It is entirely impossible to either suppress or depress the instincts, as this would involve pointless struggle against the child's nature, and if this struggle were to ever succeed, it would mean a diminishing and a suppression of the child's nature, causing childhood to be deprived of its most precious and its most important properties. It is only necessary to recall how tame and lifeless, how frail and unfit, were the sorts of people produced by the old education, which viewed the suppression of the instincts as being of paramount importance. The full force of human creativity, the most exuberant flowering of genius, is possible not in poor, infertile soil where the instincts have been done away with, but on the foundation of the most exuberant flowering and the full-fledged tensing of all its forces. The American psychologist Edward Lee Thorndike speaks of the instincts roughly as follows: "One cannot make the Niagara River return to Lake Erie and keep it there, but, by building discharge channels, it is possible to give its waters a new direction and to force it to serve our purposes, for example, to set in motion the wheels of plants and factories."

Thus it is with the instincts. The instincts constitute a vast natural force, they are the expression and voice of the organism's natural needs, but this does not mean they have to be a fearful and destructive force. Like every other form of behavior, the instincts emerged out of adaptations to the environment, but since they constitute extremely ancient forms of adaptation, it is understandable that, as the environment changed, these forms of adaptation turned out to be unsuitable to the changed circumstances; thus arose a certain incongruity, a discordancy, between the instincts and the environment.

An obvious example of such disharmony is apparent in the hitherto preserved form of the instinct of self-preservation in its fugitive and combative manifestations. The instinct of fear and flight from danger is, without a doubt, one of the most beneficial of all biological achievements in the animal kingdom. How true it is that, as the saying goes, "fear is the guardian of mankind." Were there no fear, it is not very likely that life could have reached its highest forms. It is extraordinarily useful for an animal that, whenever it encounters danger, it instinctively takes to flight. But in the last few centuries, the conditions of life have so changed that instinctive flight from danger is now not in the least an appropriate reaction for a human being. For the rabbit, it is a useful that the slightest sound will cause it to prick up its ears and make its entire body quiver; thus does it protect itself from the hunter and from the predator, but it is not always useful for a person to grow pale, to begin to tremble, and to lose his voice upon meeting up with danger. The conditions of the environment have so changed that man has to respond to danger in entirely different ways. Thus it is with anger; it is extraordinarily useful for a predatory animal that has encountered a foe to reflexively bare its teeth, for blood to rush to its head, and for it to paw the ground in preparation for an assault, but it is hardly useful for a person to clench his teeth, tighten his jaws, and make a fist when on the attack. In other words, the instincts, understood as a form of adaptation that has evolved under certain conditions, may turn out to be useful only under these conditions; as conditions change, an instinct may prove to be in conflict with the environment, and then the task of education is to eliminate this disharmony, and make the instincts once again accord with the conditions of the environment. All of man's culture as it relates to the individual himself and to the behavior of the individual constitutes nothing other than such an adaptation of the instincts to the environment.

The Concept of Sublimation

The old psychology assumed that man's psyche was limited to the narrow range of his conscious experiences. To the old psychology, therefore, all those mental phenomena that man himself was not conscious of, but which nevertheless proclaimed his presence in the realm of behavior imperiously and persistently remained incomprehensible and mysterious. Psychologists suggested calling this domain of the reactions, a domain that basically defines our behavior, the sphere of the *subconscious* for that which was *beyond the threshold of consciousness*, or that which was subliminal (from *limen*, Latin for "threshold").

Investigations have shown that the subconscious sphere derives from certain strivings, or instinctive impulses, which, because they were unable to obtain satisfaction for one reason or another, had come into conflict with other mental forces, and were exiled to the domain of the unconscious. In this way, they seem to have been prevented from having any influence on our behavior, though they have not been obliterated entirely; though they have been exiled there, they nevertheless continue to exist and continue to exert their effect on the course of man's reactions. Action thus assumes a dual character, depending on the outcome the conflict takes. If it takes protracted forms, the ousted strivings and desires have a disruptive and inhibiting effect on the reactions, and take advantage of every opportunity to once again reach conscious awareness, to burst into conscious processes, and take possession of the motor mechanism; in this case, we always have in the subconscious an enemy, a malicious and hurtful enemy that has been driven underground. The outcome of this conflict sometimes assumes the rather unhealthy forms of neurotic illness. In its main points, neurosis is a form of illness in which, as a result of the conflict between the instincts and the environment, the former are not satisfied, desires banishment to the sphere of the subconscious, and mental life becomes severely alienated. Even if these conflicts do not assume explicitly morbid form, they remain essentially abnormal, and, frankly speaking, a system of education that has nothing to say about the instincts reduces to the manufacture of neurotics. Flight into neurosis is the only means of escape for desires that remain unsatisfied and for instincts that are not employed.

Conflict may assume a second form. In this form, desires that have been dislodged from the sphere of consciousness take on higher forms, are transformed, changing into higher forms of mental energy. This case has been referred to as *sublimation*. Just as in physics, where we might study the conversion of mechanical, light, electrical, and other forms of energy, so in the psyche, the work of each of the centers in the psyche is not something closed off and insulated, but rather allows for the possibility that certain desires may be transformed into other desires, and certain reactions transformed into other reactions. The conversion of lower forms of energy into higher forms through banishment of the former to the subconscious, is referred to as *sublimation*. Thus, from the psychological point of view, the education of the instincts confronts a dilemma, whether to choose neurosis or sublimation, i.e., whether to side with the eternal collision between unsatisfied desires and our behavior, or whether to convert unacceptable desires into higher and more complex forms of behavior.

Education of the Sex Instinct

In order to explain all the problems of the instincts, let us consider as an example the sex instinct and the education of this instinct. That the sex instinct constitutes the most powerful biological mechanism for the preservation of the species, that wherever it withers, there life ceases to be, requires no special explanation. It is no less self-evident that, psychologically speaking, the sex instinct constitutes a powerful source of mental impulses, of sufferings, pleasures, desires, anguish, and joy.

The problem of sex education has always been solved in different ways, though it has assumed especially tragic forms in recent decades. Middle-class morality, on the one hand, and cultural conditions, on the other, together with the structure of the educational system, led the problem of sex education down a blind alley without producing any sort of method of solution. It is difficult to conceive of anything more appalling than the position of the sex instinct in the school of the recent past.

The sexual problem had, ostensibly, been banished from the life of the school, and moreover, was assumed to be without substance. Such neglect of sexual problems led to a struggle with every manifestation of sexual feeling, and the claim that the entire realm was sordid and foul. In response, students reacted with neuroses and unhealthy acting out, or were led to actually drive underground this, the greatest force of the human body, and placed his or her own sex education and responsibility for gaining knowledge of matters sexual in the hands of degraded servants and acquaintances. Thus did all the different types of sexual abnormality, reaching all the way down to the very roots of life in such tragic ways, find their place in the school.

There are two fundamental points we should bring up in rebuttal to the old school in this regard. First, we reject the view that childhood is an innocent, sexless period, and that, consequently, sexual problems do not exist for the child. We are also of the belief that the elimination of sex education from the overall system of educational influence, the total expunging of this realm of life from the life of the young, the brazen and intrusive prohibition imposed on these questions, was the worst of all possible outcomes. The new approach compels us, above all, to acknowledge that the state of childhood should not be conceived as entirely asexual until the onset of what is commonly referred to as puberty; on the contrary, psychological studies have shown that childhood sexuality, together with a variety of healthy and pathological manifestations of childhood sexuality, may be found in the earliest years and even at the breast-feeding stage. Masturbation in early childhood, and even in infancy, is a phenomenon that has long been an established fact in the practice of medicine. Psychoanalysis, the investigation of mentally ill adult patients, has discovered in these patients a conflict involving sexual experiences of the most remote past and early childhood.

But it goes without saying that these sexual experiences assume entirely different forms than the sexual experiences of the adult. Above all, in childhood we encounter a kind of highly developed eroticism not associated with the functioning of particular organs nor localized at strictly demarcated sites, but rather excited by the functioning of the most varied organs and associated chiefly with the mucous membranes of the body, the so-called erogenous zones. Further, the very character of this eroticism distinguishes it from the eroticism of the adult in certain ways; it assumes the form of auto-eroticism, i.e., eroticism directed at oneself, as well as psychologically healthy narcissism, i.e., the state in which erotic excitations emanate from one's own body and find their resolution there. It would have been utterly incongruous for such an important system as the sexual system to have existed entirely independently from everything else and to manifest itself all of a sudden with the onset of a certain age.

In the very next period, childhood eroticism assumes novel forms. Now it is directed towards the most familiar persons with whom the child tends to become involved with, and occurs as a complex component in the relationship between the child and his or her mother and with others. The sensation of any difference between the sexes is absent in children in the early years, though quite often we encounter childhood infatuation, often of a highly impulsive and intensive nature, which is characteristic of the most tender age. In general, it should be noted that, throughout this period in the life of the child, the sex instinct assumes concealed and latent forms, and, under ordinary conditions, itself follows the path of sublimation. Even in children at a tender age, we encounter a whole series of traits in the behavior of boys and girls that make these children seem like little men and little women. In all these instances, we are undoubtedly dealing with a sublimited sex instinct.

Far more complex is the matter of the education of the sex instinct in puberty, when awakened desires cannot find an outlet and satisfaction, and are expressed in the stormy, troubled, anxiety-ridden state of the psyche that everyone experiences in adolescence and early youth. Here sexual feelings inevitably assume the nature of a conflict, and a favorable outcome of this conflict is possible only if there is an essential level of sublimation, i.e., only if the stormy and destructive forces of the instinct are guided along the necessary channels. Understood as an object of education, the sex instinct requires adaptations to the social structure of life that would not cut into its already established forms, and the problem is not in the least one of suppressing or blunting the sex instinct; on the contrary, the teacher must be concerned with ensuring the full preservation and healthy development of the instinct. The principal divergence of the sex instinct in its educated form from the natural conditions of the environment can be seen in the fact that, in its inherited, natural forms, the sex instinct is entirely indifferent and blind, without any relation to the ultimate purpose it serves. The sex instinct of man and the animals is directed towards every individual of the opposite sex.

The principal difference that culture brings to the sex instinct is that selective, personal character which sexual feelings assume in man. From the moment the instinct becomes directed towards one definite person and seems to fade away in relation to all other persons, at that moment from an animal instinct it becomes a human instinct. Romeo and Juliet could not live without each other despite the fact that in Venice there were many beautiful young women and handsome young men, and each of them could have found a spouse, Romeo a wife of his own and Juliet a husband of her own. But Romeo had need only for his Juliet, and Juliet only for her Romeo. Such a situation would be unthinkable in the animal kingdom, and it is here that we begin to discern the human element in the sex instinct. This is why the modern psychologist must undertake a thorough reappraisal of all values in the area of sexual pedagogics.

Youthful love, which, until recently, had been thought of as being inappropriate and harmful, and therefore assumed the grotesque forms of courtship or flirtation, is, in the eyes of the new psychologist, the only means of humanizing the sex instinct. It teaches us to restrict the instinct and to guide it in only one direction, it teaches us how to build entirely exclusive relations with one other person on a sound basis for the very first time, to isolate these relations from all other human relationships, and to assign to them an exceptional and profound meaning. Love in the time of youth is the most natural and the most unavoidable form of sublimation of the sex instinct. And the ultimate purpose of sex education is solely to teach the person how to love. Disharmony between the real unemployment of love and the enormous strain love imparts is another way that the educated form of the instinct diverges from the natural conditions of the environment; in this regard, too, the goal of education is to direct the instinct not only along the line of least resistance, nor along the shortest and least troublesome path through which the most immediate satisfaction may be attained, but along a lengthy, difficult, and graceful path.

Finally, it is necessary to overcome the blindness of the instinct, to bring it into the general sphere of consciousness, to set it in relation to all other forms of behavior, and to associate it with the goal and purpose it is called upon to serve. It is in this connection that giving children anatomical, physiological, etc. knowledge of matters sexual has long been advanced as a fundamental educational measure. We understand this to refer to the process of acquainting children from their earliest years with the scientific view of sexual life. In fact, one cannot but recognize the positive educational force of providing children with information about sex. Truth always educates one to be truthful. All those stories of storks bringing babies, about infants being found beneath the bushes, show themselves to be false in the child's eyes rather quickly, cloaks the truth in a veil of mystery, arouses the child's curiosity, causes him to think of all of this as wrong and shameful, and leads him to try to find out everything on the sly, from unscrupulous and corrupt sources, dulling and tarnishing the child's mind and imagination. In this sense, acquainting the child with the truth about sexual life becomes an urgent psychological necessity, and the saying, "it's better to be a day early than an hour late," becomes the teacher's watchword here.

Placing an excessive value on sexual knowledge should, however, be rejected, since it has a limited and often provisional value. Above all, providing the child with information about sex should not be seen as a kind of radical method of sex education. A person can possess an excellent and entirely correct store of knowledge of matters sexual and be very badly educated. The instincts are too complex and subtle a thing to be struggled against and to be subordinated to this or that bit of information. Like any set of moral rules, information about sex is quite powerless in the face of genuine desires and cannot give them any necessary guidance. Knowing how one should act is still far from the same thing as acting correctly; on the contrary, very often it brings out extremely unhealthy conflicts in the child's behavior. For example, all explanations and warnings about the harm caused by masturbation, threats and the like are quite powerless in the struggle against childhood masturbation. On the contrary, it would appear that the greatest harm in this area has been the result of slipshod knowledge of sex, since threatening the child has always created a serious impasse between indomitable desire unable to find another outlet and the agonizing consciousness of guilt, fear, and shame. Not knowing how to handle this impasse, the child suffers far more from harm to his mind than from real harm. Moreover, sexual information is not always considered with the psychological interests of the child in mind; foreign manuals usually suggest subject matter for children without considering the child's natural interests. Thus, the process of reproduction in the world of plants and animals with which manuals of sex information commonly begin is usually less of a concern to the child than how his little brother was born. Furthermore, it is beyond the child's capacity to grasp such disparate processes as the growth of plants and the birth of a child in a single, general train of thought and to understand how they are connected.

Finally, it is also essential to observe extraordinary tact when providing children with sex information, since children do not, in general, understand any sort of abstract knowledge, they are unable to place all these newly acquired bits of information into a group of its own, and instead combine this information with their own ever-present instinct of curiosity and exploration. Thus, the sex information provided to children may prove to be beyond their understanding. All these facts, of course, lead us to look upon sex information with the greatest of caution, though by no means banishing it entirely. It has to be acknowledged as possessing a certain relative value and, because of psychological considerations, must be deferred to a later age, when all three dangers associated with it, such as the exclusive concern with the concrete, the inability to make scientific generalizations, and the practical application of every form of knowledge, will have diminished considerably.

Thus, together with other educational measures, sex information, when presented with a degree of pedagogical tact, may prove to be extraordinarily useful and important. The mechanism of educating the sex instinct involves the sublimation we spoke of above. It has long been noted that the internal secretion of the sex glands is associated rather closely with the higher forms of human activity, with creativity and genius. In particular, the reader is surely aware of the sexual roots of artistic creativity. The ancient Greeks understood this relationship perfectly, calling Eros not only the force of sexual attraction, but also the tension of poetic creativity and of philosophical thought. Plato expressed this most profound truth quite correctly, though in mythological form.

In Plato's belief, the basest and most exalted are equally combined in Eros, which he represented as the son of the god of plenty and the goddess of poverty: "He is poor, coarse, dirty, wallows about naked, and is always in search of the good and the beautiful—a great wizard and sorcerer." The same thought was expressed by Arthur Schopenhauer when he claimed that the greatest creative tension begins just at the moment when sexual desire matures. It is easily seen, using a purely experimental technique, that every disturbance in, and withering of, sexual feelings is accompanied by a stagnation and extinction of creativity. It is hardly remarkable that man's most creative period occurs when the sexual urges are in full bloom. Thus, the sublimation of the sex instinct, i.e., supplanting the sex instinct by other interests of higher order in the subconscious in order that it nourish creativity from its place of exile, is the principal theme of sex education. The reader surely knows how greatly sublimation relieves that special state of *Sturm and Drang*, that craving for adventure, that vast host of drives, which manifests itself in youth. In these cases, the teacher does not have to artificially create a source of sublimation in this or that sphere of knowledge, the age of youth is the age of natural creativity, and all the teacher has to do is choose a direction for sublimation.

Social relations, which also seem to be natural channels along which the sublimated sexual instinct travels, are a further source of sublimation that is no less fertile than is individual creativity. In no other period of a person's life is there found anything like the friendship and companionship, profound affection and emotional bonds, that commonly bond youths together at this stage. No other period of a person's life knows of such friendship as that of youth. And there can be no doubt that these social relations are nourished ultimately from the same source as is youthful creativity. Note, too, that sublimation is a profoundly private and inner process which might be likened to a grain that perishes in order to germinate anew.

Psychological Preconditions of Co-education

Next is the question of the particular techniques to achieve sublimation. It should be clear to the reader that techniques of moral suasion, and even the various methods of inculcating sex information, are powerless to counter any sort of powerful centers of excitation that might arise in connection with sexual activity. Against these centers it is necessary to oppose centers that are just as powerful and that act just as constantly. This may be achieved not by isolating sex education as something special, but only through the construction of a systematic framework that would be in accord with the vital concerns of youth, and that could be thought of as a system of highly coordinated "diversion cuts" that would accommodate sublimated sexual energy and give to it an appropriate direction. The goal of sex education is also to construct these channels, and this goal must, consequently, be achieved somewhat apart from all questions of sex.

The only step to take, one that is quite necessary and, moreover, social in nature, is to institute the *co-education* of the two sexes. Though it has now become the ordinary form of education in the Soviet school, co-education has yet to achieve universal recognition and still continues to encounter objections. The psychological preconditions of this system are extremely simple and clear. The first such precondition derives from the psychological rule which states that if we wish to achieve a weakening of the force of a stimulus, we have to take care to make it constant, habitual, and entirely imperceptible and see to it that it does not induce a reaction of its own. The greater the number of combinations the particular stimulus becomes part of, the easier it is for us to make it imperceptible and relatively neutral. We will stop noticing it the same way we don't notice air or an ordinary situation, and develop steady and brief automatic reactions of the greatest subtlety and discrimination in relation to these combinations.

Thus, the first goal of sex education is to dull this reaction to the face of every person of the opposite sex. But precisely the opposite goal is achieved by having boys and girls educated separately. In its desire to insulate sexual stimuli and thereby protect the instinct from being discovered prematurely, separate education emphasizes the differences between the sexes, and excludes any focus of interaction between girls and boys, concentrating all the student's attention on the differences between the sexes. From the very first year of life, boys are accustomed to look upon girls, and conversely, as if at an entirely alien being with strange interests, with whom interaction is not permitted, with whom interaction represents something unseemly, shameful, and contrived, and with whom all feelings of companionship are excluded from the outset. The very system of the old education, say in the old gymnasium, reserved for the relations between the two sexes only such forms of interaction as ballroom dances, secret courtship, and flirtation. It goes without saying that this contributed to the creation of a peculiar stifling and sexually unhealthy environment in which the sex instinct was constrained and restricted, though because it lacked any outlet or the opportunity for sensible use, manifested itself violently and graphically in the most brutal, harshest and coarsest forms.

As a result of this form of sex education, the view developed quite naturally that, for a man, any relation with a woman other than sexual relations is impossible, that a women is, above all, a female, and that every person of the opposite sex is, for this very reason alone, the most powerful stimulus of the instinct. Nowhere, not even where debauchery was the least hampered, was the view of woman so associated with the sexual element as in the monasteries. Precisely because it was extraordinarily rare, the stimulus retained an extraordinary power of influence, and the system created by this form of education was thought of, quite properly, as a system for the temptation of the sex instinct. It was also quite remarkable that the stricter the system of separate education thus created and the more isolated were the two sexes, the more acute and the more objectionable were the forms assumed by the instinct, for example, in boarding schools and equally so in the boarding schools for boys as in those for girls.

Secondly, once they were in constant interaction with each other, entering into the thousands of the most distinct and most complex relations with each other, both boys and girls learned not to react to nor notice sexual characteristics; they became accustomed to each other, rather than obsessed with each other, no longer irritable, but rather understanding. The other person's sex then came to be noticed like light, air, or warmth. Such broad and powerful channels are created and developed through which sexual excitation can drain off that the problem of sublimation is solved to an enormous degree simply by this one fact alone.

And the third, the most important, result: the possibility of achieving the principal goal of the education of the sex instinct. That is, the development of a selective function, the capacity to choose and focus one's love on one person of the opposite sex, can likewise develop in no better way than against the background of a general suppression of sexual stimuli. To this we might add that the sharing of common interests can create such a dilution of the purely sexual component of young love in the context of all the other manifestations of fondness that we end up with the most subtle, the most complex forms of sublimation. Every young man must inevitably pass through his own period of chivalry towards a young woman. Like any genuine psychological category, chivalry is an unavoidable form of sex education.

The usual argument against co-education is that there are physiological and psychological differences between boys and girls, and that these differences demand different systems of education and programs of instruction in certain instances, as used to be the case in Russia, where girls' gymnasia differed from boys' gymnasia in having their own curriculum and educational systems. It is not hard to see that these limitations were, for the most part, of a class character and sprang from entirely different sources. Above all, the fact that the middle-class school prepared boys and girls for different vocations played a role here. The educational ideal was taken from the careers that the grown-up man and grown-up woman were to follow later on in life. In other words, these differences were due to the correspondence between the school and the social environment which, as we have already seen, is the fundamental rule of pedagogics. Now, with the revolutionary reconstruction of the social structure, relationships in the school must naturally change. And since an ethics of equality in sexual life has become the fundamental rule for both men and women, for that very reason all necessity of any form of special education for women vanishes.

Finally, the purely psychological differences between boys and girls, such as different capacities for certain subjects, for example, the notorious incompetence of girls in mathematics or in activities that require assertiveness, likewise are not primarily conditioned facts, but rather are derived from the special historical role of women in which the division of social functions condemned women to the limited path of the "four K's" (*Kinder, Kuche, Kleider, Kirche*; i.e., Children, Cooking, Dress-making, Church).

However, there cannot be the slightest doubt that there nevertheless exist substantial differences in the behavior of boys and girls caused by the very differences between the sexes, and that these differences appear in earliest childhood. For the most part, all of them are more or less related to the instincts, though it is extraordinarily difficult to tell how powerful a role is played in this area by the infectious example set by the social environment as opposed to the child's tendency to imitate. For example, in games involving dolls or other manifestations of the maternal or paternal instinct, we undoubtedly encounter a more or less exact replica of all those relationships the child sees at home. Nevertheless, there undoubtedly remains a substantial psychological difference between boys and girls, though, all the same, this difference is of such a character that there is no way it may be taken into account in a syllabus or in an educational program.

The goal of the school is not at all a matter of reducing everyone to the same level, on the contrary, one of the goals of the social environment that is created in the school is to achieve as complex, as diversified, and as flexible an organization of the various elements in this environment as possible. It is only necessary that these elements not be in any way irreconcilable, and that they be linked up together into a single system. What with the wealth and flexibility of this system, all the differences between the sexes can be easily taken into account through educational measures. And since establishing relationships in the school that would be needed later on in life is the fundamental psychological premise of our educational systems, we must start by infusing the school with the network of nonsexual relationships that the child will need later on in life. This already presupposes the broadest interaction between the sexes in the school as the foundation of the educational system.

One last question remains, whether the principle of separate education for boys and girls should be maintained only from necessity, and only in part, during the transitional age of puberty, which is an especially painful period, one which boys and girls live through at different times. It is easy to see, however, that such a proposal suffers from all the shortcomings of a half-way measure and, even more, reveals its fallaciousness. In fact, if we acknowledge the healthy sexual effects of co-education, we also have to acknowledge the fact that nowhere is the demand for co-education felt as strongly and as acutely as during the critical years of puberty. Conversely, if we are in agreement that separate education of the sexes emphasizes the differences between the sexes, and excites and leads to temptation and to intensification of the sex instinct, then we will have to admit that never is the damage produced by this temptation as strong and as palpable as in these years. Thus, the distinctive feature of this period in the child's life, understood as the most critical period of sexual life, not only does not minimize, but rather intensifies, the psychological necessity of co-education.

Pedagogical Application of the Instincts

The first question that the teacher faces is the general one of direction, i.e., in which direction are the instincts to be developed. The most general rule is to inculcate an awareness of the social value of each instinct and to show students what are the different ways an instinct can be applied in the most harmless, the most civilized, and the most acceptable form. There are two approaches to the subject here, if we leave aside the pedagogics involved in restraining the instincts.

According to the first, or conservative, approach, it is necessary to overcome the instincts, i.e., a form of education is needed in which once a particular instinct has assumed harmless and peaceable forms, it becomes possible to respond to the excitations associated with it in certain artificial ways. Consider, for example, the habit of collecting things, as a harmless means of overcoming the instinct of greed and the accumulation of wealth. One might think of athletics likewise, as a means of overcoming the instincts of strife, combativeness, and competitiveness. Here the idea is to construct what might seem like safety valves for the instincts, artificial forms of activity in which an outlet for excess instinctive energy could be found.

It has been noted that such a technique for overcoming the instincts produces such good psychological results that a person who has collected much in childhood never displays either greed nor stinginess later on, and that, consequently, it is necessary to take care to create substitute forms of activity where the instinct would be directed towards innocent objects while retaining all its distinctive features. It's all a matter of what is to be the ultimate goal of the instinct, and how the instinct is directed. It is here that the heart of the problem lies, say the proponents of this view. The act of collecting retains the full force, the diversity, and the passion of the instinctive striving for the accumulation of wealth, but it is directed toward postage stamps or tobacco pipes and, consequently, is rendered harmless. In athletics, the full force of the competitive instinct is preserved, for example, the desire to vanquish an opponent, to surpass a rival, to be a source of trouble for someone else, to fight one's way forward, and to attain success by pushing others aside, but this dubious social trait is pointed in a harmless direction, since here the losses occur on the chessboard or on the croquet lawn, and competition is expressed by the best strike of the mallet or by skillfully carrying a football about.

It is, however, not hard to see that this point of view suffers from two drawbacks. In creating and cultivating artificial forms of activity of this type, we again run the risk of creating a host of curiosities and prejudices, and of ending up with a system of education that produces eccentrics. There is something pitifully frivolous from the standpoint of real life, something unwise in an excessive passion for the most innocent of pleasures, and the passionate player at pick-up-sticks or the person always on the lookout for silk embroidery to make curtain lace, though as harmless as that famous hero of Gogol's in *Dead Souls*, represents a kind of parody of life.

Meanwhile, in the case of a highly developed instinct, we inevitably obtain such forms of eccentricity as to make this clearly understood from the very start. We are thus forced to acknowledge that the principle of overcoming the instincts does not constitute a radical solution of the question. There is, furthermore, the inefficiency of such an educational principle to consider. It presupposes that the instincts may be rendered harmless, though the question is really what to do with them; it wastes the precious forces of human striving, passions, and perseverance on worthless and empty goals. Finally, the third and most important fact is that this principle far from always attains its goals. It re-educates not this or that instinct, but only its sphere of application, and the instinct itself is not only not overcome, but, like a passionate player in a game or a passionate collector of objects, often becomes more focused and more persistent, and is permanently reinforced. The result, thus, is that instead of being overcome, the instinct seems to become permanently ingrained and consolidated.

For all these reasons, a different principle is needed in the education of the instincts, not one that calls for overcoming the instincts, but one that mandates the greatest possible employment of the instincts in the process of education. From this approach, one has to speak of the construction of absolutely the entire system of education on the foundation of the child's instinctive strivings. Forms of instinctive activity also have to be developed that would contribute to pointing instinctive activity in the direction of maximally useful educational development. In this sense, the very same psychological principle underlying the education of new relationships, such as the conditional reflexes, becomes the foundation of the education of the instincts. In the course of activity and reaction, the instincts are readily transformed one into the other. And just as in the case of Pushkin's avaricious knight in whom the lust for power engendered greed, because the attainment of power was associated with the unceasing accumulation of money, so does the fundamental psychological law consist in the transformation of one instinct into another, the conversion of every form of activity from a means into an end in itself.

The psychological difference between the two principles can be understood quite easily from the examples presented above. The collection of postage stamps is, in and of itself, pointless and unnecessary, though it can become a valuable educational tool when combined with some more complex form of activity, for example, the rudiments of geography, practical international correspondence, or the esthetic appreciation of postage stamps. The habit of collecting objects, combined every time with more complex activity, thus makes it possible to transfer the instinct of accumulation from postage stamps to the geographic knowledge associated with stamps, or to transform the instinct into a sense for international relations.

It is here that we discover a genuine conquest of the instinct, in which the innate striving for accumulation and possessions begins to nourish and promote a passion for the accumulation of knowledge, or a passion to learn about the whole world. Or, to take another example, consider a chess game; the complexity of the mental combinations, the necessity for the most complicated mental effort at every stage as we search for the necessary move, becomes at first a simple tool and, initially, expresses the need to achieve some result in the game, but gradually from a tool it becomes an end in itself, and for a good chess player the purely emotional moment of struggle, victory, and defense is pushed into the background, by comparison with the pure joy of abstract thought, of finding the solution to the most intricate combinations; the satisfaction the chess player experiences from his own play is no longer a matter of mere pleasure at causing trouble for an opponent, but the far greater pleasure gained from correctly solving a problem, or from correctly finding one's way out of a difficult position. If this were psychologically untrue, then, all other conditions being equal, there would be the same level of interest in a game with a weak opponent as with a strong opponent. The general principle may be formulated in the following way. The fundamental pedagogical rule for the education of the instincts requires not just that they be rendered harmless, but rather that we make use of them, not overcoming them, but transforming them into higher forms of activity.

The Child's Interest

In childhood the basic mode of appearance of the instincts is in the form of interest, i.e., a special inclination of the child's psychic apparatus aimed at a particular object. Interests possess an all-encompassing importance in the child's life. Everything we do, even the most uninteresting, we nevertheless do out of interest, according to Thorndike, though from negative interest, out of a fear of trouble. Thus, interest would appear to be the natural motive force of the child's behavior, it is the true expression of instinctive striving, an indication that the child's activity coincides with his organic needs. That is why the fundamental rule demands that the entire educational system, the entire structure of teaching, be constructed on the foundation of children's interests, taken into account in exact fashion.

The psychological law simply says that before trying to get a child involved in some activity, get him interested in it, take care to discover whether he is ready for it, so that all the forces necessary for the activity are tensed, and the child is ready to act on his own, with the teacher left to simply guide and direct his activity. Even superficial imitation of interest clearly shows that interest is nothing other than the disposition and preparation of the organism for a particular activity, accompanied by an increase in overall vitality and a general sense of well-being. He who heeds his own interests, thus, holds his breath in, turns his ears in the direction of a speaker, does not lift his eyes from him, leaves aside all other cares, and avoids all movement, and, as the saying goes, "is all ears." This is also the clearest expression of an organism's focusing all its energies at a single point, as if transformed into a single kind of activity.

We should keep in mind an extremely critical danger the teacher encounters here. In striving to gain someone's interest in one thing or another, that person's interests may switch. There may be interest, but not the sort of interest which is needed, or this interest may not be pointed in the right direction. There is an eloquent story told in one of the American textbooks on psychology. A teacher in a public school who wished to teach geography had decided to begin by acquainting the children with regions that were nearby and accessible to them, and, moreover, were natural features, for example, fields, hills, rivers, and valleys in their environs. This the children found boring, however, and lacking all interest. It turned out their previous teacher, out of a wish to arouse their interest, had brought in a rubber ball with a hole in it and filled it with water as a way explaining the nature of geysers. This she did by cleverly concealing the ball in a sand pile and then pressing down upon it with her foot at the proper spot. As a result she succeeded in causing a stream of water to shoot through the sand to the universal delight of the children. In her explanation of volcanos, the same teacher employed a small piece of cotton dipped in sulphur and placed it in a pile of sand where she set it on fire, making it look just like the burning crater of a volcano. This aroused the liveliest interest in the children and to the new teacher they said, "All of us know this, show us better fireworks than Miss N," or "how a syringe works," said one of them to another.

This example easily shows how one interest may be falsely substituted for another. The first teacher had, undoubtedly, succeeded in arousing lively interest in the children, but it was an interest in a particular artifice, in fireworks and syringes, not in volcanos and geysers. Such interest is not only not useful pedagogically, but is even profoundly harmful. This is because it not only does not contribute to the development of the various forms of activity we require from children, but instead creates a powerful rival to these activities in the form of strong interests and, consequently, causes the child's sense of readiness, which the teacher anticipates awakening, to slacken off. It is rather easy to arouse interest in history lessons by relating anecdotes, but it is difficult to tell whether the resulting interest has to do with history, and not the particular anecdote. The interest thus aroused by such supplementary techniques not only does it not promote, but may even hold back, the development of the form of activity we require.

This is why nothing will arouse the child's attention or interest in a project if the stimulus consists in the fear of punishment or the expectation of a reward. We can be certain that we are developing in the child not an interest in sewing or arithmetic, though the child sews or counts diligently, but an interest in the candy we will have to give him as a reward, or a fear of being left without any sweets if he's wrong. It's an extremely complicated psychological problem to determining how to discover a genuine interest, and how to always take care that the student's interest not wander off from the subject and that he not get into the habit of switching his interest from one subject to another.

This, incidentally, is why rewards and punishment are, psychologically speaking, entirely inappropriate techniques in the school. Besides all the other harmful effects we will speak of below, they are also harmful in being useless, i.e., they are powerless to induce the form of activity we need, since they introduce an incommensurably more powerful interest which, we have to admit, forces the child into making his behavior coincide outwardly with what we desire, though internally he remains entirely unchanged. "Punishment educates slaves"—this ancient saying is, psychologically speaking, profoundly true, since punishment, in fact, does not teach anyone anything other than fear and the ability to guide one's own behavior in terms of fear and nothing else. That is why punishment is the easiest and most feeble of all pedagogical techniques, producing a rapid but slight effect regardless of the inner education of the instincts. In view of the child's natural aversion to pain, it is extraordinarily easy to intimidate him with the rod and thereby force him to suppress a bad habit, but this does not make it disappear, on the contrary, instead of one bad habit, yet another habit is inculcated, the new habit of submitting to fear. Thus it is with rewards. It is easy to induce a reaction if its performance is associated in the child's mind with some pleasure, but if we wish to foster in the child just this reaction, then we must take care that satisfaction and pleasure are associated with the reaction proper, and not with the anticipated reward.

Thus, the guiding principle does not reduce simply to the arousal of interest, but also demands that this interest be guided in an appropriate direction. It is always necessary to adhere to the psychological rule that requires passing from the child's natural interests, of which the child tends to have a sufficient quantity, to those interests we wish to foster. From the psychological standpoint, here we would be correct in distinguishing between new interests, the inculcation of which represents an end in itself, and interests that are inculcated to function only as a tool. Only an interest that takes root and lasts for one's entire life following lengthy reinforcement may represent an end in itself. The development and reinforcement of interests constitutes a fundamental law of education and requires on the part of the teacher the gradual implantation of this or that interest in the course of activity. Such, for example, are interests in daily life, in science, in labor, and so on.

Other interests that may happen to be of a more private or more transient nature may serve only as means for the inculcation of particular essential reactions in the course of education. Among these interests, we may cite, for example, interest in the grammar of a foreign language, in washing and other areas of hygiene, and so on. It is extremely important to arouse the child's interest in the process of washing or in the grammatical forms of the declensions until he has acquired the habit of washing or has learned how to speak the particular foreign language correctly. But as soon as this is achieved, there is no longer any need for us to be concerned about this interest, nor any need to maintain, develop, and reinforce it, and we may let it quietly fade away.

Indirect interests that are not related directly to a desired reaction, but which may indirectly serve to develop it possess an even more transient purpose. Such, for example, is the nature of Thorndike's pedagogical problems, for example, suggesting using the child's natural interest in cooking in the study of chemistry, though here it is essential that the newly emerging interest in chemistry stifle and neutralize the initial interest in cooking.

The following is a general psychological rule for the development of interest. On the one hand, for an object to be of interest to us, it must be related to something that interests us, something we are already familiar with, and, in addition, it must always include certain new forms of activity, else it will be pointless. Something that is entirely new, like something that is entirely old, is incapable of arousing our interest, of exciting our interest in some object or event. This means that in order for a student to relate to some object or event in a personal way, it is necessary to make the study of this object the student's personal affair, and only then can we be certain of succeeding. From one interest of the child's to a new interest—that is the rule.

The labor method of instruction can be of substantial assistance here. It derives precisely from the child's natural propensity towards ceaseless action, towards engaging in activities. In this method, any object can enter into a whole series of interesting actions, and in fact, there is nothing so distinctive of a child as the pleasure he experiences from his own activity. By virtue of the very nature of children's activity, it is possible to lead the child into relating to any object in a personal way, and make it his business to succeed. It is here that we see the connection of school lessons to real life, the requirement that every newly imparted piece of knowledge be linked to something already known and explain something new to the student. It is difficult to imagine anything more unpsychological than the old system of instruction, in which the child studied arithmetic, algebra, German and so on without ever having any idea at all as to what was the point of this or that subject and what might be the areas where he would have to use this knowledge. If interest was nevertheless aroused, this always occurred fortuitously, independently of the child's will.

There are three important pedagogical conclusions that may be drawn from our study of children's interests. First, all the topics in a course must be interconnected, which is also the best way of ensuring that a common interest will be aroused and that this interest will collect around a single axis. Only then may we speak of a more or less prolonged, lasting, and deep interest, an interest that will not shatter into dozens of unrelated parts, making it impossible to grasp in a unified and general thought all the different subjects of study. The next conclusion has to do with that rule which said that everything has to involve recourse to repetition, to memorization and assimilation of knowledge. But we all have come to realize how uninteresting is such repetition for children, how they dislike these lessons, even if they do not find them difficult. The reason for this is that here the fundamental rule of interest is violated and, consequently, repetition turns into mere dawdling, constituting the most irrational and unpsychological of all techniques.

The rule is to avoid repetition absolutely and to make instruction focused, i.e., to arrange the material in such a way that it may be gone over fully and all at once in the briefest and most simplified way possible; then the teacher may return to a topic, but not to just repeat what has been already gone over, but to review the same topic one more time in a more thorough and more all-inclusive form, complemented with a wealth of new facts, generalizations, and conclusions, so that topics students have already studied are repeated anew, though unfolded from a new perspective, and this new aspect is so connected with what they are already acquainted with that interest is readily aroused all by itself. In this sense, just as in science as in real life, it is only a new view about what is old that may arouse our interest.

Finally, the third and final rule governing the employment of the child's interest mandates the construction of the entire educational system in the school in direct proximity to everyday life, to teach children in such a way as to interest them, to begin with what is familiar to the child and what arouses his interest in a natural way. Froebel points out that the child obtains his first bits of knowledge on the basis of his own natural interest in life and from the lessons he receives from adults. From earliest childhood, the son of a peasant, of a merchant, or of a craftsman acquires a host of the most diverse bits of information in a natural way, in the course of observing his father's behavior. At a later stage, therefore, it is essential to always take as a starting point for the development of a new interest one that already exists, and to proceed on the basis of what is known and familiar. This is the reason why classical education, which began all at once with mythology and the ancient languages and with subjects that had nothing in common with everyday life as it affected the child, was tedious. Thus, the basic rule is that before imparting new knowledge to the child and before fostering a new reaction in him, we must be sure to prepare the ground for it, i.e., arouse the appropriate interest. For an analogy, just think of how we loosen the soil before planting seeds.

The Pattern of the Child's Interests

The development of the child's interests is closely related to his overall biological growth. *Interests* are an expression of the child's organic needs. In the very first hour of life, when the infant has only begun to learn how to control his own perceiving organs, e.g., how to move his hands, head, and eyes, there is an interest in every stimulus, whether it involve sound, light, or something else. A loud voice, a bright color, the feel of an object, all these stimuli arouse his interest. At this time, the infant grasps whatever is placed in his hand in an entirely natural way, and, since he associates everything with eating, he tries to get a taste of everything, pulling everything into his mouth.

Gradually, the child begins to learn how to walk, and movement in space, climbing, crawling, clambering about, and pushing objects about becomes the focus of his interest, and he begins to show an interest in his surroundings. The succeeding years are devoted to gaining as thorough a sense of direction in his surroundings and as discriminating a sense of familiarity with the individual elements of the environment as possible through practical activities, and by combining together all of these different elements. Spontaneity becomes the child's principal interest, along with the desire to do everything on his own and take charge of everything through his actions. Now the child is capable of working on something or other until he gets tired, to find infinite satisfaction in the course of his own simple actions time and again.

In the following period there is an expansion of interests beyond the limits of the immediate environment, since the child is already quite familiar with his entire surroundings and with the full range of maneuvers he is capable of. His interest in taking trips, in wandering off, and in truancy is aroused. A special interest in adventure, in famous travelers, and in exploits is distinctive of these years. Finally, in puberty there is a heightened interest in oneself, the child again becomes a philosopher and lyric poet as he had been earlier when he would ask an infinite number of questions. His own experiences, the problem of his ego, now engrosses all the adolescent's attention, to be replaced in the time of youth with an expanded and heightened interest in the world and in the most radical questions of being, which now obsess consciousness. In youth, one's eyes are always wide open to the world, which underscores the greater maturity of youth towards life.

The Psychological Value of Games

But children's games are very nearly the most valuable of all tools for the education of the instincts.

The popular opinion is to look upon games as a form of idleness, as a kind of fun that only takes up time. It is rare to see any value whatsoever in games, at best one may think of games as a natural weakness of childhood which only helps the child kill time for awhile. Meanwhile, quite some time ago it was discovered by means of careful observation that games are not something fortuitous, but arise unavoidably at all stages of civilized life and among the most diverse peoples and, thus, represent an intrinsic and natural feature of human nature. Moreover, games are inherent not only to man, but are also engaged in by young animals and, consequently, this fact must possess some kind of biological import. Games must be needed for something, must possess some sort of expressly biological purpose, otherwise they could not have come about and become so widespread. Several theories on the nature of games have been proposed by researchers in an attempt to unravel this thought. According to one such theory, games are simply the discharge of accumulated energy in a young person who does not have any other outlet or means of using this energy for his natural needs. In fact, the young animal, like the human child, is kept from participating in the struggle for existence, from the building of a life, he has nothing on which he could expend the energy accumulated in his organism, and so undertakes a series of unnecessary and pointless movements, runs around, romps, jumps up and down, and all this provides an outlet for the accumulated energy.

Thus, even this theory sees in games not an accidental whim, a pastime, but an important vital necessity. It is, in this sense, a step forward from the popular view. But it still far from exhausts the meaning of games, in this theory games are only a valve, only an orifice, through which unused energy escapes. But this still does not answer the question, what is the function of such an expenditure of energy, and is it a good thing.

It is this question that a second theory provides an answer to. This theory perceives a biological utility to games, in that games would appear to be the natural school of the young animal's education. If we take a look at games, it is not hard to see that games include not only useless and unnecessary movements, but also movements that are associated with the future activity of an individual animal who has developed the skills and habits proper to this activity, skills and habits that will prepare it for life and establish and give exercise to necessary aptitudes. Games are the natural school of the animal. The kitten playing with a ball of yarn or with a dead mouse its mother has brought back learns how to capture live mice and so on. This, the biological value of games, the understanding of games as representing a kind of school and preparation for future activity, is fully confirmed by the study of man's games.

The child is always playing, he is a playful being, but his games always have a larger meaning. They are always exactly appropriate to his age and interests, and encompass all those elements which lead to the development of essential habits and skills. The first group of games are those which involve individual objects, such as rattles, or those in which objects are flung about and caught. And while the child is occupied with his objects, he is learning how to look about and how to listen, how to throw objects about and how to push them away, and how to grasp objects. The games of the next period, such as hide-and-seek, running, and the like, are associated with the development of the ability to move about in one's surroundings and to orient oneself. Without any overstatement, one could say that nearly all of our most fundamental and most characteristic reactions are created and develop in the course of the games we play as children. It is this which is the meaning of the element of *imitation* in children's games; the child deliberately copies and assimilates what he sees in adults, thereby learning about relationships, and develops his earliest instincts, instincts that he will have need for in his future activity.

One psychologist has declared that, "If you wish to know which of two girls will be a better mother, take a look and see which of them plays with her doll better and for longer periods of time." By this he wished to underscore the educational value of playing with dolls for the development of the maternal instinct. It would be wrong to think that in playing with dolls, the girl is learning to be a mother in same the sense in which a cat playing with a dead mouse is learning how to catch a live mouse. The relationship between game and experience here is far more remote and far more complex, and it is entirely possible that the future mother will neither retain nor remember any of the movements she used with her dolls. Undoubtedly, however, what is being put together here are the basic lines of development, the basic features of the girl's future inner experience, features that will help her subsequently carry out in real life what now occupies her in play. In playing with dolls, a girl learns not how to relate to a real live child, but rather what it feels like to be a mother.

This is how to view those elements of imitation that are brought into games; that is, they promote the child's active mastery of various aspects of life and, along the same lines, give a sense of discipline to his inner experience. Other games, so-called building games, i.e., those involving working with materials, teach us how to make our movements precise and sure-footed, develop thousands of the most valuable habits, and diversify and multiply our reactions. These sorts of games teach us how to set ourselves a particular goal and how to organize our movements so as to guide ourselves to the realization of this goal. Thus, these games provide the first lessons in systematic and rational activity, in the coordination of movement, and in the ability to guide one's own organs and control them. In other words, they are the guides and teachers of our external experience, just as the former games serve as guides of our inner experience.

Finally, the third group of games, called *conventional games*, which arise from purely conventional rules and from actions that are associated with these rules, constitute a kind of advanced school of games. They organize the higher forms of behavior, involve the resolution of rather complex problems of behavior, require effort, guess-work, quickness, and resourcefulness, and the concerted and coordinated efforts of the most diverse capacities and forces.

No one game repeats another exactly, but each one of them presents ever newer situations that change from one moment to the next, requiring ever newer solutions. Bear in mind that these types of games represent the greatest school of social experience. In a game, the child's effort is always limited and regulated by the aggregate of moves made by all the other players. Every game problem includes, as an indispensable condition, the ability to coordinate one's behavior with the behavior of others, to enter into active relations with others, to attack and to defend oneself, to harm and to assist, and to determine in advance the result of one's course of action relative to the complete group of all the players. Such a game is a vital social and collective experience of the child's, and in this sense it constitutes an entirely irreplaceable tool for the inculcation of social skills and habits.

Note that, in general, it can hardly be said that all is well in present-day pedagogics as regards the education of the social instincts. The family constitutes too simple a social unit with too small a number of familiar elements, and also involves fully established forms of relationships between its members. It is, therefore, capable of creating in the heart of the child lasting and profound social relations, through relations that are extremely limited in scope, teaching the child how to be a citizen of a little social world by virtue of spontaneous relations that are highly intimate and are deeply engraved in the child's personality. The family teaches only the most intimate and most familiar of social relationships, it educates someone to be a family member, whereas the present epoch confronts the enormous problems involved in educating a citizen of the world in view of increasingly more complicated international relations. Nor is the school classroom appropriate in this sense, since it likewise consists of just a few elements in which social relationships assume fixed and frozen forms in no time, in which one rapidly gets accustomed to relationships with each other that also do not trip one up or lead to new reactions, and in which all relationships develop in a given mould, one that is barren and monotonous. The school body is not a broad enough arena for the development of the great social passions, and is even too narrow and insignificant a school for the social instincts. Meanwhile, education confronts two enormous problems. It is, first of all, necessary to educate the social instinct at a vast, worldwide scale. Psychologically, such a goal may be achieved only through an enormous expansion of the social environment. We have to break down the walls of the home on behalf of the classroom, break down the walls of the classroom on behalf of the school, break down the walls of the school on behalf of the association of all the schools in the city, and so on, right on through the development of children's movements that extend throughout the entire country, or even the development of international children's movements, such as the Pioneer or Communist youth movements. It is in these movements, and only in these movements, that the child may learn how to respond to the most distant stimuli, how to establish relationships between his own reactions and events thousands of miles away, and how to coordinate and relate his own behavior with the behavior of enormous masses of people, say, with the international worker's movement.

The other goal of public education consists in the development and polishing of particularly subtle forms of social interaction. In fact, social relations in the present epoch have become vast not only in terms of scale, they are also vast in terms of degree of differentiation and complexity. Formerly, social relations were confined to a small group of stereotypical relationships, and the course of man's social behavior encompassed more or less completely the ordinary rules of everyday courtesy. Together with the growing complexity of life, the individual now finds himself involved in increasingly more complicated and more highly diverse social relations, he is a member of the most diverse social groups, and therefore the full multiplicity of modern man's social relations cannot be confined to any sort of pre-set collection of skills and habits. Rather, the goal of education is to develop, not a definite quantity of skills, but particular creative capacities for rapid and skillful social orientation.

Starting with the most barren and the shallowest of relations, such as those which arise between passengers in a streetcar, right up through the most profound and the most complex relations, for example those that arise in the deepest forms of love and of friendship, man must exhibit a genuine creative skill in establishing relations with another person. Love and friendship involve just as much creativity in the development of social relations as do political and professional education. It is precisely because of this refinement, finish, and diversity of social relations that we can learn how to play. By repeatedly throwing the child into ever newer situations, subordinating him to ever newer conditions, games force him to vary the social coordination of his movements in infinite ways and teach him such a degree of flexibility and elasticity, and such a wealth of creative skills, as does no other field of education.

Finally, it is here that the last feature of games—the fact that, by subordinating all of behavior to special conventional rules, games are the first medium to teach the child rational and conscious behavior—manifests itself particularly clearly and conspicuously. Games are the child's first school of thought. Every form of thinking arises as a response to a particular difficulty, as a consequence of a new or difficult encounter with the elements of one's surroundings. Wherever there is no such difficulty, wherever our surroundings are fully known to us and our behavior proceeds effortlessly and unimpeded, as if it's simply a matter of adjusting to our surroundings, there is no thinking, there wherever one looks are gears and linkages turning. But as soon as the environment presents us with any kind of new and unanticipated position on the board [kombinatsiya] that requires in our ways of behaving likewise new moves [kombinatsiya] and new reactions and quick reorientation of our activity, there thinking arises, as a special anticipatory stage of behavior, as an internal ordering of more complex forms of experience whose psychological essence reduces ultimately to choosing, from out of the set of all the possible reactions that present themselves to us, only those which are needed in light of the basic goal which behavior is called upon to achieve.

Thus, thinking is always a kind of solution of a new problem of behavior through the selection of essential reactions. The moment of "set" [ustanovka], i.e., the element of anticipatory reaction by means of which the individual sets himself into a certain pattern of behavior—this is the essential moment here. The entire mechanism of selection involves nothing other than an internal, and concealed, reaching out [proektirovanie] of behavior towards certain ultimate results which thereupon force the individual to discard certain patterns of behavior and adopt others. Thus, thinking arises out of a clash of reactions and out of a selection of some of these reactions under the influence of anticipatory reactions. But it is just this clash and just this process of selection which makes it possible—once, that is, certain rules are introduced into a game and the possibilities of behavior are, thereby, restricted, where, in addition, the child's behavior is given the task of attaining a definite goal, all the child's instinctive capacities being strained to the utmost and his interest being stretched to the highest degree—that it becomes possible to induce the child to discipline his behavior in such a way that it obey certain rules, that it point in the direction of a single goal, that it solve certain problems deliberately.

In other words, a game is a rational and appropriate, methodical, and socially coordinated system of behavior or consumption of energy, subordinated to definite rules. Thus does it disclose its complete analogy with the consumption of the adult's energy in work, the features of which fully coincide with the features of a game. The only difference is that the results which, in the labor process, are expressed in a definite, objective outcome, which one also has in mind ahead of time, in a game are expressed in a certain conventional affective satisfaction, which is resolved subjectively within the individual player himself, in the form of pleasure which he gains from winning a game. Thus, notwithstanding all the objective differences that exist between play and work, which would even lead us to consider them polar opposites, they possess absolutely the same psychological nature. This underscores the fact that games are the natural form of work in children, a form of activity which is inherent to the child, as preparation for his life in the future.

A psychologist has told of how the natives living near one of the English colonial settlements would watch in amazement as the Englishmen would kick a soccer ball about until they were exhausted. The custom among the natives was for the men to do nothing, though for small change they would usually perform errands for the colonists. On this occasion, one of them walked over to an Englishman who was playing soccer and offered to play in his stead for a few shillings so that he wouldn't get all tired out. The native didn't understand the psychological difference between a game and work, that is, the subjective effect of the game, and was deceived by the utter outward resemblance between playful activity and work.

---

[1]See too, Vygotsky's article, "*The Biogenetic Law*" written around the same time as the present book and published in the edition of *The Great Soviet Encyclopedia*, then being compiled. -- trans.

Chapter 6

EDUCATION OF EMOTIONAL BEHAVIOR

The Concept of Emotion

The science of the emotions or feelings constituted the most undeveloped chapter in the old psychology. This aspect of man's behavior proved to be more difficult to describe, to classify, and to relate by means of particular laws than did all the other subjects. Nevertheless, there are entirely valid views on the nature of the emotional reactions which may be found in the old psychology.

William James and Carl Georg Lange were the first to obtain results here, the former emphasizing the broad physical changes that accompany feelings, and the latter noting those vasomotor changes with which they are accompanied. Independently, the two researchers came to the conclusion that the ordinary conception of feelings is the product of a profound delusion, and that, in fact, emotions occur in an entirely different way than is usually conceived.

Ordinary psychology and everyday thinking distinguish three components in the feelings. The first, the perception of some object or event, or a representation of it (an encounter with a thief, the recollection of the death of a loved one, and so on), let us call A, the feeling thereby induced (fear, sadness) we will call B, and the physical expression of this feeling (trembling, tears), C. It was believed that the complete course of an emotion was represented by the sequence ABC.

If we look carefully into any feeling, we may easily notice that it always has its own physical expression. Strong feelings always seem to be spelled out on our face, and once we look at someone we can tell without any explanation whether he is angry, frightened, or at peace.

All the physical changes that accompany a feeling may be easily divided into three groups. First is the group of mimetic and pantomime movements, special contractions of the muscles, chiefly of the eyes, mouth, cheekbone, arms, and trunk. This class constitutes the class of emotional motor reactions. The somatic reactions, i.e., changes in the activity of certain organs associated with the most important vital functions of the organism, such as changes in respiration, in heart beat, and in circulation, form the next group. The third group consist of the group of secretory reactions, such as tears, perspiration, salivation, the internal secretion of the sex organs, etc. The physical expression of every feeling is formed from these three groups.

James distinguishes the same three components in every feeling listed above, though in the theory he suggested these three components occur in a different sequence. Whereas the ordinary schema of the feelings establishes a sequence of three components *ABC*, i.e., perception, feeling, mimicry, the true situation, James suggests, is more in accord with a different formula, *ACB*, i.e., perception—mimicry—feeling.

In other words, James suggests that various objects possess the ability to induce in us directly, in a reflex pathway, various physical changes, and that feeling is, in and of itself, now the second component in the perception of these changes. An encounter with a thief, he suggests, induces in us, reflexively, trembling, dryness in the throat, pallor, heavy breathing, and other manifestations of fear without recourse to any feeling. The very feeling of fear is nothing less than a collection of just these changes, as recognized by the organism. To be frightened denotes a sensation of one's own trembling, one's own heart beat, one's own pallor, and so on. In nearly the same way, the recollection of the death of a friend or relative reflexively induces tears, causes one's head to sink down, and so on. Sadness reduces to the sensation of these manifestations, and to be sad means to perceive one's own tears, one's own bent posture, one's own drooping head, and so on.

The common saying is that we cry because we are in distress, we argue because we are irritated, we tremble because we are frightened. It would be more correct to say, according to James, that we are in distress because we are crying, that we are irritated because we are arguing, and that we are frightened because we are trembling. Thus, what had hitherto been considered a cause is really the consequence, and conversely, the consequence turns out to be the cause.

To see that this, is in fact so, consider the following reasoning. First, if we induce various external expressions of some feeling artificially, the feeling itself will be sure to emerge without delay. James suggests as an experiment to try to assume an expression of sadness upon awakening in the morning, speaking in a low voice, keeping your eyes down, taking quicker breaths, arching your back and neck very slightly, in a word, assuming all the signs of sadness—and by nightfall you will be filled with such anguish that you won't know what's gotten into you. Teachers are well aware how easily a prank turns into reality in children, how two boys who had begun by making believe they were fighting, suddenly, when their struggle was at its height, and without any animosity towards each other, began to get angry at each other and cannot say whether they are still playing a game, or whether it was no longer a game. Just as easily does a child who is making believe he is frightened suddenly begin to actually experience fear. And in general, every external expression contributes to the onset of the corresponding feeling, a runner easily becomes frightened, and so on. Actors are well aware of this fact, and know when a particular posture, intonation, or gesture will induce in them a strong emotion.

The converse law supports this thesis even more convincingly. One only has to overcome the physical expressions of an emotion, and the emotion itself quickly vanishes. If we keep ourselves from trembling when we are frightened, force our heart to beat evenly, and assume a normal facial expression, the very feeling of fear vanishes. Suppress the expression of some passion and it fades away. One psychologist has told how every time he feels an attack of anger coming on, he flattens his palms out as much as he is able to and spreads his fingers apart until they hurt. This would paralyze his anger every time, because it is impossible to be enraged when one's hands are spread apart, since anger denotes tightened fists and mouth shut tightly. If we were to mentally eliminate from the emotions, as if performing a subtraction, all physical changes, then, as can be easily seen, there would be nothing that would remain of the feelings. Take away from fear the symptoms of fear and you stop being afraid.

There are two facts that are obvious objections to this point of view. If understood correctly, however, they not only do not contradict, but even confirm this approach. First is the well-known circumstance that various reactions often are not absolutely connected in any way with an emotion. For example, the eyes can be easily made to produce tears if we grate an onion, though this does not in the least mean that sadness follows upon these tears. It is easily observed that, in this case, we are inducing only a single, isolated symptom, which, in and of itself, is powerless to induce an emotion, but which would certainly induce it if it were encountered in the necessary combination with all the other symptoms. It is not enough to induce tears in the eyes in order for sadness to appear subsequently, because sadness consists not in a flow of tears, but, even more so, in a whole series of internal and external symptoms which, at this moment, are absent.

Finally, the other objection is that any one feeling is easily induced by means of the internal administration of intoxicants introduced into the blood. Without assuming any of the artificial expressions of a feeling, one need only drink a certain amount of alcohol, or take a certain amount of morphine or opium, in order to induce a host of complex feelings. But it is easily seen that, through the intake of these substances, we are acting upon the very fount of the emotional reactions. We are varying the chemical composition of the blood, varying the entire circulatory system and all those internal processes that are associated with the blood, in particular, internal secretion, and, accordingly, we obtain a distinct emotional effect in the organism without any difficulty.

Thus, everything leads us to assert that emotion is, in fact, a certain collection of reactions which is connected, by means of the reflexes, to particular stimuli.

James fully identifies the schema of the emotions with the schema of behavior and of conscious experience that underlies everything we do. Feelings do not arise by themselves under ordinary conditions. A feeling is always preceded by a particular stimulus, a particular cause—whether internal or external (A). What compels us to be frightened or to be happy is, thereby, the stimulus the reaction always begins with. There then follows a series of reflexive reactions, whether motor, somatic, or secretory (C). Finally are the feedback reactions, the return of one's own reaction back to the organism as a new stimulus, the second-order perception of the proprio-ceptive field, which also constitutes what was formerly called the emotion itself (B).

The subjective nature of feelings is thus not hard to understand, i.e., the fact that a person who is experiencing a feeling and a person who is viewing its external expression will have entirely different ideas of this feeling. This is because, in this case, the two observers are focusing on two different components of the same process. The person looking from outside focuses on component C, i.e., the emotional reaction in and of itself. The person looking from within focuses on the proprio-ceptive stimulus emanating from this reaction, component B, and here, as was explained above, other nerve pathways are involved, and, consequently, different processes.

Biological Nature of the Emotions

That the emotions arise on the basis of the instincts and constitute closely related branches of these latter is not difficult to see. This has led certain researchers into considering instinctive emotional behavior as a unitary whole.

The instinctive roots of the emotions can be seen especially clearly in the most primitive or elemental, or "lowest" sensations. Some researchers here ascribe the very same reactions at times to the instincts and at times to emotions. Consider, as an example, two elementary emotions, anger and fear, and their possible biological meaning. It is not hard to see that all the physical changes that are accompanied by fear possess a biologically explicable origin.

There is every basis for supposing that all those motor, somatic, and secretory reactions that occur as part of an emotion, as an integral form of behavior, once constituted a collection of useful and adaptive, biological-type reactions. Thus, undoubtedly, fear was once the higher form of a precipitous and sudden escape from danger, and in animals, as in man sometimes, it still bears quite unmistakable traces of its origin. The mimetic reactions of fear usually involve an expansion and preparation of the perceiving organs, whose purpose it is to put one on one's guard, to make one extraordinarily wary and sensitive to the slightest changes in the environment. Eyes wide open, nostrils flaring, ears straining—all these features denote a guarded relation to the world, an attentive listening for danger. Next a group of muscles becomes strained as if preparing for action, as if being mustered in preparation for jumping, running, and so on. Trembling, which is so typical of fear in man, constitutes nothing less than a rapid muscular contraction, a kind of adaptation for unusually rapid running. In animals, trembling when accompanied by fear turns directly into running. The somatic reactions of our body also have the same meaning and connotation of running from danger. Pallor, the cessation of digestion, diarrhea—all denote a flowing of blood away from those organs whose activity is not of vital and paramount necessity and importance for the organism at the present moment, and a flow of blood towards those organs which, now have the final say. This, in fact, recalls the "mustering of forces" which is observed when the blood, this provender of our organism, shuts down and halts the activity of those organs which seem to be in the background and which are associated with the placid activity of the organism, and throws the full force of all its reserves at embattled sectors, i.e., those which are to be rescued from danger without delay. Respiration, similarly, is altered, becoming deep, spasmodic, and adapted for rapid running. The secretory reactions associated with dryness of the throat and so on seem to point to a similar blood flow.

Finally, recent investigations on animals have shown that the emotions also induce changes in internal secretion. We know that the chemical composition of the blood is altered in a startled cat. In other words, we know that the most intimate of all internal processes are adapted to the basic goal of the organism, i.e., escape from danger. Together with the foregoing, these results lead us to define fear as a mustering of all of the forces of the organism for the purpose of running away from danger, that it is an *inhibition* of running, and to understand fear as a hardened form of behavior that arises from the instinct of self-preservation in its defensive form.

It is easily shown in an entirely analogous way that anger constitutes the instinct of self-preservation in its offensive form, that it constitutes another group of reactions, another form of behavior, an offensive form of behavior, and that anger consists in the mobilization of all the forces of the organism for attack, that it is an *inhibition of fighting* which arises from the instinct of self-preservation in its offensive form.

However, it is not hard to see that both fear and rage in the form in which they are now encountered in man constitute extraordinarily attenuated forms of these instincts, and one is left with the thought that, in the path of development from the animal to man, the emotions would appear to be on the wane and have not progressed, but rather atrophied.

Fear and anger in a dog are more powerful and more expressive than is the anger of a savage; in a savage these sensations are more impulsive than in a child; and in a child they are more striking than in an adult. Hence, we easily arrive at the general conclusion that, in the system of behavior, the emotions function like vestigial organs that once possessed a significance of their own, but now, as a consequence of the altered conditions of life, are condemned to extinction and constitute an unnecessary and, at times, a harmful element in the system of behavior.

Come to think of it, in the context of education, feelings constitute an unusual exception in the following sense. It is desirable for the teacher to augment and reinforce all the other forms of behavior and reactions. Just imagine there was a way for us to increase a student's memory or understanding by a factor of 10—this, of course, would make the job of education 10 times easier. But just imagine for a moment, if you will, that we could increase a child's emotional capacities by a factor of 10, i.e., that we could make him 10 times more sensitive and that he would thereupon go into ecstasy at the slightest pleasure, and sob and go into hysterics at the slightest distress. Then, of course, we would obtain a highly undesirable type of behavior.

Thus, the ideal of emotional education would appear to consist not in the development and reinforcement of the emotions, but, on the contrary, in their suppression and attenuation. Since the emotions are biologically useless forms of adaptation, because of altered circumstances and of altered conditions of the environment and of life, they are consequently condemned to extinction in the process of evolution, and the man of the future will not know of the emotions in the same way that he will not know of other vestigial organs. Feelings are man's blind gut. Such a view, which asserts that the emotions are entirely unnecessary is, however, profoundly mistaken.

Psychological Nature of the Emotions

From simple observation, we know how the emotions complicate and vary behavior, and how far an emotionally gifted, refined, and educated person towers over an emotionally uneducated person. In other words, even everyday observation underscores a kind of new meaning that the presence of emotions brings to behavior. The very same behavior, when emotionally tinged, assumes an entirely different character than its lifeless forms. The very same words, though pronounced with feeling, act on us in a different way than when they are pronounced colorlessly.

What novelty does emotion bring to behavior? To answer this question, it is necessary to recall the general character of behavior as sketched above. From our point of view, behavior is a process of interaction between the organism and the environment. Consequently, in this process it's as if there were always three forms of this relationship, and that these three forms, in fact, alternate. The first case is that which occurs when the organism senses its superiority over the environment, when the goals it sets for itself and the demands placed on behavior are achieved and satisfied by the organism without any difficulty and without any strain, when behavior proceeds without any internal impediment, and optimal adaptation is accomplished with least expenditure of energy and forces. Here the organism dominates the environment.

The second case occurs when weight and ascendency are on the side of the environment, when the organism experiences difficulties and considerable stress in adapting to the environment, when there is always a feeling of disharmony between the extraordinary complexity of the environment and the organism's poor defences. In this case, behavior proceeds with the greatest consumption of forces, with maximal consumption of energy and with minimal adaptation.

Finally, the third possible and genuine case occurs when there is a degree of equilibrium established between the organism and the environment, when neither side is preponderant, but the two seem to be balanced in this conflict.

These three cases together serve as a basis for the development of emotional behavior. Just on the basis of the origin of the emotions from the instinctive forms of behavior, it is apparent that they would appear to be the result of the organism's own estimation of its relationship with the environment. And all those emotions that are connected with the sensation of force, contentment, and so on, what are known as the *positive sensations*, should be placed in the first group. Those emotions which are associated with the feeling of depression, weakness, and suffering—the *negative sensations*—belong to the second group, while it is only the third group in which there is relative emotional neutrality in behavior.

Thus, emotion should be understood as a reaction that occurs at the critical and catastrophic moments of behavior, as points of disequilibrium, as the ultimate end and outcome of behavior, having a direct impact on the forms assumed by subsequent behavior at every moment.

Interestingly, emotional behavior is extraordinarily common, and, for all intents and purposes, even in our most primitive reactions it is not hard to discover an emotional component.

The old psychology taught that there is an emotional tinge to every sensation, i.e., that even the simplest experience of all the colors, all the sounds, all the smells inevitably possesses a special perceptible tinge. As regards tastes and smells, everyone knows that very few of them are neutral, emotionally indifferent sensations, that every smell, like nearly every taste, is, most certainly, either pleasant or unpleasant, is a cause of pleasure or displeasure, involves satisfaction or aversion.

This is somewhat more difficult to discover in the visual and auditory stimulations, though here, too, it is not hard to show that every color, every shape, likewise every sound, possesses a unique, intrinsic tinge or sensation. We all know that some colors and shapes are soothing, while others, conversely, excite us; some induce tenderness, while others repugnance; some make us happy, while others are a cause of suffering. It is only necessary to recall the entirely self-evident emotional value of the color red, this customary companion of every uprising, passion, and rebellion, or the color blue, this cold and peaceful color of distance and dreams, to be persuaded of this circumstance.

Come to think of it, it is only necessary to think a bit about where such forms of linguistic expression as a "cold color" or a "warm color," a "high sound" or a "low sound," a "soft voice" or a "hard voice" come from. Color, in and of itself, is neither warm nor cold, and likewise sound, in and of itself, is neither high nor low, and, in general, does not possess any spatial shape. However, everyone knows what is meant when we speak of the color orange and say that it is a warm color, and speak of a bass voice and say that it is a low, or, as the Greeks put it, a "thick" sound. Obviously, there is nothing in common between color and temperature, or between sound and magnitude, but apparently there is something that unites them in terms of emotional tone, something that tinges both impressions. A warm tone or a high sound denotes that there is some resemblance between the emotional tone of a color and temperature. The color orange, in and of itself, has nothing warm about it, though in its effect on us, there is something that recalls the effect of warmth. Recall that we defined an emotional reaction as an evaluative, secondary, feedback reaction of the proprio-ceptive field. And the emotional tone of a sensation denotes nothing less than the involvement and participation of the entire organism in each individual reaction of an organ. The organism cannot be indifferent to what its eyes see, it either identifies with this reaction or opposes it. "Thus," says Münsterberg, "'pleasure' or 'displeasure' does not, in fact, precede action, but is itself an action that leads to the prolongation or cessation of a stimulus."

Thus, understood as a secondary reaction, an emotional reaction is a powerful guide of behavior. It is in an emotional reaction that the purposefulness of our organism manifests itself. Emotions would not be needed if they were not purposeful. We saw that emotions arise in an instinctive pathway from the most complex and most vivid movements. Once they had been the guides of behavior in the most difficult, the most fateful, the most decisive moments of life. They arose at the highest points of life, when the organism had triumphed over the environment or had come close to destruction. At every turn, the emotions act as a ruler of behavior.

Now, under altered conditions, because they are not necessary, the external forms of movements that accompany emotion have attenuated and gradually atrophied. But their inner role as guides of all of behavior, what had been their initial role to begin with, still remains. It is just this element of purposefulness in the emotions which constitutes the most important feature in the study of its psychological nature. It would be wrong to imagine, as some believe, that emotion seems to be a purely passive experience of the organism, and does not itself lead to any sort of activity.

On the contrary, there is every reason for believing that the most correct theory of the origin of the psyche is that theory which associates the origin of the psyche with the emergence of what is referred to as *hedonist consciousness*, i.e., with the primitive sensation of pleasure or displeasure which, as the second component of a feedback reaction, affected the reaction, either by obstructing it or by stimulating it. Thus, the primordial regulation of the reactions arises from the emotions. The emotion associated with a reaction guides and regulates it, depending on the overall state of the organism. The transition to a passive type of behavior undoubtedly occurred on the basis of the emotions. In precisely the same way, there is every reason for supposing that the reactions of pleasure and displeasure, which arise earlier than all the other reactions, are primitive forms of the child's purely mental behavior.

This purposeful character of the emotional reactions is most easily understood on the basis of the three-dimensional theory of the feelings proposed by Wundt. Wundt suggested that every feeling has three dimensions, and in each dimension two directions. A feeling may occur (1) along the axis of pleasure and displeasure; (2) along the axis of excitation and suppression; or (3) along the axis of stress and resolution.

It would seem to be readily apparent that stress coincides with excitation, and suppression with resolution. This, however, is not so. If a person is angry for some reason, his behavior is characterized by an extraordinary degree of stress and tension of every muscle and, moreover, an extraordinary suppression of all reaction. In precisely the same way, the expectation of a prize or the anticipation of a verdict turns into the joyful excitation associated with the utter resolution of all kinds of stress.

It is because there are three dimensions to every emotion that feelings are essentially purposeful. Every emotion constitutes an urge to action or a rejection of action. No feeling can be indifferent and without outcome in behavior. Emotion is also the inner guide of our reactions, a guide that strains, excites, stimulates, or obstructs this or that reaction. Thus, the emotions still function in the role of inner guide of our behavior.

If we do something or other with joy, the emotional reaction of joy does not point to anything other than the fact that we will strive to do the same thing later on. If we do something or other with distaste, this will mean that we will try in every way possible to cease performing these tasks. Thus, the novel component which emotion contributes to behavior is wholly reducible to the organism's regulation of every one of its individual reactions.

That there exists a concerted diversity of emotional reactions, which involves all of the most important organs of our body in the course of each isolated reaction, thus, should be entirely understandable to the reader. Experimental investigations have shown that, according to recordings of respiratory movements, cardiac beat, and pulse rate, the curves produced in these recordings, which express the course of the most important organic reactions, respond submissively to the slightest stimulus and seem to quickly adapt themselves to the subtlest variations in the environment.

It is not without reason that the heart has long been thought of as the organ of feeling. In this regard, the conclusions of exact science are in full agreement with the ancient view of the role of the heart. Emotional reactions are, above all, reactions of the heart and of circulation; and if we recall that respiration and blood determine the course of absolutely every process, in all our organs and tissues, we an understand why the reactions of the heart could serve as the inner guides of behavior.

"We owe all the emotional side of our mental life," writes the Danish psychologist Lange, "our joys and sorrows, our happy and unhappy hours, to our vasomotor system. If the impressions which fall upon our senses did not possess the power of stimulating it, we would wander through life unsympathetic and passionless, all impressions of the outer world would only enrich our experience, increase our knowledge, but would arouse neither joy nor anger, would give us neither care nor fear."[1]

Education of the Feelings

"Education always denotes a change." If nothing changes, then nothing has been taught. What are the educational changes that must be introduced into the feelings? Above, we saw that every feeling is nothing other than the mechanism of a reaction, i.e., a particular reaction of the organism to some stimulation from the environment. Consequently, in its general outlines, the mechanism for the education of the feelings is precisely the same as for all the other reactions.

By connecting together various stimuli, we can always form new relations between an emotional reaction and some element of the environment. Thus, altering all those stimuli a reaction is associated with is the first step in education. Everyone knows that the fears we experience in childhood have no analogue in later life. That which has caused us to fear and scared us becomes safe, though on the other hand, we learn to fear many objects and things that we had previously related to with trust.

How does this transfer of fear from one object to another take place? The simplest mechanism is that of the education of a conditional reflex, i.e., the mechanism by which a reaction is transferred to a new stimulus, which occurs every time this new stimulus coincides with the unconditional stimulus of an innate reaction.

If, for example, some event which a child is frightened of is accompanied each time by certain other circumstances, these circumstances will, in and of themselves, be capable of subsequently inducing fear in the child. The child will be scared to go into a room where he had experienced something frightening even once, he runs away from all those objects which were present when he was frightened. Hence, the first rule for the education of the feelings: Try to so organize the child's life and the child's behavior in such a way that he encounters those stimuli between which such transfer of feelings is to be created as often as possible.

At first the child will respond with fear only to the onset of his own troubles, but suppose that every time something unpleasant threatens his friends, his mother, or his sister, this is also associated with personal pain for the child. After a short period of time, a new relation will have been formed in the child, and he will respond with fear to impending troubles and sufferings that do not personally affect him in the least, but threaten those close to him. Thus out of a narrow, self-centered sensation of fear there is created the foundation for broad and profound social feelings.

In precisely the same way, we can easily lift out of the narrow circle of personality all the self-centered feelings, i.e., teach the child to respond with anger not to the wrongs done to him personally, but to the wrongs done his own country, his own social class, or his own craft. It is this possibility for the broadest possible transfer of feelings which also constitutes the surest guarantee of the education of the feelings, which may be expressed as the possibility for the creation of entirely new relationships between the individual and the environment. This is why there can be no unacceptable or undesirable emotions, from the teacher's standpoint. On the contrary, the teacher must always start from what are thought of as the lowest or self-centered feelings, understanding them to be the most primitive, the most basic, and the most powerful of all feelings, and just on the basis of these feelings, lay the foundation of the emotional structure of personality.

The division of the sensations into lower and higher, self-centered and altruistic, should, therefore, be dropped, since absolutely every sensation may be pointed in any direction by teachers and associated with any stimulus. One can teach the child to be frightened of a little pimple on his face or of a spider on the wall, and train him to be frightened of general calamities, of failing his favorite subjects, or of the misfortunes that have befallen those close to him. And what we have said of fear we could just as well have said of all the other feelings. All the emotional reactions can be related with the most diverse stimuli, and this relation may be brought into existence only by creating conflict between different stimuli in the student's personal experience.

In other words, here the educational mechanism reduces to a special organization of the environment. Thus, the education of the feelings is always, basically, a *re-education* of the feelings, i.e., a variation in the direction of an emotional innate reaction.

There is one more psychological mechanism for the education of the feelings, which is inherent only to the emotional reactions and which has its roots in the distinctive features of the constitution of these reactions. According to our understanding of this mechanism, the path pointed out above is not the only way for a relation to form between a reaction and some event. It is also possible for the feeling of, say, fear, to be associated with a stimulus that had not been connected with an unconditional stimulus of fear in the child's experience, though it had been connected with the sensation of pain, with displeasure, and so on in his experience.

It is only necessary to create what is known as a *preventive reaction*. Thus, the first time a child sees a lit candle, he will unsuspectingly try to touch it with his hands, but once he's gotten burned, he will begin to be frightened of fire and will respond to a flame brought near him with a sharply expressed fear. In this case, a new reaction is locked in, although not through the establishment of a conditional reflex, but in an entirely different way—through the creation of an independent relation between two emotions in which the strongly experienced emotion of pain induces the emotion of fear. In other words, the emotional effect of a particular event, of a particular reaction, becomes the cause for the establishment of a whole series of other emotional relations. If you would like a child to be afraid of something, then relate the approach of this something with pain or with suffering for the organism, and the desired fear will arise all by itself.

Thus, the emotions have to be considered as a system of anticipatory reactions that inform the organism as to the near future of his behavior and organize the different forms of this behavior. For the teacher, therefore, the emotions become an extraordinarily valuable tool for the education of various reactions. No form of behavior is so vigorous as when it is associated with an emotion. If you would like to induce in a student certain desirable forms of behavior, therefore, always be sure that these reactions leave an emotional trace in the student. No moral sermon educates like real pain, like a real feeling, and in this sense, the apparatus of the emotions seems like an expressly adapted and subtle tool by means of which behavior may be influenced effortlessly.

Emotional reactions turn out to have a substantial influence on absolutely all forms of our behavior and on all the components of the educational process. Whether we wish to help students achieve a better memory or whether we wish thinking to proceed more successfully—in either event we must take care to stimulate the particular activity emotionally. Experience and research have shown that an emotionally tinged fact is remembered more strongly, more firmly, and longer than one that is neutral. Every time you tell a student something, take care to engage his feeling. This is needed not only as a tool for better recall and better assimilation, but also as an end in itself.

Education in pre-revolutionary times rationalized and intellectualized our behavior in infinite ways, resulting in that frightful hardheartedness, in that utter absence of all feeling, which became an inevitable trait of every person who passed through the educational system. In modern man, everything is mechanical to such an extent, his individual impressions are so associated with concepts, that life passes in tranquility, neither engaging nor affecting his psyche, nor tinging his relations with the emotional, and this joyless and untroubled life, without serious catastrophes, but also without great joys, creates a foundation for that fastidious gradation of feelings which, in literary language, has long been known as narrow-mindedness or Philistinism.

Everything that we lost as a consequence of this education, the spontaneous sensation of life and, incidentally, the lifeless, uninspired method of teaching all the different subjects played no small role in this disengagement from the world and in this destruction of feelings. Who among us has not thought of what an inexhaustible source of emotional stimulation is concealed in an ordinary course of geography, astronomy, or history, all we have to do is think of ways of teaching these subjects that go beyond all dry logical schemata and make of teaching not only an object and labor of thought, but also a labor of feeling.

Emotion is no less important a tool than is thinking. The teacher must be concerned not only that students think about and learn geography, but also feel deeply about it. Such a thought usually does not come to mind for one reason or another, and teaching that is emotionally felt is a rare visitor to our schools, and is associated, for the most part, with an impotent love for one's own subject on the part of a teacher who doesn't know of any way of imparting this love to his students and, therefore, usually has the reputation of being eccentric.

Meanwhile, it is precisely the emotional reactions that have to serve as the foundation of the educational process. Before communicating a particular piece of knowledge, the teacher should induce the appropriate emotion in the student, and take care to associate this emotion with the new knowledge. Only new knowledge that has passed through the student's senses may be inculcated. Everything else is lifeless knowledge that diminishes every vital relationship to the world. Of all the subjects taught in school, only in the teaching of literature, and there only to an insignificant degree, was the presence of an emotional component recognized as an essential element of the educational process in the classroom.

The ancient Greeks said that philosophy begins with wonder. Psychologically, this is true with regard to all knowledge, in the sense that every bit of new knowledge must be preceded by a certain sense of craving. A certain degree of emotional sensitivity, a degree of involvement must, of necessity, serve as the starting point of all educational efforts.

There is a short, though profoundly meaningful comic story of Chekhov's that may serve as the best example of the sterile indifference we spoke of earlier.

In this story, an elderly official who had never studied anything would recollect the meaning of all the punctuation marks from experience; he knew that a colon is placed before a listing of pages or references, that a comma separates a list of names, that, in other words, in his life and his experience there were always times whose emotional meaning was represented by these punctuation marks. In all his years of work only the exclamation point had never turned up even once; from his wife, he learned a rule she had memorized in her boarding school, that the exclamation mark is used to express delight, enthusiasm, anger, indignation, and other feelings. But it was just these feelings that were missing in the life of the official, and the feeling of infinite grief for the life he had so foolishly led, his resentment and indignation, forced him to experience a strong outburst for the very first time, and, in the office supervisor's book of congratulations, he wrote three large exclamation marks following his signature.

If you would prefer that your students not repeat the pitiful life of Chekhov's official, take care that delight, indignation, and other feelings do not pass them by in life, that there are exclamation points in their lives that are just a little bit larger.

In our society, there has developed, for one reason or another, a one-sided view of the human personality, and everyone, for one reason or another, thinks of natural gifts and talent as applicable only to intelligence. But one may not only possess a talent for thought, one may also possess a talent for feeling. The emotional aspect of personality has no lesser a value than all the other aspects, and constitutes a subject and a concern of education just as much as does the mind and the will. Love can involve just as much talent and even genius as the discovery of the differential calculus. In both, human behavior presents exceptionally and monumental forms.

The extreme and falsely exaggerated sensitivity that must be rigorously distinguished from feeling is another result of emotional education, though no better than an extreme result. By "sensitivity," we should understand all those forms of the emotional reactions that are observed when emotion is not associated with any action and when everything without exception is resolved in the internal reactions that accompany it. To give an example of a false feeling, James points to those sentimental Russian plantation owners who would cry in the theater while watching some sensitive drama without it ever crossing their mind that their coachman was out in the street freezing in the 40 degree weather. As much as emotion is powerful and important for action, so is sentiment sterile and of no value.

As regards the education of the emotions in the proper sense of the term, here the essential pedagogical task is to teach the child to become ruler of his emotions, i.e., to teach him to incorporate the emotions into the general network of behavior, to make them intimately related to all the other reactions and not burst into the course of these reactions in a disruptive and disorderly fashion.

The ability to master one's feelings through psychology means nothing less than the ability to master their external expression, i.e., the reactions associated with them. Feelings are conquered, therefore, only through the mastery of their motor expression, and he who learns not to make a grimace and wince when tasting something disagreeable or disgusting conquers disgust itself. Hence that extraordinary power over the education of the feelings that belongs to the development of conscious movements and the control over these movements.

A coward who strikes an attitude of pride and approaches a foe boldly, openly and with a warlike demeanor has thereby already conquered his cowardice. We know that famous warriors such as Peter the Great and Napoleon were as scared of mice (and insects). Consequently, they knew of the feeling of fear, and emotional reactions were natural to them. However, in a battle they could stand under fire without trembling because they were able to master their fear.

Such a mastery of the emotions, which constitutes the task of every form of education, might at first glance appear to consist in a suppression of all feeling. In fact, it denotes only the subordination of feeling, in which the feelings are bound up with the other forms of behavior and guided in the appropriate directions. One example of such rational employment of the feelings we might cite are the intellectual feelings, i.e., feelings such as curiosity, interest, wonder, and the like which arise in immediate association with intellectual activity and which guide this activity in most explicit fashion, though, in and of themselves, these feelings possess an extraordinarily imperceptible physical expression, confined for the most part to slight movements of the eyes and the face.

Games, which we spoke of as constituting the best educational mechanism of the instincts are, in addition, also the best means of disciplining emotional behavior. The child's games are always emotional, there are always strong and vivid feelings in these games, though they teach the child not to follow emotions blindly, but to make them conform to the rules of the game and to the ultimate goal of the game. Thus, games are the first forms of conscious behavior, arising on the basis of instinctive and emotional behavior. They are the best tool for the integrated education of all these diverse forms of behavior and for the establishment of the proper coordination and interdependence between them.

---

[1]*The Emotions,* translated by Istar A. Haupt from the German translation by Dr. H. Kurella of the Danish original, New York, Hafner, 1967, page 80.

Chapter 7

PSYCHOLOGY AND PEDAGOGICS
OF ATTENTION

Psychological Nature of Attention

Traditional psychology defined attention as the form of activity wherein we are able to divide up the complex composition of impressions that reach us from outside. We then identify in this flux the most important variable, focus on this variable with the full force of activity and, thereby hasten its penetration into consciousness. Thus the particular distinctiveness and clarity with which this segment of our impressions is experienced.

However, the old psychology also knew that, in acts of attention, we encounter phenomena that are not all of the same "psychic" order. Attention begins most often and, in its very development, originates out of a whole series of manifestations that are purely motor in nature. One need only take a look at the simplest acts of attention to see that these acts begin every time with particular set reactions that involve movements of different perceiving organs. Thus, if our intention is to attentively scrutinize something, we assume the appropriate stance, place our head in a certain position, and adjust and focus our eyes as required. The adaptive and directional movements of the ears, neck, and head are of no lesser importance in the act of attentive listening.

The meaning and function of all these movements inevitably reduces to the placement of the perceiving organs, which are responsible for the most important tasks here, in the most convenient and appropriate position. However, these motor reactions of attention involve more than the above reactions of external organs of perception. The entire organism turns out to be permeated with these motor adaptations to the perception of external impressions. It has, in fact, been shown by experimental investigation that even the least troublesome acts of attention are accompanied by changes in the curves of respiration and pulse rate.

Even the most intimate process of the organism are adapted to impending activity. But these active motor reactions constitute only part of the story. A second, no less important element consists in the cessation of all other movements and reactions not associated with the impending activity. The reader surely knows from personal experience how darkness is conducive to attentive listening, how the inactivity and state of rest of organs then not in use help to focus attention and the work of the principal organ. From the psychological point of view, the cessation of a reaction or its inhibition represents just as much of a motor reaction as does every purposeful movement. Thus, from the motor standpoint, attention is characterized by the adaptive movements of the internal and external organs and by the inhibition of all other activity on the part of the organism.

However, those acts of attention in which the first part of this picture is entirely absent play the greatest role in our life. This happens in those instances when it is a question of what is known as "inner" attention, i.e., when the object towards which the force of our attention is directed is not in the world external to the organism, but constitutes part of the reaction of the organism itself, which in this case serves as an internal stimulus.

From the reactological point of view, phenomena of attention must be understood no differently than as a particular system of orienting reactions, i.e., preparatory reactions of the individual that cause him to place his body in a desired position and attitude and prepare it for impending activity. From this point of view, orienting reactions are absolutely no different than any other reaction. The same three essential components that arise in the full course of any reaction may be discovered and demonstrated in them quite easily.

The first component is apparent in the presence of an appropriate stimulation, impetus, or impulse, however it is expressed, whether in some external impression or internal stimulus, an uttered word, desire, emotion, and so on. No orienting reaction could ever arise without such a reference point.

Next is the component of central processing of the impulse. We can always tell whether this component is present on the basis of the diversity of forms assumed by these reactions, even though they are all induced by the same impetus, depending on the diversity and complexity of the states in which the central nervous system is found. It is only necessary for one excitation to end up in one group of sources of excitations, and it will induce one effect; if the arrangement of these sources is altered, the effect achieved by the very same excitation will be totally different.

Finally, there is the third component of a reaction, its responding effect, which is always realized in an act of attention through a series of movements of external or internal organs, in a series of somatic reactions of internal organs, or in internal secretion. A set reaction, in this sense, is the most customary reaction of the organism, except for the fact that in human behavior it bears a special role—that of laying the groundwork of our future behavior. Such preparatory reactions of orientation may, therefore, be called *pre-reactions*.

Description of Orientation

Set reactions have to be described from several directions. First, the aspect that makes it possible to distinguish between different set reactions is the *capacity* of these reactions, i.e., the very quantity of simultaneous stimulations that may be incorporated into the functioning mechanism of our behavior as part of a given orientation. According to Wundt's calculations, our consciousness can grasp from 16 to 40 simple impressions simultaneously, whereas attention is capable of preparing our organism to respond simultaneously to far fewer impressions—from 6 to 12 impressions of the same type. The selective character of the set reactions, which, out of the full range of our behavior, pick out just a small variable of this behavior and, it would appear, places it together with all the other conditions for a reaction, despite everything to the contrary, becomes perfectly clear.

It should be noted that the extent of an orientation is not a biologically invariant, constant magnitude. It exhibits very great variability depending on sex, age, and individual circumstances, but principally as a function of the level of practice, habits, and experience of the particular person. Even for one and the same person, the range of possible orientations is not something constant, but may vary depending on the general state of his organism. Concepts of limits and of boundaries of the orientation capacity of the individual, however, constitute among the most valuable achievements of the psychology of attention and brings this study into the realm of providence, making it possible to always determine and take into account in advance the possibilities of our behavior.

The factor of *duration* is the second component characteristic of orientation. In fact, the act of orientation displays an extraordinarily unstable, wavering, seemingly oscillatory state, as is apparent from the simplest experiments. If we focus our eyes on a single point or letter for a prolonged period as attentively as possible, we will notice quite easily that our initially strong attention begins to gradually attenuate; a spot which was perceived initially with the greatest distinctness and clarity begins to grow dim before our eyes, becoming indistinct and obscure, drops out of our vision, re-emerges, flickers and seems to twinkle before our eyes, though all the external conditions that define the course of the stimulations have remained exactly the same. Obviously, the variations in the results must be ascribed to changes in certain internal processes, particularly the process of orientation.

Strange as it may seem, an orientation will last for an extraordinarily insignificant period of time, in most cases hardly exceeding several minutes; subsequently, a kind of rhythmic fluctuation of orientation sets in. Orientation vanishes and reappears if behavioral conditions require that it be maintained for a prolonged period of time. Thus, orientation manifests itself as if in fits and starts, in a broken line, rather than as a straight line, regulating our reactions by means of shocks and allowing them to proceed by inertia in the intervals between one shock and the next.

Thus, a rhythmic character is the fundamental law of our acts of orientation, forcing us to take account of all the pedagogical requirements that are thereby implicated. Urbanchich's simplest experiments confirm this conclusion in its entirety. In these experiments, a subject was asked to listen to the ticking of a clock with his eyes closed and to indicate with the words, "nearer" and "farther," those cases when it seemed to him that the ticking of the clock had become stronger, accordingly weaker. In every case without exception, the same result was obtained: By turns, the subject pronounced the words, "nearer" and "farther," alternating correctly, since he was always under the impression that the ticking was now becoming stronger, now becoming weaker, and it seemed to him as if the clock was approaching, accordingly moving away from him, at a uniform rate, though all the time the clock was suspended in a fixed position from some frame never changing its position.

Again, it is evident that the reason why the sound became stronger or weaker must be sought not in external processes, but in the internal processes of orientation. In this case, we are dealing with an entirely pure form of rhythmicity or undulation in our orientation, which, since it is directed towards a uniform and continuous series of stimulations, perceives them not as an uncoordinated series of entirely similar stimulations, but as a unified, undulating unity with its own points of rise and fall.

Accordingly, we should now consider the last distinctive feature and function of orientation, i.e., the way in which it manifests itself in the role of unifier and guide of external impressions. Since our attention is rhythmic, we are inclined to introduce rhythm into all external stimulations, and to see a rhythm at work in all external stimulations, whether or not they, in fact, possess a rhythm. In other words, we perceive the world not in its divided up, chaotic form, but as a connected and rhythmic whole that combines together smaller elements into a group, and these groups into new, large formations. We can now understand what one psychologist meant when he said that it was because of attention that the world is perceived as if it were verse in which individual syllables were combined together into metric feet, these latter into hemistiches, the hemistiches into verse, the verse into strophes, and so on.

Internal and External Orientation

From the qualitative standpoint, empirical psychology described attention as both voluntary and involuntary. *Involuntary attention* was usually considered to consist in those acts that were in response to certain external stimuli that attracted us by virtue of their remarkable force, interest, or expressiveness. If, sitting in a quiet room, I become all ears upon hearing the report of a gun shot, this may readily serve as the best example of such involuntary attention. Here the cause of my set reactions is found not in the organism, but in phenomena that occur outside it, in the unexpected force of a new stimulus that takes possession of the entire free field of attention, and pushes aside and inhibits all of our other reactions.

Psychologists refer to those cases when concentration is focused not outside the organism, but within it, when the individual's own experience, action, or thought becomes the subject of attention, as *internal* or *voluntary attention*. As an example of voluntary attention, just recall how it is when you are concentrating on one of your own thoughts, trying to recall or imagine something, or when you are involved in some project, whether reading a book or writing a letter, and set about preparing all the organs that would be needed for this project entirely consciously and voluntarily.

For a long time, it seemed that there existed an inherent and fundamental difference between the two types of attention, and that this difference was fully exhausted in the difference between the physiological nature of the second type of attention and the mental nature of the first type. Psychologists were wont to characterize this first type as inner will, as a pure act of volitional effort without any direct relation to physical manifestations. Meanwhile, the same experimental investigations demonstrated that, in voluntary attention, we are dealing with the very same somatic reactions of respiration and circulation as are observed in the second type of attention. Moreover, these acts are accompanied by the very same cessation of extraneous movements, the very same delay in activity, as occurs in external attention, and the only difference between the two is that, in the first type of attention, there are no clearly expressed adaptive reactions of the external organs.

But this difference is explained quite clearly and completely by the difference in the object at which attention is directed in the two cases. It is entirely understandable that, in the case of attention which is excited by an impression that comes from outside, the organism will respond by readying the appropriate organs of perception through which this impression is to be brought to consciousness. It is just as understandable that, in these reactions, there is not the slightest need whatsoever for orientation to focus on external stimuli, and instead it focuses on internal stimuli, which we perceive from the proprioceptive field, as well as from the interio-receptive field, whereas external stimuli are perceived from the exterio-receptive field.

Language usually engraves this analogy in the sorts of expressions that are used to denote such acts of internal attention. When we recall something earnestly and raptly, it is as if we are listening to words that are resounding within us, and in precisely the same way strange sounds and voices can confuse us as, for example, when we listen attentively to someone speaking or to music. Here language reinforces the complete analogy that exists between the adaptive movements of the ears and the adaptive movements of the proprio-ceptive nerve pathways in the first and second types of attention. The presence, in the latter case, of a certain inner stimulus that proves to be capable of inducing the very same effect of an orienting reaction as does an external stimulus is the only essential psychological difference.

We can be sure of making no mistake if we agree that the difference between the two types of orientation reduces to the difference between innate or unconditioned and acquired or conditioned reflexes. Concentration and its simplest, elementary forms constitutes, as is shown by observation, an unconditioned reflex that manifests itself in the very first days of an infant's life and possesses absolutely all the typical features of the attention we observe in an adult. But like every unconditioned reflex, the reflex of concentration may be subjected to education and re-education. If a stimulation that induces this reflex is always accompanied by still another foreign stimulation, then, as a result of numerous repetitions of the two stimulations occurring simultaneously, a new relation will have been formed in the cerebral cortex between the second neutral stimulus and the simultaneously accompanying reaction. Now a conditioned reflex has been formed, which will function with mechanical regularity and will be induced now by the new stimulus just as precisely as it had been previously induced by an unconditioned reflex.

Consider how a reflex of concentration is induced in a child always by means of impressions reaching it from its nursing mother. If the system formed by these stimuli occurs simultaneously with stimulations of the eyes produced by the child's own reactions or from the child's own unsatisfied cries, then as a result of lengthy training only a single sensation of the eyes or a single cry will be sufficient for all of the child's reactions to focus on feeding, on the intake of nourishment, even though its mother is not at all present at the particular moment.

Thus, an external orientation that is induced by an external stimulus has now entered a second phase, and become an inner orientation, since it has become subordinated to an inner stimulus.

Attention and Distraction

Distraction is usually taken to mean the direct opposite of an act of attention. And in fact, if we were to understand by acts of attention the organism's state of readiness in anticipation of the approach of certain stimulations, then distraction would, of course, denote the utter unexpectedness of an approaching stimulation and the organism's complete lack of adaptation to responding to this stimulation. Thus, if we are attentive to foreign words, we respond to them at once with an appropriate and meaningful answer; if we listen distractedly, we either do not respond at all or respond after some delay, inappropriately.

However, this notion requires a major corrective. In fact, from the psychological point of view, it is necessary to distinguish between two entirely different aspects of distraction, which are no less incompatible than is attention and distraction. Distraction can, in fact, spring from a low level of attention, from an inability to collect oneself or to concentrate and focus one's orientation on some one single object. Therefore, it may refer to a certain suspension and derangement of the entire mechanism of our behavior and, in this sense, when any sort of marked features are present, it assumes an explicit pathological character and must be deemed unhealthy.

However, the distraction that teachers generally have to contend with, which also manifests itself at every step of a normal person's life, constitutes an essential and useful companion of attention. Above we explained the value that orientation acquires when it restricts our behavior to a certain narrow path. The meaning of an orientation always reduces to a constriction of the course of reactions, which, because of their quantity, gain in force, quality, and clarity. This, quite naturally, presupposes a constriction in our behavior to such an extent that the whole series of stimulations that impinge upon us remain neutral and do not excite any reaction on our part.

To be attentive to some one thing inevitably presupposes being distracted with regard to everything else. The relationship here assumes the wholly mathematical character of a direct proportionality, and we can say quite frankly that the greater the force of attention, the greater the force of distraction. In other words, the more precise and the more highly perfected an orientation to some one reaction, the less adapted is the organism to other reactions. This psychological law of the relationship between attention and distraction finds its most brilliant confirmation in well-known anecdotes of the absentmindedness of scholars and, in general, of anyone occupied with one particular thought. The absentmindedness of the scholar, the absentmindedness of the scientist, always denotes an exceptional degree of focus of his thoughts on a single point. In this sense, from the scientific point of view, it would be correct to speak, not of the education of attention and the struggle to overcome distraction, but of the proper education of both attention and distraction together.

Biological Value of Orientation

The biological value of orientation is best revealed if we consider the demands out of which it arose. The more complex the organism, the more manifold and the more subtle are the forms of its relationships with the environment and the higher are the forms assumed by its behavior. The edifice formed out of what is known as personal experience, that is, of conditioned reflexes, and built atop innate or inherited experience, is the basic complication that distinguishes the behavior of the higher animals. In fact, 99% of the behavior of a spider or of a butterfly is determined by inherited instinctive forms, and only 1%, roughly speaking and approximately, is determined by the personal relationships established by the individual. This relationship changes into its opposite the moment we move from the lower animals to the higher.

In the complex composition of man's behavior, barely one-hundredth of all reactions are innate, unaffected by any individual influences of personal experience whatsoever. The biological sense of this superstructure lies in the "preliminary," or "signal" adaptation of the organism to the approach of those events that have not yet occurred, but which will have to inevitably occur because of known features. In its higher forms, this *signal* or *preliminary form of adaptation* to future changes in the environment turns into reactions of attention or orientation, i.e., it is related reflexively with those reactive impulses that lead the organism to the most perfected state of readiness.

Thus, according to the rigorous definition given by Karl Groos, an orientation may be defined, from the biological point of view, as the anticipation of an impending event, as a tool in the physical struggle for existence by means of which the organism is able to respond with essential movements not at the very moment the danger is impending, but rather far in advance of its approach.

In its complex forms, man's behavior seems to be divided into two parts. Because of the enormous quantity of already developed organic reactions and the exceptional complexity of the ways they are brought together and combined, there arises the necessity for special control over the course of these reactions, for the organism's control over its own behavior. Internal stimuli that arise from the proprio-ceptive field and which lead the organism into combat readiness for every possible reaction is, above all and quite naturally, such a controlling and regulative reaction.

This is why we have every right to make comparisons between attention and the organism's internal strategy. Attention, in fact, serves as a strategist, i.e., a director and organizer, a guide and commander of the battle, without, however, participating directly in the combat itself.

All the features of orientation established above may be readily explained from this fundamental point of view. It is quite understandable that, in order to maintain the functional unity of our organs, it becomes biologically inevitable for the organism to develop a certain narrow groove for the orienting reactions and to restrict the scope of these reactions in order to ensure the operational unity of the most diverse organs of our body. The exceptional short-term nature of the orientations also becomes understandable, since an orientation represents an extraordinary risk for the organism precisely because of its narrow scope. By preparing the organism for combat in one arena, it weakens it and demobilizes it in all other arenas, and if orientation were not so skittish and not so precipitate, it would place the organism in the greatest of danger time and again, against which the organism would be entirely powerless to resist.

It is biologically necessary for one's orientation to focus first on one reaction and then on another, encompassing by dint of its organizing effect all the aspects of our behavior. Such is the nature and rhythmic character of our attention, which should be taken to denote nothing less than a rest for attention, a rather essential need for the prolonged functioning of attention. The rhythmic character, thus, must be understood not as a principle of abridgement of attention, but, on the contrary, as a principle of prolongation of attention, since, by saturating and interposing the functioning of attention with moments of rest and respite, rhythm preserves and maintains the energy of attention, making it ultimately inexhaustible and infinitely engrossed over as long a time as possible.

Finally, the last point that has been discovered in the nature of attention, in the course of unraveling its biological import, lies in the fact that an orienting reaction has to be understood as a continuously prolonged effort of the organism, and not at all as a momentary manifestation of its activity. In this sense, those thinkers are correct who have declared that attention functions like a motor, in bursts, retaining the force of the impulse from one burst to the next. Thus, an act of attention must be understood as continuously annihilating itself and continuously reappearing, as if dying away and flaring up from one moment to the next.

Educational Value of the Orientations

Without fear of overstatement, one may say that orientation is the first condition where it becomes possible to affect the child through education. Certain teachers even suggest reducing the entire process of education to the development of certain forms of orientation, and thus claim that every form of education is an education of attention above all, so that the various modes of education differ from each other only by the nature of those acts of orientation that are to be fostered.

In a certain sense, this is entirely correct, since in education we are always dealing not with movements and actions that possess a purpose and goal in and of themselves, but with the development of skills and habits for future functioning and future activity. If that's the case, our task is not so much a matter of summoning up particular reactions in and of themselves, but only of educating the essential orientations. The call of education is to introduce a degree of coordination, meaningfulness, and direction into the chaotic and uncoordinated mass of the newborn's movements. The full range of behavior of the adult differs from the newborn's behavior solely by the presence of this component. It is, therefore, clear that the fundamental principle of education lies in the selection of those most essential and most important reactions that have to be preserved, that should be thought of as being of paramount importance, around which other reactions of lesser value group and take shape, bearing in mind that, ultimately, those reactions that are not at all needed by the organism will be inhibited and suppressed.

But it precisely these three functions, of identification, grouping, and delaying, that the mechanism of orientation implements. In order to explain the pedagogical importance of attention, it is usually observed that a mother who is entirely indifferent to every possible noise will awaken at the slightest sound from her child, just like a miller who will not be aroused by the loudest thunder and rumbling of a storm, but who will awaken to the slightest murmuring of a stream of running water. In other words, usually for this purpose we tend to refer to those facts and circumstances when orientation makes it possible to identify those influences of the environment that are biologically of the greatest importance for the organism, even though, in and of themselves, they defer to other influences in terms of force.

Development of Attention

The infinite capacity of attention for development makes orientation no less valuable as a subject of education. If the various capacities of a child and an adult are compared, in no realm will we find such an enormous and vast difference as in the realm of orientation. In the earliest years, attention is nearly exclusively reflexively instinctive in nature, and only gradually, through lengthy and complex training, does it turn into voluntary orientation guided by the most important needs of the organism and, in turn, guiding the full course of our behavior.

The child's interest, as the most frequent form of manifestation of involuntary attention, thus, assumes extraordinary pedagogical importance. The child's attention is directed and guided nearly entirely by interest, and, therefore, the phenomenon of distraction in a child always has its natural source in a "divergence," pedagogically speaking, between two paths, the path followed by the child's natural interest and the path mapped out by those tasks given to the child as required tasks.

This is why the old school system, in which the divergence between these two paths was taken as the foundation of psychological wisdom, was, more than anything else, compelled to resort to outside measures in its organization of attention, was compelled to evaluate students' attention by means of special grades and, for all practical purposes, was quite powerless to develop the essential forms of orientation.

If we let the child follow his own interests and develop accordingly, this will unavoidably entail a process whereby he follows his own whims and needs, and we will end up with the same result as that produced from the relationship of a horseman to his horse. To many teachers, this seems like a rejection of any control over, and guidance of, the educational process. Their reasoning is, roughly speaking, as follows. If the child is to be guided by his own interests, what, then, should the teacher do? He is useless if he blindly follows behind the student who is pursuing his own interest; he can be harmful if, standing ahead the child, he tries to divert this interest and paralyze its force of action.

This apparent difficulty may be resolved, essentially, and in the most painless way, in educational psychology if we begin with the only correct standpoint, that education means neither simply following the organism's natural inclinations nor a fruitless struggle against these inclinations. The path of scientific education lies between these two extremes and requires combining these two extremes together into a unified whole. Education cannot be conducted in any way other than through the child's natural inclinations; in all its strivings, education proceeds by taking as its starting point precisely these inclinations. But it would be an admission of impotence if the calling of education were to lie in this goal and this meaning alone. In fact, it intervenes actively in these natural inclinations of the child, brings them together, grouping them in whatever way one might wish, protecting some of them, stimulating some of them at the expense of others, and, in this way, introduces the spontaneous process of the child's inclinations into the organizing and shaping channel of the social environment in the school.

The question as to the role of the teacher in the development of the child's interests is in precisely the same state. On the one hand, the psychologist is forced to acknowledge the omnipotence of this law and, following Thorndike, to affirm that this principle has universal value, and that the most uninteresting thing we do, ultimately, is when we do something, while nevertheless from interest, still from negative interest, i.e., when we strive to avoid unpleasantness.

From this point of view, teaching in general is possible only inasmuch as it relies on the child's own interests. There can be no other form of teaching. The whole question has to do with how far this interest may be directed along the path of the actual subject being studied, and not involve recourse to the influence of rewards, punishments, the desire to please, and so on, all of which are alien to it. But this acknowledgement of the omnipotence of the child's interest can hardly be taken as condemning the teacher to impotently following in the tracks of the child's interests. In organizing the environment and the child's life in this environment, the teacher intervenes actively into the processes by which the child's interests evolve and acts upon them in precisely the same way he influences all of the child's behavior. His rule, however, must always be: Before giving an explanation, arouse interest; before asking the child to do something, get him ready it; before resorting to a reaction, prepare an orientation; and before communicating some new information, induce the anticipation of this new information.

Thus, from the subjective standpoint, orientation manifests itself for the student, above all, in a certain anticipation of an impending activity.

Psychological Value of Anticipation

From everyday life, it is easy to see that anticipation assists behavior when some event is impending. For something to be unanticipated denotes, for the most part, the absence of readiness and the inadequacy of a reaction. However, only by virtue of rigorous psychological experiments has it been possible to discover the genuine nature of anticipation and to get a true idea of the limits of its value for education.

Experience demonstrates that, for all intents and purposes, anticipation reduces always to some preliminary readiness of the appropriate working organs, that anticipation represents a kind of mustering of the organism for a future action, that it is even an already commenced action that has not, however, been brought to fruition. These nascent actions Binet has referred to as *mental stances*. In precisely the same way as a stance arises as a result of certain movements and serves as a starting point for subsequent movements, these mental states of anticipation arise as a result of certain reactions and create a foundation for the emergence of subsequent states.

In measurements that have been made of the duration of a simple reaction, it has been possible to establish the following extraordinarily interesting fact. Every person exhibits three entirely distinct types of reaction in a simple response to some simple stimulus, and these reactions differ sharply from each other, depending on the person's preliminary orientation.

The most ordinary type of reaction is usually referred to as a *natural reaction*. This is the reaction that is made when movement is performed in accordance with the orientation that is the most customary to, and the most distinctive of, the particular person. It is encountered whenever we do not intervene actively in a subject's orientation and do not organize this orientation in our own way, as a function of the goals of some experiment. Experience has shown that, in these cases, there is a mean time of reaction that is characteristic of each person, i.e., a customary mean duration of orientation, which manifests itself in an ordinary, natural rate of movement in this person's walking, speaking, or writing. In other words, in these cases we seem to induce a natural orientation that forms and develops in this person over the course of a number of years, becoming an inalienable part of this person's temperament and character.

The reader surely knows that each one of us has his own customary manner of speaking, his own customary rate of walking, his own customary rate of gesticulation and speech. However, this natural orientation may be made to deviate sharply from the individual's own mean rate in either direction if, by means of preliminary instructions, we induce a new orientation in the subject.

If before such an experiment, we ask a subject to respond not in his customary way, but possibly more quickly, as soon as he perceives an external impression, and, meanwhile, ask him to direct all his attention at the responsive organ itself, say, his fingers, which is to make the responding movement, we will obtain an extraordinarily noticeable effect every time. This effect will manifest itself in a very appreciable drop in reaction time, due to the fact that the preliminary orientation to the corresponding movement that we have induced has already produced all the essential nerve excitations needed to complete this movement, and only the very movement prior to the onset of the signal is delayed. Once the signal has been given, the delay is eliminated and the reaction is performed vigorously and strenuously.

This same law is taken into account in an elegant way in the pedagogics of military science, when, in the course of instruction, the attempt is made to develop movements that are as rapid and as exact as possible, through recourse to a subdivision of commands, i.e., essentially stimuli, into two parts, into the "executable command" and the "preliminary command." In the course of teaching, these two parts of a command are separated from each other, often by an interval of several minutes, in order to foster in the soldier a fully distinct movement of orientation and a distinct movement of the reaction itself. When the command, "Forward," is given, the soldiers remain in place, though they know that now they will have to move; they carry out on command only the act of orientation, preparing the groups of muscles that will be needed for the movement, mobilizing them, and this is expressed outwardly in a special straining, in a special readiness to move at every moment, that turns rapidly into active movement as soon as the executable part of the command, "March," is given. Only through such a deliberate subdivision of orientation and movement itself does there develop a maximally exact and perfected reaction.

One might ask whence arises this abridgement of time that occurs in such a muscular reaction or, in other words, in an orientation to the muscular part of a movement. It is perfectly evident that it occurs due to the part of the processes that have been completed in preparation for the actual orientation, and if the motor orientation reduces the time of the muscular reaction, this will mean that it performed part of this work on its own, and that the muscular reaction now proceeds under the control and guidance of this orientation.

We find full confirmation of this result in the opposite case, when an orientation of a diametrically opposite nature is induced. This will occur whenever the instructions require the subject to direct all his attention not to the responding organ, but to the perceiving organs, when we ask the subject to carefully listen to or look at a stimulation, and not respond before perceiving it clearly and before being conscious of it. With such a sensory orientation guiding all the preparatory functions to the first perceptual component of the reaction, we obtain the extraordinarily pronounced effect of an overall retardation of a reaction by comparison with the mean time of its natural form.

This retardation of movement is induced, undoubtedly, by the delaying action that every foreign orientation exerts on a reaction. In this case, the orientation was directed wholly to the perceiving organs, and was naturally delayed and retarded by the reaction of the hand.

Thus was the entirely genuine influence of orientation on the course of subsequent reactions demonstrated by experimental investigation. Experimental psychology has shown that the duration, force, and form of every movement is wholly predetermined by preliminary orientation.

An experiment with two objects of equal weight but different size testifies to the effect of orientation in a simple and graphic way. If two objects of the same weight are lifted one after the other using the same hand, first the larger one and then the smaller one, because of our impressions, it will seem to us that the larger one is most certainly the lighter of the two, no matter how many times the two objects are shown, right before our eyes, to balance each other on a scale. In other words, even exact and certain knowledge is powerless here to refute the illusion and, consequently, the source of this illusion must be sought not in the actual process of weighing, but in the preliminary orientation that is performed unconsciously by virtue of the acquired habit—prior to the process of weighing.

Orientation in this sense can be understood by noting that when we see a large object in front of us, we orient ourselves, make ourselves ready for the act of lifting a heavy weight, we seem to allocate a considerable motor impetus, produce a more significant dispatch of energy, than happens when we see a small object in front of us. Accordingly, the same weight in one case calls up an insignificant muscular effort, and in the other case a more significant effort, and, without any change in magnitude, the same object may appear to us to be at times smaller, at times larger, depending upon our orientation.

These experiments all demonstrate essentially one thing, that every form of behavior is determined and controlled by orienting reactions that quite clearly precede it, though the influence of these reactions is not always expressed directly, but sometimes indirectly, in reactions that follow upon it.

Pedagogical Conclusions

The most important pedagogical conclusions that should be drawn from research on orientation may be reduced, basically, to a general formula. According to this formula, the teacher must attend not only to the student's ongoing and explicit reactions, but also to the unseen, submerged orientations that precede these reactions. Thus, the teacher must not only observe the student, but must also make conjectures at every turn as to what is happening in the student, whether seen or unseen.

In order to ensure successful teaching and learning, the teacher must not only maintain all the conditions necessary for the proper development of the reactions, but, what is far more important, also maintain the proper orientation. We might say, in complete agreement with psychological theory, that in education the principal emphasis must be precisely on orientation. Accordingly, the teacher has to determine at every turn whether the subject matter he has introduced is in accord with the fundamental laws of activity of attention.

Above all, this subject matter must be arranged and presented in such a way as to be in accord with the narrow range of the orienting reactions and, in terms of the nature of its effects, not be in contradiction with the duration of these effects. According to the simplest and most commonplace rules of pedagogical civility, a lesson should not last too long nor should the teacher talk a mile a minute. Essentially, these rules express, in most primitive form, the very same demand for a correspondence between subject matter and the student's adaptive reactions.

It is extremely important to organize the subject matter in such a way that it also correspond to the rhythmic functioning of our orientation. The simplest observation of the errors made by children when taking dictation when they are distracted, but not ignorant of the rules of orthography, reveal a wave-like, rhythmic character, in the sense that if the dictation is subdivided into equal time intervals, each such segment will exhibit, in succession, an increase or decrease in the number of errors.

It is extraordinarily important to so organize the lesson from the standpoint of pedagogics as to subdivide the subject matter so that the most critical and the most important points will be reached just as the force of attention rises, and that the least important parts of the presentation, those which do not suggest something new, occur as the wave of attention is falling.

Further, the subject matter itself must incorporate a degree of give and take and allow for smooth development, i.e., it must be presented in a connected form that would make it possible for all of its parts to be perceived as a unified whole.

Finally, the last and most important rule requires, on the part of teacher, the same attitude and the same concern for attention as for distraction. That teacher is profoundly mistaken who sees in distraction his own worst enemy, who does not understand the simple truth that it is precisely the student who is most distracted in his class who may, in fact, be his most attentive student.

The secret of turning distraction into attention, for all intents and purposes, lies in turning the arrow of attention from one direction to another. It is achieved by the general pedagogical technique of transferring interest from one subject to another, by creating a link between a pair of topics. This is also the principal means for the development of attention and for the conversion of involuntary external attention into voluntary attention.

The teacher must take care to create and develop in the student a sufficient quantity of internal stimuli associated with all the different orienting reactions. Once this has been accomplished, he may be certain that attention has become one of the internal mechanisms of our behavior and is functioning in accord with these mechanisms.

Thus the absolute necessity of taking into account the fundamental orientation of education, that which has been termed in the pedagogical literature of recent years the *orientation towards goals* of every educational act. Since the new psychology takes the educational process itself out of the hands of the teacher and places it in the hands of the student, for that very reason it is essential to also transfer the awareness of the goal of this act from the teacher to the student. It is not only essential for the student to educate himself by his own natural actions, but that the teacher guide and regulate the factors that define these actions, and likewise is it essential that not only the teacher, but the student as well, be conscious of the goal of these actions.

The meaningless and pedagogically destructive orientation towards examinations that was common of our Tsarist schools may serve as the simplest example of the import of such a fundamental orientation towards goals in the educational process. Examinations, which were usually left for the end of the school year, because of their very ephemeral status in the system of instruction and because of the consequences for the students that were associated with them, became such a natural orientation towards goals, despite the best wishes and hopes of the teachers. And once the better teachers saw to their sorrow that in the secondary school students would study to pass examinations, and would pass examinations in order to obtain diplomas, they were powerless to combat this tendency, since they could not suggest in place of this natural orientation towards goals any other orientation, and accordingly, were defenseless in the face of the natural and elemental force of this orientation.

It is extremely important to note here that orientation plays a decisive role even in such apparently mechanical and "passive" processes as memory and memorization. Experience demonstrates that memorization occurs quite differently and yields entirely different results depending on what sort of tests the person is subjected to afterwards. And if subjects know that they will only have to reproduce everything all at once when asked about what they have studied, they will study using one method; if they know that they will be making choices from among what will be reproduced before them, they will study using quite a different method. Thus, the decisive point in the educational process is an awareness of what is the goal of the different actions and what is the purpose of learning the material, moreover, by virtue of a preliminary orientation, this ultimate goal proves to be the most important guiding influence on the educational process.

The pedagogical value of anticipation involves not only a "loosening" of the soil and a preparation of the ground for the perception of new knowledge, but also, and far more importantly, to the development of the proper direction to be imparted to the newly emergent reaction. Indeed, it should be perfectly clear to the reader that the process of education reduces ultimately to the development in students of a certain quantity of reactions and of other, more complex forms of behavior. Thus. whether the direction of these reactions coincides with the direction they are meant to function in is decisive for the success or failure of this process. If I store in my memory thousands of useful bits of knowledge, but am unable to make use of any of this knowledge at the appropriate and required time, this knowledge becomes like a burden to me, and not only is it of no use within the system of behavior, but can be truly harmful, because it takes up space and keeps us from establishing and developing other reactions that are less fruitful, though more correct in terms of direction.

What has been referred to in the popular pedagogical literature as the "lifelessness" of the school essentially denotes this very error in the fundamental orientation towards the goals of education. The greatest sin of the Tsarist school was that none of the people involved in it had any answers when they were asked why study geography and history, mathematics and literature. Those who think that the Tsarist school did not provide one with very much knowledge are mistaken. On the contrary, it imparted an uncommonly great quantity and abundance of knowledge, particular the schools on the European model. But this was only an abundance of knowledge that always lay buried, an abundance that none could make the proper use of, because the fundamental orientation towards goals of this knowledge was to pass by life, and this orientation turned out to always be utterly antagonistic to life. Like a polished gem in a wasteland, this knowledge was unable to satisfy the simplest and most vital queries of the average and unassuming student.

From personal experience, the reader should have no trouble recalling that virtually the only application he has been able to make of the knowledge he acquired in the school was to give a more or less correct answer on an examination. The knowledge of geography has yet to help anyone get a sense of direction in the world outside or to enlarge the set of impressions we gain when traveling, and the knowledge of astronomy has not helped anyone experience the magnitude of the heavens any more strongly or more vividly.

Hence the two requirements, that absolutely all subject matter and absolutely all educational material be impregnatured and saturated through and through with such an orientation towards goals, and that the teacher possess at every moment exact knowledge of the path along which a new reaction is to function, become of fundamental pedagogical importance.

Attention and Habit

Habit and attention are antagonistic relations, and wherever habit has taken root, there attention vanishes. The reader surely knows how everything new, everything we are not accustomed to, engages us, and how we are often unable to tell what is the color of the wallpaper in a room or what is the color of the eyes of someone we meet every day.

In its very meaning, the effort of attention must be one of particular stress and must be truly in earnest whenever behavior overflows the bounds of habit, and we confront problems that are especially complex and difficult to deal with. Accordingly, habit is usually termed the foe of and a respite from attention, and until recently a contradictory and dual attitude towards the two dominated the field of educational psychology.

In fact, the pedagogical value of both these processes is so clear and so self-evident that neither should ever be renounced in favor of the other, but instead we must search for ways and methods of reconciling the two, of unraveling the genuine interrelation between attention and habit in a psychologically correct way. Attention, in fact, ceases to function as soon as behavior becomes habitual, but this not only does not denote an attenuation of attention, but, on the contrary, tends to be associated with an amplification of its activity.

This becomes perfectly understandable if we recall the essential circumscription of attention and the fact that, at every turn, it gains in force what it loses in amplitude. By making entire actions mechanical and subordinating these actions to the autonomous workings of the lower nerve centers, habit fully liberates and relieves the work of our attention and, thus, induces what would appear to be a relative exception from the law of differential inhibition of foreign reactions in the presence of a basic orientation.

We mentioned earlier that every orientation inhibits the course of foreign reactions. It would be correct to add that this holds except for the automatic and habitual reactions. One can engage in conversation rather intently while continuing to walk down the street just as one can carry on a discussion when doing complex needlework. The extraordinarily important psychological value of this exception from the law of inhibition becomes perfectly obvious if we bear in mind how much our behavior gains in diversity and scope once there arises, in parallel to our chief central orientation, a series of parallel, partial orientations to habitual actions.

Strictly speaking, this phenomenon should not be understood as an exception from the general psychological law, but rather as an expansion of this very principle. Both habitual actions and entirely automatic deeds require for their initiation and cessation the participation of an appropriate orientation, and if we wish to do needlework entirely oblivious of the fact, attention will nevertheless be needed if we are to work for awhile, then stop, then pick up the work, and then put it aside, i.e., the onset and termination of automatic actions can in no way be realized without an appropriate orientation.

Moreover, this orientation—the preliminarily adopted direction and rate of a reaction—will manifest itself in the continuation of absolutely the entire course of a habitual reaction. Thus, we have every right to speak not of a single orientation of our organism, but of a series of simultaneous orientations, one of which is the dominant orientation, and the others subordinate to it. This psychological observation is fully in accord with results found in the physiological study of the existence of dominant and subdominant focuses of nerve activity in the central nervous system.

Physiological Counterparts of Attention

Only recently have physiologists succeeded in discovering in the nervous system phenomena that, without question, are related to the act of attention. The study of what are called dominant excitations of the nervous system that has developed quite recently belongs in this field.

According to the basic results of this study, it has been established that some of the excitations that arise in the nervous system prove to be so powerful that they assume the role of dominant excitations, suppressing all other excitations or deflecting the direction of these excitations, or, finally, attracting them to itself and becoming augmented thereby. Such a fundamental excitation is usually called a *dominant excitation*, and all other foci in the nervous system are referred to as *subdominant excitations*.

An extraordinarily important fact has been discovered in this area, that when a dominant excitation is associated with an instinctive act, the basic focus of the excitation is amplified every time there arises a foreign stimulation in the nervous system. The act of the embracing reflex in the frog, the act of defecation and swallowing in the horse, sexual excitation in a female cat isolated from male cats when in heat, all constitute such types of natural dominant excitations which have been studied with laboratory precision.

It has turned out that all these acts become amplified when there is a foreign stimulation present. Thus, if, during the action of the embracing reflex, a frog is pinched, pin-pricked, or stimulated by acid or by an electrical current, the foreign stimulation not only does not weaken the embracing reflex, but even reinforces it. Thus, in the simplest nerve organizations, the act of attention proves to be constructed in such a way that not only does it induce an inhibition of the reactions conjugate to it, but even turns out to be capable of being amplified accordingly.

The extraordinarily interesting case where a sensory dominant and a motor dominant have been experimentally created separately in a prone frog is very nearly the most important of all results for psychologists. Here physiological analysis penetrates so deeply into the nervous system that it seems to turn into an attempt to distinguish between the roots of the two types of attention, sensory attention and motor attention, embedded in it.

It turned out that if a dominant excitation of the motor centers of the rear right leg is induced artificially in a frog, for example by means of phenol, the frog will respond to every stimulation emanating from any point on its body using just this leg. But if a dominant excitation of the sensory centers of the same leg is induced, when any point of its body whatsoever is thereupon stimulated, a licking reflex will be activated with mechanical precision, but always directed at the spot associated with the dominant stimulation of the centers, i.e., the rear right leg, even if it was the frog's belly, or its back, or its neck, etc. that had been stimulated.

Thus, it was established that a sensory dominant will preserve every other reflex, but will alter their course and deflect it towards the spot that was stimulated the most; whereas a motor dominant will cause the motor organ associated with it to present itself whenever other organs must begin to function in the normal course of the reflex.

The study of analogous phenomena, carried over to the case of human beings, cannot, of course, boast such ideal precision, which is possible and can be realized only in subjects of laboratory experimentation. It might even seem that the results achieved by physiologists go counter to the facts established by psychologists. It would appear paradoxical to assume the possibility of acts of attention that not only were not weakened by foreign stimulation, but, on the contrary, become reinforced thereby. That this view is correct is confirmed, however, by a whole series of observations that have yet to be collected into a single psychological law.

A rather curious circumstance was noted by M. Rubinshtein in his story of the construction of a facility at one of the universities in a large European center. In the eyes of the builders, the edifice had to be ideally adapted for educational purposes, and accordingly, they sought to exclude every feature that might serve as a foreign stimulus during classroom lessons. Basing their approach on the traditional view of attention, they assumed that, by eliminating all extraneous influence, they would thereby help stimulate attention.

In accordance with this plan, the building was constructed without any protruding or angular shapes, even the corners in each room were cleverly concealed, and each wall imperceptibly turned into and become the adjacent wall in such a way as to preclude spatial shape from ever having any effect on the students. Other details were similarly designed, and all the different parts of the structure were painted throughout, everything whatsoever having to do with education, from the very first step all the way up to the dome, whether classroom furnishings or student uniforms, or whatever, in a soft, monotone, neutral gray.

It turned out that the building, which was to reflect the latest word in the psychological study of attention, produced results that were in utter contradiction with what had been expected. It was generally and universally acknowledged by students and teachers that the surroundings not only did not contribute to stimulating attention, but, on the contrary, acted as a depressant, and even in the most interesting lectures and classes, absolutely none of the students could keep from falling asleep no more than a few minutes after having assumed a fixed and attentive attitude.

Obviously, the lack of foreign stimuli proved destructive to the act of attention, and the relationship that has been established by physiologists turns out to be true for psychologists as well, since the act of attention apparently requires certain subdominant stimuli by means of which it may be nourished. In other words, one can be attentive only when stimulations that tend to distract us are reduced to a subordinate position relative to what is our principal concern, though are by no means eliminated entirely from the field of our consciousness, instead continuing to have an effect upon us.

Psychologists have long known how great is the effect of orientation on our overall system of functioning, which, in terms of the thrust and content of lessons, students may not even take notice of, and may have to remain unaware of, while at work. Even if the color of the walls in a room are changed from blue to yellow, a person who is involved and absorbed in some activity, whether speaking, reading, or writing, will have no idea at all as to this change, even if it is now possible to find objective manifestations of the changes that have occurred in the altered nature of his activity. A person will speak differently if surrounded by blue walls than if surrounded by yellow walls.

Meumann has been able to demonstrate that the process of memorization occurs best not in absolute and deathly silence, but in lecture halls where muffled and barely audible noise reaches one's ears. Practical experience long ago established the stimulating influence of weak, rhythmic stimuli on our attention. Immanuel Kant wrote of a remarkable psychological case of an attorney who had the habit, while making complicated legal speeches, of playing with a long thread, holding it all the time in his hands in front of him. An attorney for the opposing side who had observed this little weakness of his, made off with this thread without being noticed, and, according to Kant, by this cunning move, entirely deprived his opponent of the ability to present a coherent argument, or, more properly, the capacity for psychological attention, since, in making his presentation, the attorney now jumped from one topic to another.

Titchener established that voluntary or secondary attention arises out of a conflict between involuntary or primary forms of attention and associated nascent, though incompatible motor stances. Thus, the mechanism of struggle for the total motor field underlies attention and, in general, all the higher, conscious forms of behavior that arise out of biological necessity, as a tool for the solution of conflicts between reactions and as a means of conferring a unity on behavior.

The pedagogical conclusion that follows thereby complicates even further the teacher's problems, requiring him to not only guide the basic task the student is now entrusted with, but also all those extraneous circumstances expressed in the student's orientation, attitude, school uniform, even the scenes he sees out the window, which, as subdominant excitations, are far from neutral in the general work of attention. One writer has declared that, for a Russian, everything depends on orientation, a Russian will inevitably be the tough guy in a bar and will be entirely incapable of doing evil when surrounded by severe and austere architecture. This observation is, undoubtedly, of the same order, though expressed only in rough and overstated form.

The Overall Function of Attention

To characterize the pedagogical value of attention in its entirety, it is necessary to point to the integral, holistic character that distinguishes it. Without exaggeration, absolutely every aspect of the picture of world we perceive and every aspect of our own view of ourselves depends on the functioning of attention. In this regard, attention when altered slightly at once changes the picture radically, without, however, producing any sort of physical changes in the environment around us.

To illustrate this result, one usually refers to figures that reveal the existence of fluctuations of attention in graphic ways. If a square is drawn inside another square, and the figure constructed in such a way that lines connecting the vertices of both the squares have been drawn in, and if we then look at this figure, focusing on it as long as possible, the figure will seem to possess three distinct views, depending upon the fluctuations in our attention. At times it will seem to us that the front plane is represented by the small square and that what we have before our eyes is a truncated pyramid with its small base turned towards us. But no matter how hard we try to keep our eyes in this position, after several minutes our switched attention will show us the same picture, but in reverse perspective. It will look like a room or a box that is receding from us, with the large square now in the foreground, and the smaller square misinterpreted as being foreshortened, as four walls receding far off into the distance. Finally, in the third view, the entire figure is turned towards us with its own true side and appears to entirely lie in one plane, as one square inside another square.

Whereas in this case we are dealing with a natural fluctuation of attention and, accordingly, natural changes in the picture we perceive, the same holds true whenever we cause our attention to switch by artificial means, and, accordingly, alter the pattern of the environment as perceived by us. To look at one and the same object with attention directed differently means to see it in an entirely new view.

An observation of extraordinary importance for psychology was made when it was noted how wondrous and unusual is the picture we get of an ordinary and familiar room or some spot if we throw our head down and suddenly look at it from an entirely novel point of view. Thus, there is a degree of psychological truth in that popular tale of the sage who declared that the human soul that has migrated after death to other bodies lives in another world: "You see the world once as a merchant," he said to his fellow citizens, "you see it another time as a seafarer, and the very same world, with the very same ships, will seem to you to be something entirely different."

Attention and Apperception

As a result of the prolonged functioning of attention proceeding constantly in the same direction, all of our experience is formed and develops in this very same direction. This phenomenon has been termed *apperception*. By this term, we understand all the preliminary elements of experience that we bring to external perception and which defines the way in which a new object is perceived by us.

In other words, apperception denotes nothing less than the participation of our previous experience in the formation of current experience. If, in looking at objects lying in front of me, I not only see and am conscious of their sensible qualities, their color, shape, and so on, even though these qualities act on me by virtue of the direct force of the things lying in front of me, I possess, above all, a vivid idea that this is a hat, this is a briefcase, this is an ink-well, and so on, all of which occurs by virtue of this very same act of apperception, i.e., by virtue of already accumulated experience and of previous acts of attention.

Apperception may be likened quite properly to a railroad switch by means of which a train is transferred from one track to another. If the course of our thoughts and perceptions is determined wholly by the order of the objects in front of us, on the one hand, and by the laws of our associations, on the other, it would be correct to liken the decisive role played by both these factors to the tracks that guide the movement of our psyche. But the free activity of our apperception and our attention also functions like a switch that makes it possible for thinking to select one of a set of possible paths. Thus, attention is properly defined as the relative freedom of our behavior, as the freedom to choose and to limit ourselves.

Apperception, thus, would appear to be the accumulated capital of attention. But, in turn, it accumulates and forms a new reserve of our behavior, which has long since been referred to as *character*. Thus, the stages in this three-level formation of experience exist in the following sequence: attention, apperception, character.

For the teacher, this means nothing less than an even greater role for attention in education, since now attention is considered not as a means of facilitating a particular educational or classroom activity, but proves to be extraordinarily important as an end in itself. It never functions without leaving a trace, rather every time it leaves behind it a result. The set of results is collected into apperception, which strives to guide our behavior. Character is formed by the collection of apperceptions working together, which the subtlest educational measures are powerless to overcome. Thus, by guiding attention we take in our hands the key to the formation and the development of personality and character.

Chapter 8

REINFORCEMENT AND RECOLLECTION OF REACTIONS

Concept of the Plasticity of Matter

Plasticity constitutes one of the fundamental and primitive properties of every form of matter. Every substance is more or less plastic, i.e., possesses the capacity to change and vary the structure and relative position of its molecules under the effect of various types of influence and to retain the imprints of these changes. Iron, wax, air, all are plastic, but are subject to such influence to varying degrees and retain the imprint of these influences to varying degrees. These phenomena reach deeply into the primary properties of every form of matter and are rooted in processes that are inherent to inorganic nature. Thus, one could say that the roadway recalls how wheels have traveled on it, since it retains the impression of those changes in the relative position of its molecules that were produced as a consequence of the pressure of the wheels. In this sense, one could also say that rocks and plants remember. Thus, plasticity may be taken to mean the following three properties of a substance: (1) the capacity for its molecules to alter their relative position; (2) the capacity for it to retain the imprints of these changes; and (3) the predisposition to the repetition of these changes. Thus, the ruts produced in the roadway help to create a new path for the wheels, just as a sheet of paper that has been folded in the right place possesses the tendency to repeat the bending at the very same place when the merest effort is made. Our nerve matter is, in all likelihood, the most plastic of all the forms of nerve matter known in nature. Consequently, it can develop like nothing else the capacity to undergo changes and to store the imprints of these changes and a predisposition to these changes, which is what constitutes the foundation of memory.

Psychological Nature of Memory

When we speak of memory, in the ordinary understanding of the meaning of this term, we have in mind two entirely different processes. Even the old psychology distinguished two types of memory, *mechanical memory* and *logical* or *associative memory*. By mechanical memory was understood the capacity of the organism to preserve the imprint of multiply repeated reactions, and to generate the appropriate changes in the nerve pathways. This process psychologists likened quite properly to tracks in a roadway, and spoke of the "patterning" of tracks as the foundation for the accumulation of individual experience. The sum total of personal habits, skills, movements, and reactions that are accessible to us constitutes nothing less than the result of such a process of forming patterns. A multiply repeated movement seems to leave an imprint in the nervous system and facilitates the passage of new sensations through the same pathways.

The value of such patterning of nerve pathways may be established most easily by means of a rather simple experiment with a chronoscope, a special clock used in psychology to measure the rate of a reaction that is accurate down to 0.001 part of a second. Let us try to measure how long it takes to respond to some number that follows a given number. For example, a subject who is shown the number "17" would have to call out "18." Then suppose the experiment is so arranged that the subject must respond to a number presented to him by calling out, not the next number, but the preceding number, i.e., in this case he has to call out "16." It turns out that the former case requires one-third less time to respond than in the latter case. This is because the reaction is this much more habitual for the organism and is performed along patterned paths, whereas the act of responding in reverse order is less habitual for the nervous system and is more difficult to perform; the greater time needed for the reaction to run its course is an objective indicator of this degree of difficulty.

Associative memory is the other form of memory. The study of associations has long been the foundation of psychology, numerous psychologists referring to every relationship between, or combination of, reactions as an association. But it is always only an association of representations that is the general concern. Meanwhile, we would be equally justified in speaking of an association formed by absolutely every movement. Thus, by the term, *association*, we will understand a relationship between reactions in which the approach of one reaction inevitably causes the other to appear. In its simplest form, the study of associations anticipated the study of conditioned reflexes, which are basically a special case and variety of associations. We would be correct in thinking of conditioned reflexes as an instance of incomplete association in which a relation is formed not entirely between two reactions, but rather between the stimulus of one reaction and the responding part of the other reaction. Psychologists have distinguished three types of association, by analogy, by contiguity, and by contrast. There is no real need for such distinctions, since they express more of a logical distinction in the course of our thinking than a psychological feature that might be distinctive of every process. The old psychology always knew that the establishment of an association depends on experience, and that association denotes nothing less than a nerve-based relationship between reactions that is formed on the basis of a relationship given in experience. Thus, the old psychology also knew that the entire wealth of personal behavior arises out of experience.

Of considerable interest in this connection are psychological experiments involving the comparison of the two types of memory for the purpose of determining which is the more essential and useful; in these experiments, identical and uniform material was learned in two distinct ways, first by means of mechanical repetition, and second by establishing a logical relationship between the elements learned. Then a comparative evaluation of the rate of success of each method was carried out, and the experimenters were able to show that logical memory is related to mechanical memory, quantitatively, as 22 is related to 1. In other words, experimental investigation demonstrated that, all other conditions being equal, material is assimilated and recalled 22 times better and more successfully if memorization is done by a logical technique, by drawing connections between the newly studied material and material previously assimilated.

The simplest way of reproducing the experiment would be to take 100 words of approximately equal difficulty that have been chosen in advance, and to present them to subjects either verbally or in writing separated by given intervals of time, and then count how many words the subjects recalled after a single reading. With words of average difficulty, usually only around 10 words are recalled, and not even in the correct order or sequence. Next a second series, also of 100 words, and of the same degree of difficulty, is presented with the same pauses between the words, through this time the subject is asked to select in advance a collection, again of 100 words, that he knows well, in which the order of the words is familiar to him. For example, geographic names, the names of his friends by grade, the names of relatives, of historical figures, of authors, and so on are all well known in terms of their sequential order. The subject is then asked to establish an association between every one of the given words and each of the words in the selected system that occurs at the corresponding spot in the sequence.

For example, suppose that a series of Russian authors from Lomonosov to Mayakovskii is selected as the basis; the first word presented to the subject, say *ryba* [fish], is matched with Lomonosov; the subject searches for a relation between the two words and finds it in the fact that Lomonosov was the son of a fisherman. A relation is similarly established between the second name and the second word, and so on. Now it usually turns out that the subject is able to reproduce all 100 words presented to him in the correct order, from the first word to the last word, and from the last word to the first word, to recall a word given its position in the sequence and, given a word, to recall its position. All 100 words are recalled without any difficulty and are retained in memory in full and in exactly the right order; if, nevertheless, there are some mistakes, these will usually not amount to more than 2 or 3 out of the entire series. This experiment makes it clear that to recall denotes, for all intents and purposes, either one of two different processes, either the simple drilling in of a reaction, the patterning of a pathway, or it may denote the repeated establishment of a new relation between something that had already been learned earlier and has to be learned anew. It is this latter case that is of especial importance to the teacher. Pedagogical conclusions must be drawn for each form of memory separately.

Structure of the Process of Memory

What we usually call memory does not in the least constitute something uniform, but, in fact, incorporates a series of complex components. According to the old psychology, there were four such components, the first of which was referred to as the actual consolidation of a reaction, i.e., the presence of a nerve trace from a given sensation. For all intents and purposes, this component was viewed as probably inherent to absolutely every sensation that passes through our brain.

The investigation of the subconscious sphere of our dreams, fantasies, and so on has shown that none of the representations and impressions that we perceive vanishes without a trace, rather everything seems to be stored somewhere in the realm of the subconscious and reaches consciousness anew, though with an altered structure. There is a famous story often told by psychologists about an illiterate woman who, when delirious, began to recite lengthy quotations from ancient Greek and other ancient European languages she had no knowledge of. It turned out that, before her illness, the woman had worked for a priest, as a servant, and, while sweeping the rooms, overheard the priest reading the Bible in these languages, though never actually listened to him, however. In her normal state, of course, she could never repeat even a single word of the priest's, to this extent the traces of these sensations were inconsequential and weak in her. However, she had nevertheless retained them in her memory, and they proved to be strong enough to emerge and manifest themselves in her delirium. This example shows that no sensation that reaches our nervous system vanishes, everything is retained and, under certain conditions and in certain circumstances, may be recalled.

By virtue of the second component of the process of memory, a subject will recall a learned movement or utter a desired word in response to a given signal. Thus, if a subject reads some poem out loud several times, keeping the book in front of him and his eyes on the page, the moment when these reactions are recalled will be understood to refer to the moment when these reactions are able to emerge from the subject in the absence of the corresponding stimuli, i.e., when the poem can be recalled in the absence of the book. But we are perfectly well aware that no reaction is possible in the absence of stimuli, consequently the act of recollection, which denotes, basically, a reaction, is always also in need of particular stimuli for its appearance. What, then, will serve as these stimuli in this case? Obviously, it all comes down to the fact that the process whereby the reaction is recalled is subordinated to an internal stimulus as its basic impetus. All the various parts of the recollected reactions are then linked up so that the response to one reaction serves as the stimulus of a succeeding reaction. This may be seen quite easily in the rather simple example when we have forgotten a line in a poem. When we then start to read the poem from the very beginning, the preceding line itself then reminds us of the missing line. Thus, the second component involves the formation of a relation between an inner stimulus and a given group, between a reaction, on the one hand, and the individual members of a group, on the other.

The third component in the process of memory is the moment of "recognition," the moment when we become aware of a recollected reaction as of something that has already happened. In this case, what happens is that a new reaction is adjoined to a recollected reaction, this new reaction seeming to identify the recollected reaction as something that happened before. Finally, in last place is a component that basically constitutes an entirely new reaction all over again, that is, the moment of localization, i.e., finding the place and time and a relation between circumstances in which the given reaction occurs. It should be perfectly clear to us why each of these components may exist entirely separately from all the others. That is, entirely distinct types of memory activity are involved here.

Types of Memory

For a long time memory was thought of as a general property of the nervous system that functions the same way in everyone. Subsequently, observation demonstrated that in each individual person, memory functions roughly in accordance with a particular type, depending on which forms of those reactions the person makes use of in his own life have occurred the most frequently. Psychologists began to distinguish between several types of memory, and began to speak of *visual memory* whenever a person is most likely to make use of his own visual reactions or recollections. In a similar vein, psychologists have established the phenomena of *auditory memory* and *motor memory*, and also speak of mixed forms of memory, e.g., *motor-visual, auditory-visual,* and other forms of memory. This difference between the various types of memory may be made most obvious using the last example, where we spoke of learning a poem by heart. People with different types of memory will learn the same poem in the most diverse ways. One person may find it easiest to memorize a poem by reading it out of a book, silently. He will assimilate it through his eyes and, subsequently, in reciting it, will recall on what page it was written. Some people may be able to point out, ten years later, in what corner of the page in a book a particular word may be found—it is this which the term, "visual memory," denotes. Others have no choice but to listen to a particular poem they wish to learn by heart, they learn easiest by ear, and in their reading of a poem it may strike an observer that they seem to be listening to the inner sound of a word and will recall the intonation with which it had been uttered, the timber of the voice, and so on. A curious feature is that when the former type of individual is involved in reciting something, he will screw up his eyes and will seem to be scrutinizing, whereas when a person belonging to the latter type tries to recall something he will engage in movements that recall the act of listening. It is said of Mozart that, like all other great musicians, he possessed an astounding auditory type of memory. At the age of 14, he only had to hear a complex symphony once and this would be sufficient for him to recall it from memory.

Finally, the third type of memory is that of memorization, not through the eyes or the ears, but through natural movements involving muscular and kinesthesia sensations arising thereby. In learning this same poem by heart, people whose memory is of this type will inevitably have to write it out, or will have to say it to themselves, even if silently. When trying to recall something they have forgotten, they will produce motor speech reactions, and the very act of recollection will occur at the very tip of their tongue or right on their lips. We say that a word is "on the tip of our tongue" or, when trying to recall the spelling of some word, we entrust the task to our hand, the movement of our hand and of our fingers bringing to mind the spelling of the word.

Bear in mind that each of the individual types of memory is encountered only very rarely in pure form, for the most part the various types occur in mixed form, with no one type of memory causing another type to cease functioning. On the contrary, these other types may be utilized as the occasion arises. But the pure neutral type, i.e., the memory that operates equally well in all three types, is just as rarely encountered. Usually, two of the three types of memory are present in combined form and together hold sway and are dominant. The choice of type of memory apparently derives from a whole series of reasons, though principally from the overall structure of our perceiving organs and the method of recollection the individual is most accustomed to.

The pedagogical conclusions that may be drawn from the study of the different types of memory reduce to the rule that the teacher make use of a variety of different paths for the purpose of training memory. The greater the diversity of paths a particular reaction is guided along in its entry into the nervous system, the more firmly will it be retained. The best method is to apply all the different techniques of recall one after the other, as, for example, in studying a foreign language, where students will see a word written out in front of them, will hear it pronounced, will repeat it to themselves and will write it out—thus is accuracy and ease of assimilation ensured. Nevertheless, it is useful for the teacher to recognize the type of memory each student possesses and to resort to just this type as often as possible.

Individual Features of Memory

Like all other forms of behavior, the reinforcement and recollection of reactions does not constitute something unchanging, but varies strongly depending upon age, sex, and features particular to the individual. In particular, memory tend to be distinguished in terms of rate and strength of recall. James compares the memory of different people to wax and jelly, since in both cases a desired impression is obtained quickly and easily thanks to the plasticity of matter, but whereas wax retains an impression, in the case of jelly any impression fades as quickly as it is created. Moreover, memory varies in terms of volume, i.e., number of reactions reinforced, in terms of duration, i.e., length of time reactions are retained, in terms of accuracy, and so on. These aspects are far from being of equal significance in all the different types of reinforcement.

It is sometimes important for us to obtain prolonged recall, though not one that is especially precise, while at other times, on the contrary, it is necessary for us to possess a capacity to recall that is as accurate as possible, though not especially prolonged. It is especially important for the teacher to always be cognizant of precisely which form of recall he envisions obtaining on the particular occasion, since, as we will see below, it is this which governs the character and results of recall.

Memory does not develop in children all at once, and in the earliest stages the child is, as Stern puts it, a being that exists in the present. Memory begins to develop in children somewhat later on, though immediate recall nevertheless proves to be more elusive in children than in adults. After performing an experimental investigation of memory involving the recollection of meaningless syllables, Ebbinghaus found that, from the age of 8 to 10, children can recall only two-thirds as many syllables right after having heard them as can teenagers 18-20 years old. Analogous results were obtained by Binet in an investigation of the memory of students in three grades in school. The responses produced by students in the lowest grade were incorrect 73% of the time, those produced by students in the middle grade were incorrect 69% of the time, and those produced by students in the highest grade were incorrect 50% of the time. According to all the results, memory should be thought of as growing and developing in childhood, reaching its high point at the age of 25, according to Meumann, but thereafter beginning to slowly diminish.

Limits of Memory Training

The question naturally arises whether it is possible to improve the nature and force of human memory through educational measures. Since memory is based on the well-known plasticity of our nerve matter, it goes without saying that the natural forces of memory cannot be increased or decreased in any way other than through methods that lead directly to the attenuation and renewal of the nervous system. Severe anemia, the presence of intoxicants in the organism, and an overall slackness of the nervous system are associated, obviously, with an attenuation in memory just as every form of nourishment, amplification, and reinforcement of the nervous system restores memory. It is for this reason that James, for example, is absolutely certain that the natural qualities of our memory cannot be improved by any sort of exercises.

There can be little doubt, however, that recall may be easily improved by means of exercise and education. Meumann found that, as a result of several weeks of exercises involving the recall of meaningless syllables, one of his subjects, who had initially required 56 repetitions in order to recall 12 syllables, after the exercises needed only 25 repetitions, while a second subject who had at first required 18 repetitions, after the exercises could recollect after only 6 repetitions. Recall is an activity and, as such, it may be improved through exercise, for example, special habits and skills for recall may be developed. Indeed, the first step in the training of memory is precisely to improve recall. Moreover, memory may always be improved and strengthened in particular ways, though this does not denote an increase in the natural capacity of memory. Recall that, psychologically speaking, memory denotes a relationship that may be established between a pair of reactions. The greater the quantity of associations we possess, the easier it is for us to establish a new association and, consequently, the higher the quality of our special type of memory.

It should be noted that what has previously been thought of as memory constitutes a complex and aggregate form of behavior, beginning with a simple reaction and ending in complex mental reflexes. Accordingly, by means of special exercises we can improve both individual aspects of this form of behavior as well as the very fundamental mutual connections between its different parts. It is in this way that a special memory may be developed in man, i.e., the ability to reinforce and recall those types of reactions that prove to be, first, the most vitally necessary and, second, the ones that are the most frequently exercised. We can always rouse the memory of a librarian who knows tens of thousands of books from their cards and knows the place of each of them on the shelves, or the memory of a pharmacist for all his test tubes and measuring cups, or the memory of a physician for the symptoms of a disease. But in all these instances we are dealing with a new phenomenon.

Interest and Emotional Tinge

Investigations of memory have demonstrated that memory functions best and is the most intensive whenever it is attracted and guided by a particular interest. We learn best that which we look upon with the greatest of interest. We may think of interest as internal attraction, an attraction that guides all our efforts in the investigation of an object. Psychologists are quite correct in comparing the role of interest in recall to the role of the appetite in the absorption of food. Experiments performed on dogs have shown that whenever food intake is accompanied by a strongly stimulated appetite, where the dog's eyes and sense of smell also participate in the process, food intake is associated with rapid secretion of gastric juices and by rapid digestion of the food and its complete absorption. Whenever such preliminary stimulation of appetite is prevented, for example, when food is introduced directly into the dog's stomach through an opening, food absorption occurs slowly and sluggishly, though the food remains just as nutritious. Obviously, appetite plays an enormous role in the sense of preparing the organism for digestion and in stimulating its activity. When learning a new reaction, according to psychologists, interest exerts precisely the same type of preparatory effect on our organism. The reader surely knows the extraordinarily enhancing effect that interest produces in the psyche. Someone without a great capacity for scientific subjects in school and who is unable to learn any sort of rule will prove to be extraordinarily talented and capable in a sphere of activity that stimulates his interest.

It is curious that in real life, say in business or in stamp collecting, a student will be fully capable of engaging in various manipulations or in performing calculations that he was not able to perform when in school. Once his interest has been aroused, he will recall a whole set of geographic names or a collection of pictures, whereas in school he couldn't remember the name of the capital city of any country at all. Above all, here it's all a matter of demanding that interest always be coordinated with recall. If it is the teacher's wish that something be learned well, he should take care to make it interesting. From this point of view, the Tsarist school was counter-psychological, since it was uninteresting in just this way. The other role interest serves is that of a unifying function with regard to all the different elements of the subject matter. Interest creates a permanent direction by serving to accumulate recollections, and, ultimately, is the mechanism of choice, in the sense of selecting impressions and combining them into a unified whole. That recall is oriented towards ends, as a function of interest, is, therefore, of extraordinary importance. Investigations have shown that every act of recall is performed under the guidance of a particular orientation of this process. In their experiments on recall, psychologists refer to this as the *influence of differential orientation*. Experiments have shown that the results of recall depend to an enormous degree on the instructions that are given at the start of the experiment.

These instructions explain to the subject what is required of him, what are the goals that his recollection must aim for, and what sort of tests he will be subjected to afterwards. Accordingly, the instructions produce a whole series of orienting reactions that are expressed in the adaption of recall to the goals of memorization. This is even more convincing proof that memory is only one of many types of activity, that it is a form of behavior.

Aall's experiments demonstrated that the duration of our recall is influenced by the fundamental orientation, i.e., the seeming intention to retain what we have learned for a particular length of time. He told his subjects to learn the material by heart, first warning them that they would be questioned about part of what they will be studying the next day, and about the rest of it four weeks later. All questions relating to both parts of the material were then deferred for four weeks, and the results showed that the children were much better at retaining that which they had been told, when actually learning the material, they would have to recall at this point; they did much worse with material they had been told they would be tested on the next day. Experiments performed by other researchers have demonstrated that, depending upon orientation, the same material may be learned in terms of meaning, without any recall of the individual words, or only by literal memorization, without capturing the meaning of the entire text as a whole.

Hence the need for an extraordinarily important pedagogical conclusion, that students have to be made aware of the point of what they are learning and of the constraints that will be imposed upon the material subsequently. The greatest sin of the Tsarist school was not that there was little that was memorized there, but that memorization was performed in unneeded and fruitless directions, i.e., the point of memorizing something was always to respond to the teacher in an examination, all memorization was adapted only to this goal, and, accordingly, memorization turned out to be unfit for other goals.

The last factor that guides memory is the emotional tinge of what is recalled. Experiments have shown that words that are associated with certain personal experiences are recalled far more often than are emotionally neutral words. Those of Peters and Nemechok, who collected 15,000 responses, showed that elements are retained most often in our memory that are tinged by an emotionally positive reaction. Nothing is so recalled as that which was once associated with pleasure. It is this which expresses the biological striving of the organism to retain and reproduce experiences associated with pleasure. Hence the pedagogical rule which demands a certain degree of emotional concern to guide the presentation of all subject matter.

The teacher must forever take care not only to prepare the appropriate mental powers, but also the appropriate forces of the senses. Do not forget to always stimulate the student's sense if you want something to take root in the student's mind. We often say, "I remember that because it struck me when I was a child."

Forgetting and Incorrect Recall

Forgetting, i.e., the disappearance of those relationships that had become established in us as transient relations, is, in and of itself, a fact of the highest degree of biological and psychological utility, as it is directly responsible for the extraordinarily diverse and flexible forms of our behavior. The ability to forget what is not needed, to discard what is superfluous, to disrupt relations once they have already accomplished their purpose—this ability is just as essential a part of our behavior as is the formation of new relations; there is the well-known aphorism of Themistocles, who, in response to the suggestion to remember, is supposed to have said, "Teach me rather how to forget."

Unfortunately, teachers do not always place a high value on the useful and healthy value of forgetting. They lose sight of the fact that memory is not simply the granary or warehouse of the nervous system to be used for the retention of learned reactions in the form in which they were learned. Rather, it involves a creative procedure of processing perceived reactions, moreover it nourishes all the spheres of our psyche. This demands the wholesome development of the child's memory, in such a way that it not be overburdened with material, with an over-abundance of detail, with an excessive store of trivialities, with recall that goes further than is necessary, and that it not become clogged up.

Otherwise, we lose all power over recall, and it assumes the power to control us, whereas the basic pedagogical rule prescribes that memory assume a subordinate, auxiliary role in our behavior as a whole, and for this to happen it is necessary to banish from memory all those reactions that are not needed and that have become uncoupled. Everything in our memory that we do not make active use of, turns into a harmful and burdensome load, ballast, which the teacher has to expel.

Thus, forgetting is not always an evil, but is sometimes even a blessing, and the business of pedagogical tact is to find those limits within which recall and forgetting could work together and in harmony, like a pair of opposing, though collaborating functions. Incorrect memory, i.e., the establishment of false and unneeded relations and reactions, represents a far greater danger, from the pedagogical point of view. Chekhov's satirical story, "A Horsey Tale," of the family whose last name "sounded like 'horse'" is the best illustration of such instances of incorrect recall. Because of an association or relation that had been established accidentally between the last name "Ovsov" and the word, "horse," when there was a great need to recall this name, it was forgotten, and the most varied words that came from thinking of all the objects associated with a horse would come to mind, though not the last name. That would appear by chance, when the need for it had passed, and this comic misunderstanding occurred because memorization had been established in an entirely different plane from recall. Now, if we wish to avoid such comic mishaps, we must never leave everything to chance and allow accidental associations to form.

The selection of these associations must always be under the teacher's control. And he must always have an eye towards the future activity of recall in which associations between reactions will be discovered out of necessity. It may be said without exaggeration that wherever school learning is not guided by real life, there will always be false and incorrect relations, and though knowledge is acquired, it will remain unused in the course of activity. If we could find a way of using in the course of our behavior all the knowledge we have acquired in school, we would easily confound all the shortcomings of education. But here the tragedy of circumstance is apparent, that our knowledge is formed always at the same time as the mechanism by means of which it is subsequently put to use. In other words, every time we recall something, we have to be cognizant of what use we will make of this something, and accordingly, actually reinforce the reaction. We remember things one way for an examination and another way for life. The entire realm of mnemonics, i.e., of all the artificial systems of recall based on establishing a relation between a desired word and various numbers or other conventional symbols, is one such instance of incorrect recall. In the psychological literature, there is a strongly negative attitude towards mnemonic devices because of their artificiality, complexity, and arduousness.

Meanwhile, the value of these mnemonic rules must be considered as a function of their efficiency and the degree of economy they introduce. Of course, mnemonic schemas are very often entirely haphazard, fragile, and alien, and one should not rely on them as a means of reinforcing reactions. But neither should one forget that, for all intents and purposes, every system of alphabetization, of numeric and conventional ordering, etc. is precisely a mnemonic rule by means of which a series of external signs may be related to inner reactions. The inventors of alphabets, of numerals, and of symbolic syllabaries were great creative thinkers in the realm of mnemonics. Mnemonics is, without doubt, based on the general psychological law of association, upon which all study of reading, writing, arithmetic, language, and so on is, in general, constructed.

Münsterberg is entirely correct when he says that to enrich one's mental life, it is far more essential to know how to easily put together concepts than to posses an extensive store of concepts. The 26 letters of the English alphabet is sufficient to compose all of Shakespeare's plays. Thus, the economic principle of our memory manifests itself in the infinite diversity of those conventional systems by means of which such complex spiritual values as the plays of Shakespeare may be stored and transmitted in concise and convenient form. It's all a matter of how efficiently and how cleverly mnemonics accomplishes this task. Hardly anyone could have any doubt as to the enormous economy of thought the alphabet has created. In popular mnemonic techniques, the complexity of the necessary associations very often do not shorten, but on the contrary, even lengthen the path of recollection. Instead of a single simple path, a mnemonic technique often creates a whole set of roundabout and indirect paths that only hamper recall. The harm of such mnemonic techniques should be perfectly clear.

Psychological Functions of Memory

Memory plays the same role in the overall economy of our psyche that is played by capital in the world economic system. Like capital, it denotes a certain quantity of accumulated goods created not for immediate use, but for subsequent production. In other words, memory denotes the use and participation of previous experience in current behavior; from this point of view, memory, whether at the time a reaction is consolidated or when it is recollected, constitutes an activity in the rigorous sense of the term. In the consolidation of a reaction, this activity is expressed in that artificial orientation to a particular reaction assumed by the organism by virtue of which the reaction is realized under orienting conditions that ensure its consolidation. If we were to suddenly lose our memory, our behavior would assume a fragmentary and uncoordinated character; one day would have no relation to the next, nor one deed to another. Our behavior would constitute, in the full sense of the term, a chaotic mass of uncoordinated reactions without any sort of general pattern.

However, the presence of memory does not, in and of itself, produce any additional benefits for spiritual life, and very often children who are mentally handicapped or who are entirely abnormal are distinguished by phenomenal recall, which, however, since it is not harnessed, remains entirely pointless. Such instances seem like a kind of experiment that has been specially designed by nature for the purpose of demonstrating how little is contained in a single memory. There are imbeciles who can recall thousands of different dates, passages, and so on, but prove to be unable to read any word at all. The most important pedagogical principle is still to relate the work of memory with all the other forms of our activity. We have seen that the process of association, the principal source of our memory, underlies all the major processes of our behavior. It is through association that memory should be linked to all the other aspects of our behavior.

Memory Techniques

Memory constitutes a sphere of activity in which productivity can be evaluated more easily than in any other activity. It is for this reason that pedagogics possesses a whole series of rules for the well-being of memory and for memory techniques. Above all, the requirement that the student learn everything as a whole, so as to grasp the meaning that unites an entire unity, as opposed to studying topics piecemeal, is the fundamental condition of every effort at the reinforcement of complex forms of reactions. Meumann suggests the value of an intermediate method in which an entire topic is subdivided into parts after each of which there is a pause. The content of each of the smaller units is brought together in this way, and the distribution of repetitions becomes extraordinarily important. In fact, repetition is the fundamental method for the consolidation of reactions.

It is of interest, above all, that there is a limit to repetition beyond which it ceases to have any effect, becoming useless and even harmful, since it exhausts the full force of any meaningful reaction, making the material meaningless. The distribution of repetitions is, moreover, extremely important. It is not at all immaterial whether students produce their repetitions one right after the other or with pauses in between one repetition and the next.

The psychological conclusion demands a distribution of repetitions such that some of them should be produced at a later time, separated from the first repetition by a pause. It should also be emphasized that every person has his own customary rate of response, and that any change in this rate, either speeding it up or slowing it down, weakens the force of recall. Finally, rhythm plays a decisive role in the learning process, unifying some of the material, conferring on it a sequential symmetry, and, finally, organizing the various elements into a unified whole. If it is recalled that the entire role of memory reduces to a cohesive activity, it becomes easy to understand the advantages supplied by rhythm, which specifies the form of such cohesion ahead of time.

Recollection of Reactions: Two Types of Recall

The recollection of a reaction constitutes just as much an activity as does reinforcement, being only a later stage of the very same process. In traditional psychology, two types of recall are usually distinguished, the first of which is called *recollective imagination* and encompasses all those instances when reactions reproduce (recollect) everything the organism, in fact, experienced; *creative* or *constructive* or *formative imagination* is recollection that recalls a certain form of experience that was not experienced in actuality. It is precisely the criterion of actuality or reality that makes it possible to distinguish memory from fantasy, reactions of recall from reactions of imagination. Meanwhile, this criterion must be seen as being quite wrong for a number of reasons, for example, there can be no exact recollection of former experience, nor can there be any absolutely exact recollections, recall always denotes a certain reworking of what has been perceived and, consequently, a certain distortion of reality. And conversely, the images of fantasy, no matter how complex they seem to be, always comprise elements, and even relationships, between these elements, that have been borrowed from reality and, thus, there is no essential difference between fantasy and recall. One might instead speak of a quantitative rather than a qualitative difference. The images of fantasy may also be directed towards reality, for examine, when I imagine what will happen tonight, or when, in my imagination, I induce a picture of something I have never seen, say of the Sahara desert—in all these cases imaginative behavior is directed towards objects that are no less real than when I recall the picture of my native city or remember what happened yesterday.

Thus, the only difference between the first set of reactions and the second set lies not in their degree of reality, but exclusively in their relationship to our experience. Some reactions form a realm that was once part of our experience, while others were never part of our experience. No mistake in memory is without basis and haphazard, rather it is always motivated by some extraordinarily important internal impetus. Thus, we now distinguish between recollections that are deliberately distorted, on the one hand, and fantasy, which serves as a cloak for certain undesirable recollections that have passed beyond the threshold of consciousness. In general, it would appear that memory is linked in most intimate fashion to the subconscious, and that it basically comprises aspects of behavior that take shape not only in the realm of consciousness; such are our recollections of childhood, which constitute, as is demonstrated by psychoanalytic study, just such forms of half-fantasy, half-memory.

The Reality of Fantasy

Fantasy, which is usually defined as experience that is contrary to reality, is essentially rooted entirely in the individual's real experience. Investigations of the most complex products of mythological creativity, religious traditions and beliefs, legends, and fantastic imagery and fictions show that a person who is under the greatest stress of some fantasy cannot think of anything he would not have experienced in his own life. When we imagine a fantastic being, a centaur or a siren, of course we are dealing with an image of a half-horse, half-man or an image of a half-fish, half-woman. But the aspect of unreality is found here in the combination of the elements in these images, in their ensemble, while the elements out of which horse and man, fish and woman, are formed are, in and of themselves, given in real experience. No one could ever create a representation that would have absolutely no relation to reality whatsoever. Even such remote and irreal images as the images of angels, the devil, Koshchei [figure from Russian folklore—trans.], and others are basically formed out of more complex combinations taken from a real collection of elements. Thus, every aspect of fantasy is, without exception, rooted in reality. A further source of reality in fantasy can be seen in the system of our internal experiences, chiefly desires and emotions, the course of which is determined by the very combination of real elements into fantastic groupings.

Though fantasy is usually thought of as the most capricious, the most inconceivable, and the most groundless of all forms of behavior, nevertheless it is just as rigorously contingent and just as rigorously deterministic at each of its points as are all the other functions of our psyche. The question only has to do with the fact that the causes responsible for its functioning lie deep within man and often remain undisclosed to consciousness. Hence the illusion of apparent spontaneity and the aspect of *ex nihilo* in the work of imagination. But this is only the result of our ignorance of the motivation responsible for this work; basically, one has only to think of all those desires that remain unsatisfied in life. It is these desires that are the true sources of fantasy, and they are responsible for the second principle of the reality of fantasy. This law may be formulated thus: Regardless of whether a cause is real or unreal, the emotion associated with it is always real. If I cry over the fictitious hero of a novel or if I am frightened of a strange monster that comes to me in my sleep, or, finally, if, in an affected state, I hallucinate a conversation with a brother who is long gone, in all these instances the causes of my emotions do not, of course, exist in reality, but my fear, my grief, my compassion remains an entirely real experience regardless. Thus, fantasy is doubly real, on the one hand, by virtue of the material it comprises, and on the other, by virtue of the emotions associated with it.

Functions of Imagination

From the foregoing, it is not hard to understand that the fundamental function of imagination lies in the organization of those forms of behavior that have not occurred even once in the individual's experience, whereas the function of memory lies in the organization of experience for those forms of behavior which, roughly speaking, repeat what has been experienced before. Accordingly, in imagination we find several functions, each with an entirely distinct character, though these functions are closely related to the basic function of situating behavior in accordance with novel conditions in the environment.

The first function of imaginative behavior may be termed the *sequential function*, and it is of the greatest importance for the teacher. Everything we get to know out of what we have not experienced we get to know by means of imagination; specifically, if we study geography, history, physics or chemistry, astronomy, any science whatever, we are always dealing with the cognition of objects that are not given to us directly in our experience, but which constitute the most important achievement of mankind's collective social experience. If the study of the different subjects is not confined simply to relating anecdotes about these subjects, but strives to penetrate through this verbal shell of their description to their very essence, it must inevitably deal with the cognitive function of imagination and must make use of all the laws governing the activity of imagination.

This means, first, that no single construction of a fantasy should be presented before the teacher has made sure that all those elements out of which the required understanding of the new subject is to be constructed are present in the student's personal experience. If we wish to arouse a vivid picture of the Sahara desert in the student's mind, we must find absolutely every element out of which this picture has to be constructed in his real experience, in rough outline, wasteland, sandyness, vastness, aridity, heat—and all of this has to be brought together, though ultimately everything depends on the student's immediate experience. This, of course, does not mean that each of these elements must be taken directly from immediate perception. On the contrary, much may be borrowed from the student's experience, cultivated and reworked in the process of thinking, though in undertaking the construction of a new type of concept, we must nevertheless first prepare all the material that will be needed for this construction, no matter where it comes from.

This is why familiarity with the student's available store of experience is a necessary condition of pedagogical work. It is always necessary to know the soil and the material which we intend to build on, else we run the risk of putting up a flimsy structure on shifting sands. Therefore, the task of determining how to convey new material that is not part of the student's past experience in the language of his own experience becomes a matter of the greatest concern for the teacher. James presents an interesting example that may serve as a good illustration of what we are speaking of here.

Suppose we wish to tell the class the distance from the earth to the sun. There are, of course, several methods we could use. We could simply tell the students how many versts [Russian traditional land measure equal to 3500 feet—trans.] separate the earth and the sun, though, note, such a method hardly serves the purpose. First, we will obtain as a result a naked, verbal reaction, i.e., a verbal symbol; we will obtain not clear-cut knowledge of the fact we require, but only knowledge of the formula which is denoted by this fact. We would, therefore, not penetrate down to the very essence of the fact. There is a rather striking confirmation of this circumstance. When the value of Soviet currency dropped and children had become accustomed every day to dealing with enormous "astronomical" figures, many teachers noticed that when it was time to talk to children about real astronomical numbers, this produced an entirely unexpected effect. Thus, a little boy who had heard that the length of the earth's equator was 40,000 versts, declared, "But that's so little, that's how many rubles it takes to buy a cup of sunflower seeds." The understanding of large numbers was so compromised in the student personal experience that they could not at all understand why they were working with such numbers when it was a matter of representing vast distances, since they had gotten the impression that these numbers referred to insignificant magnitudes. In every case, even if we get around this adverse impression, it's all the same, any one number, in and of itself, says nothing to a student's imagination except for having been deposited in the student's memory. That teacher is following the most correct path who, in his effort to create a true representation of the magnitude of this distance, takes care to convey it in the child's own language. James presents such an explanation that, speaking both psychologically and pedagogically, is the most reasonable. "Suppose we tell a student, 'Imagine that someone shot at you from the sun, well what would you do?' The student, of course, will say that he would get out of the way. To this the teacher might object that there was not the slightest need to do so, that he could `without any worry lie down and go to sleep in his room, and again get up the next day, live peaceably until he comes of age, learn a trade, reach my age—and only then will the bullet begin to come close to you, and only then will you have to get out of the way.' Thus, you see how great is the distance of the earth from the sun." A picture would be formed in the student out of entirely real events that had occurred in his personal experience, and would lead him to measure the magnitude in units that were entirely accessible and comprehensible to him. The speed of a bullet's flight and the enormous duration of an entire life, by comparison with the moment when one has to get out of the path of a bullet—all this the student knows quite exactly, and a picture constructed on the basis of this material will be entirely rigorous knowledge for him, will, in fact, turn into fact. This example shows what are the general forms imagination has to assume in order to lead to the cognition of reality. Imagination must always proceed on the basis of the known and familiar in order that we understand the unknown and unfamiliar.

The second law of fantasy requires that we take care not only as regards the material, but also ensure that this material be properly coordinated. The law of reality of fantasy asserts that the emotion associated with our construction will always be real. It is, therefore, essential to arouse emotion, and in conveying different representations to a student, we must not only be concerned with the material, but also take care to arouse the appropriate emotion in the student.

The *emotional function* is a further function of imagination; specifically, absolutely every emotion possesses its own definite expression, and not only an external expression, but also an internal expression, and that fantasy is, consequently, the mechanism which directly carries out the work of our emotions. From our knowledge of the struggle for the general motor field, we know that far from all the impulses and desires found in us are satisfied. One might ask about the fate of those nerve sensations that arise entirely naturally in the nervous system, but do not obtain any satisfaction. It goes without saying that they assume the character of a conflict, a conflict between the child's behavior and the environment. Illness arises out of such conflict when the individual is under great stress, expressed in the form of neurosis or psychosis, if, that is, there is no outlet for this conflict, i.e., if it is not sublimated and if it does not turn into any other form of behavior.

This is the reason why sublimation, i.e., the socially higher realization of unrealized potentialities, is also the responsibility of imagination. In games or in lies, or in tales, children find an infinite source of experience, and fantasy reveals itself, thus, as a kind of new door through which our demands and strivings may come to life. In this sense, there is a profound psychological meaning to children's lies; and this is something which the teacher must keep a close eye on.

The emotional function of fantasy imperceptibly assumes a new function in games, that is, the organization of those forms of the environment by means of which the child develops and exercises his natural inclinations. It would appear that the psychological mechanism of games is entirely the work of imagination, and that we could almost draw an equality sign between games and imaginative behavior. Games are nothing less than fantasy in action, and fantasy is nothing less than an inhibited and suppressed, undisclosed game. Therefore, in childhood imagination bears a third, or *educational*, function, the purpose and meaning of which is to organize the child's everyday behavior in such a way as to give it a chance to exercise and develop for the future. Thus, all three functions of fantasy are fully in accord basically with its psychological property, with the fact that it is a form of behavior directed towards forms that have not yet occurred in our experience.

Education of Imaginative Behavior

The usual view is to assume that fantasy seems to be present in the child in a far more vivid and far richer form than in the adult. Such a view is most certainly mistaken in several respects, for example, the fact that, as we have seen, real experiences are the principal source of imaginative behavior. Since the child's reserve of imagery drawn from real life is extremely impoverished, his imagination must, undoubtedly, function weaker and poorer than in adults. Hence, it is clear that imaginative behavior also has need of development and education, just like everything else.

The first task of education in this sense is, as we have already seen, to assign to imagination responsibility for the very same functions as are assigned to memory. That the child's fantasy has yet to become differentiated from his memory is, therefore, a distinctive feature of the child's imagination. Both arise out of the recollection of reactions and both forms merge together in the child, for two reasons. First, all of the child's experience still has the appearance of uncertainty, underdevelopment, and roughness, and, consequently, every act of recollection in a child will be, to some degree, distorted and inexact. Despite all good intentions and despite the best wishes, the child is unable to recall all the details of his real experiences exactly. Everything produces an incidental distortion of needs, depending on whether the child was unaware or, on the contrary, filled in details under the influence of his feelings.

Such filling in of details, such outright lies, will always be present, even in an adult's recollection. Experiments on the testimony of adults and children are highly indicative and instructive in this regard; these experiments have shown that it is impossible to obtain an exact and detailed description from any eyewitness, no matter how carefully he observed the event and no matter how honestly he strives to demonstrate what he saw. Numerous elements which he introduces out of thin air and which he will piously attest to will be present in his testimony. In experiments with children, some picture is usually given or a story is read with various details omitted, and when the children are subsequently asked about this story, they usually fill in details on their own. The same thing happens with adults if they are present at a deliberately created squabble or an incident and are then asked for the details of what happened. It turns out that not only will there be gaps in each person's memory and, consequently, the events will now assume a somewhat distorted form in the testimony of the eyewitnesses, but each of the eyewitnesses will, on their own, fill in details out of things that did not happen and thereby distort the facts.

Such involuntary distortions of our memory manifest themselves particularly clearly in children, and though the psychological nature of the two forms of behavior are the same, nevertheless each has its own special function in real behavior. The teacher's task, therefore, becomes one of constructing as rigorous a segregation of fantasy from reality as possible. Here we find, above all, the struggle against children's lies, which should scarcely be understood in the same way as adult lies, i.e., as offenses against morality.

The child's lie has as its source the inner truth of emotional experience. Children lie, and this is a general law of the child's behavior, even when this lie is not of any benefit for them and is not a necessity for them, by virtue of the fact that their emotional life is overly excited; as a consequence of the fact that passion is, as Sechenov had remarked upon some time ago, the distinctive property of childhood; by virtue of the fact that at this age there has yet to develop in the child any restraining force that would control the child's behavior. The child's fantasy has no knowledge of limits or of self-control, and is highly impulsive in the sense that it obediently realizes every one of his emotional desires. Therefore, the child will quite often relate not what, in fact, happened, but what he would have liked to have, in fact, seen. Thus, nothing so reveals the child's desires, strivings, and wishes as does the child's lie. James is entirely correct in calling the child's lie, a "sincere deception," and Hall emphasizes that the child's lie is, chiefly, fantastic and heroic and, rarely, self-centered. In fact, every lie produced by a child has its source in the child's over-emotional state, the child naturally strives to exaggerate the emotional weight of an event, to make everything that happens seem "heroic" in accordance with his heightened passions. There are other childhood lies that are direct echoes of desires, as also happens in adults; the child lies just as unconstrainedly and just as naturally as he dreams. Every childhood lie has to be interpreted and a reason for it found, and only then may we evaluate this act and respond to it correctly. We can say precisely the same thing about childhood fantasy, the child's belief in all those fantastic beings their nurses frighten them with, and his trust in whatever nonsense an adult might happen to say to him.

We will speak of the harm of such fantasizing at length in the chapter on esthetic education. The greatest and most relentless struggle against such underdevelopment of a sense of reality is, therefore, needed, and the education of fantasy must, above all, proceed through the development of a respect for reality. It is necessary to foster in the child the greatest respect for reality, though by reality we should not understand that little world which surrounds the child. Here we are concerned with the greater reality that surrounds us unless we wish to create a philistine, and conformist. There can be no denying the fact that isolation in the narrow circle of one's most immediate interests creates in the child, and in the adult as well, a narrow outlook, a bird's eye view of life, narrow-mindedness and complacency.

There is no way we can achieve respect for the larger reality unless we go beyond the narrow limits of personal experience, and this can be accomplished by means of imaginative behavior. Consequently, the struggle for reality should denote not the abolition of fantasy, but only that fantasy be kept within its natural banks, in the channel of its own natural functions, and that imaginative behavior be strictly isolated and rigorously defined. In other words, fantasy should be allowed to function, but one must not forget that one is only fantasizing. The danger in imaginative behavior is only that it is capable of reconciling all conflict between reality and dream, which, therefore, presents the danger that real struggle will be avoided and that one will yield to the temptation of resolving every difficult situation in a dream. Extraordinary devotion to dreams will lead us away from the real world, will weaken and paralyze our capacity to exert an active influence on the world, will destroy the capacity to correctly choose the necessary reactions in the organism, and will contribute to the development and survival of socially harmful and fundamentally unstable reactions. As a servant, imagination is extraordinarily useful, but as a master, it is harmful, because, as one psychologist has put it, it is like fire.

Another task of the education of imagination is to develop the positive functions that are the responsibility of fantasy. Children's games form the sphere in which fantasy finds its most complete expression and where it proceeds wholly without overflowing its own natural banks. And not only does it not undermine the sense of reality in the least, but, on the contrary, it develops and exercises all those skills and reactions that tend to develop this sense. We all know how infinitely varied are the roles that different objects may assume in children's games. The room may serve now as a forest, now as the deck of a ship, now as a lounge, one and the same chair may, with equal success, stand for a horse, a train, and a dining table. But a game is entirely without risk in that, though it excites entirely real emotions and reproduces entirely real elements of the environment, it nevertheless remains, frankly speaking, a game, and does not draw the child away from life even to the slightest, but, on the contrary, develops and gives the child practice in those capacities that will be needed in life. Interestingly, games are so strongly associated with fantasy that children prefer simple and crude toys to expensive and elaborate ones that leave no room for their fantasy and that require the greatest caution when they become part of playful activity. An expensive toy requires a passive attitude on the child's part and is not an object that could serve as good material for the development of fantasy. Gaupp writes that in no other period of his life, does the child learn as much as in the years of children's games.

It is not without reason that Kornilov took as the epigraph to his study of the psychology of children games with dolls the words of Rabindranath Tagore. "'How did I get to where you found me?' asked the baby of its mother. She answered, half-crying, half-laughing, pressing the little one to her breast, 'You were hidden in my heart in the guise of a desire, my darling. You were present in the dolls of my children's games.'"

Chapter 9

THINKING AS AN ESPECIALLY COMPLEX FORM OF BEHAVIOR

The Motor Nature of Mental Processes

Thinking is among the most difficult and least worked out of all psychological problems. It is only recently that psychologists have undertaken the study of these questions and have attempted to comprehend all the specific features of these questions by experimental techniques, and thus it can now be distinguished from all other forms of behavior. Until the most recent decades, the dominant conviction was that thinking constitutes, basically, only a combination of ordinary associative processes, of the highest and most complex order, i.e., that it is a simple relation of verbal reactions.

However, careful self-observation performed under experimental conditions and subject to precise measurement has already demonstrated that the composition of a mental event is incomparably more complex and that it encompasses numerous components that are inherent to it alone. It is because of these components that thinking cannot be reduced to the simple and free flow of images. In parallel with these subtle self-observations, suggested and developed chiefly by the Würzburg school of psychology, studies have also been made of the motor nature of mental processes, i.e., the perception of those objective manifestations of thinking that are accessible to external check and assessment. Both types of investigation have arrived at the same results, though from different directions, and both have led to a new approach to the study of thinking from which present-day psychology proceeds, as if from a starting point.

That aspect of thinking by virtue of which it comes to be viewed as part of behavior, as an ensemble of the organism's motor reactions, is, above all, perfectly clear to the psychologist of today. Every thought associated with movement induces on its own a certain preliminary straining of a corresponding muscular system that tends to be expressed in movement. If it remains only a thought, then since this movement is not brought to fruition and is not fully disclosed, it remains concealed in an entirely tangible and effectual form.

The simplest observations show that a powerful thought about an impending action or deed manifests itself quite incidentally in posture or gesture, as if it was a preliminary and preparatory effort we intend to carry through. In a very simple experiment, a subject was asked to sit down in between two objects of some kind with his eyes shut, one object to his right and the other to his left. He was asked to think hard of either one of these objects. If he was conscientious in doing what he had been asked, he usually did not have to make any special effort to move his eyeballs beneath his eyelids, or to strain his neck muscles in order to correctly guess precisely which object to think of. The movement of the subject's eyes and the straining of his muscles always occurred in the direction his thinking was aimed at. They seemed to betray the hidden thought, making it possible to guess it with unfailing accuracy, as if we were reading.

In another experiment of the same type, usually carried out in a school setting, a subject had to hold a weight suspended from a thread in one hand with his eyes shut, and to try to imagine that the weight is swinging from right to left. After several minutes, the result is that the weight is actually set in motion, moreover, in precisely the direction being thought of, though the subject himself usually has no awareness of the movements he is producing. He continues to claim he is holding his hand perfectly immobile, indeed, that the movements are occurring not through the "voluntary" efforts of his hand, but basically involve his fingertips, which is where he holds the thread. These extremely subtle movements could remain, in fact, imperceptible to the subject himself.

The technique of reading the thoughts of other people, a technique that psychologists borrowed from conjurers and stage performers, but which, like must else, derives from the stage, has gained entirely indisputable recognition and meaning for science. Essentially, in this technique one of several people is given the task of thinking of a more or less complex movement or series of movements, for example, playing a note on the piano, taking an object from one of several hundred people present and giving it to someone else, writing down a desired word, carrying an object about, opening the window, and so on. As a control, the instructions are usually first written down on paper. The mind reader usually suggests to the subject whose thoughts are to be read that he think as hard and as intensely as possible, as if to stimulate his thinking, and then carries out what the subject is thinking of by means of simple operations, usually without making any mistakes and without any problem. There usually occurs a kind of process of comparison with the subject's muscles that is quite reminiscent of genuine reading, i.e., the perception of a system of known external signs that can be interpreted subsequently in terms of their true meaning. The reader usually places his hands on the subject's shoulders, has him stand in front of him, and determines, without any difficulty, the direction in which the planned action is to be carried out. If he moves in the wrong direction, he brushes against the resistance of the subject's muscles, and, conversely, once the required direction has been ascertained, the subject's muscles betray an obvious compliance, as if in agreement with the actions to be performed. In precisely the same way, his muscles betray him at the moment he stops or turns around because this compliance of his muscles ceases, and the reader decides to turn around or stop from a series of new guiding movements.

By means of such palpitation and fingering of stressed groups of muscles, the reader recognizes precisely what sort of movements the subject's muscles are getting ready for, and usually arrives at extraordinarily complete and complex forms by working out these techniques in detail. We need only note that, by means of this technique of muscular contact, an entire piece can be played on the piano, a complex arithmetic operation written out, or objects passed around a crowded theater. In all these cases, we are dealing with a genuine muscular reading that fully justifies the claim of one American psychologist that we think with our muscles. By this the psychologist only wished to say that absolutely every thought is realized, to one degree or another, in muscular tension, and that absent such muscular movement, thought does not exist.

It is remarkable in this connection that the stronger and the more focused the thought, the clearer and more complex is its motor character. The person who is thinking hard is not content with those silent words that he says to himself. He will begin to move his lips, sometimes beginning to whisper, and at times will begin to loudly talk to himself. Actors are well aware that a monologue justifies itself psychologically, in the sense of constituting a preliminary acting of a scene when in deep and intense thought. This mood of thoughtfulness on its own then turns imperceptibly into loud speech. Usually, this is noticeable in children who are absorbed in the solution of some difficult problem, and begin to help their thoughts along with their lips, their forehead, cheeks, and tongue all beginning to take an active part in carrying out the operations of addition and subtraction.

All those phenomena of automatic writing that have engaged the interest of countless observers at so-called spiritualistic seances belong to this group of observations. That in all those efforts to summon the souls of departed ones we are dealing with the undoubted existence of automatic writing, something even the participants at the seances remain unaware of, is hardly open to doubt after all the careful tests carried out by numerous scientists. But the very same motor nature of our thoughts manifests itself here, as may be discovered also by means of the simplest experiments. During the most smoothly running seance, one need only ask the "spirit," i.e., basically, the participants in the seance themselves, a question they hold divergent opinions about, or a question the participants hold obviously false ideas about, in order to obtain, in the former instance, a confused and contradictory answer, and in the latter instance, a clearly false answer.

If you were to first tell the participants that your wife died in Canada two years ago, even though she is in good health and living in Europe, you may be certain that, in response to your question about your wife, the spiritualist table will tap out the words, "Canada" and "death" to you. Countless experiments of this type have shown that the answers are directly dependent upon the expectation that has been prepared and put into effect. The very course of a spiritualistic trance involves nothing less than an extraordinary tension of the muscular system in the fingers and in a permanent numbness of these muscles until the fingers are no longer accessible to our consciousness, becoming, conversely, extraordinarily susceptible to the automatic excitation of thought. The hands of those present at a seance are usually clasped together, so that any trembling or movement begun at one end spreads easily and seems to turn into a general movement.

That every thought of a movement induces that very movement is an instructive truth that has long been established in psychology. In fact, if a perfectly normal person were to be asked to walk on a board lying on the floor in some room, it is likely he would have no difficulty agreeing to such a request, and would perform the experiment without the slightest risk of failure. But just imagine the same board were suspended from the sixth floor of one house to the sixth floor of another, or was placed over a precipice somewhere in the mountains, and the number of safe trips across the board will be quite minimal. The difference between the two cases is explained by the fact that, in the latter case, the traveler will possess an entirely vivid and clear idea of the depth and of the possibility of falling, something which, in fact, happens in nine cases out of ten.

This is also the basis for the psychological value of hand-rails on bridges that have been built across rivers, a device that has also never been explained by psychologists. In fact, almost no one ever notices that the handrails on bridges have saved people from falling, by what is said to be the physical force of their presence, i.e., in case someone walking across a bridge actually tilts, the handrails will return him to a stable position. People usually walk alongside the handrails, nearly touching the rails with their shoulders, without leaning over the handrails in the least. But just remove the handrails or allow people to walk across an unfinished bridge, and accidents will inevitably occur. What is most important is that no one will have the courage to walk that close to the edge of the bridge. The effect of the handrails is purely psychological in this instance. They banish from consciousness the thought or idea of falling and thereby supply an unswerving direction to our movements. This phenomenon is of the same order as vertigo, or the wish to jump when we look down from a great height, i.e., strive to realize the thought, the idea, which grips consciousness at such times especially vividly and powerfully.

This is why the worst of all pedagogical techniques is to insistently and earnestly introduce into the mind of the student an awareness of those deeds he must not do. Telling him, "don't do that," is already an incitement to carrying out this deed, simply by virtue of the fact that it introduces into the student's mind the thought of this deed, and, consequently, the inclination to carry it out.

Thorndike was quite correct in emphasizing the harm of those moral injunctions that are common in textbooks on ethics used in the French secondary schools. The real effect of all those descriptions of unethical actions the teacher would wish his students to avoid only brings to the mind of the student a certain urge and yearning to perform them. This is why, Thorndike concludes, it is extraordinarily damaging to present, as the authors of these textbooks have done, detailed explanations and accounts as to why it is wrong to commit suicide. Literature knows of uncounted examples of those instances and situations when a powerful fear or fright of something induced just that action associated with this apprehension. The fear of Prince Myshkin, in Dostoyevskii's novel, *The Idiot*, that he might break an expensive vase at a ball makes him do just that, with the very sureness of a sleep-walker, i.e., the thought that was in his consciousness all the time was brought to fruition in action. There is no better way of inducing a child to break a glass than to tell him over and over, "Now look, don't break it," or "You'll break it, I'm sure of that."

If we move on to broader and more complex forms of behavior, we are forced to admit that the motor nature of thinking is not confined to this group of facts. Here we find what in psychology have been referred to as *idiomotor acts*, i.e., conceptions of movement that are quickly realized in movement itself. A second group of phenomena of the same type are known as kinesthetic sensations, which have been discovered and developed with especial thoroughness in recent decades, principally by the American school of psychology. Psychologists call *kinesthetic sensations* those sensations and experiences that are associated with the natural movements of various organs in man and that seem to make the individual aware of his own actions. Our entire musculatory system, all our joints and tendons, and nearly all our tissues are permeated down to the deepest layers by the finest nerve branchings. These nerve branching let us know of the movement and position of our organs just as distinctly and precisely as our external organs tell us about the position and movement of objects in the external world. Kinesthetic sensations are nearly always associated with the proprioceptive field we spoke of earlier.

As shown by psychological analysis, these kinesthetic sensations are the most essential aspect of our thinking and even of our volitional acts. In order to perform some movement, the image or recollection of the sensations associated with these movements must first be present in our consciousness. Thus, psychologists are generally in agreement that every voluntary movement must first occur involuntarily in order to induce the appropriate kinesthetic reaction, i.e., the appropriate internal sensation. Only subsequently, through the renewal of this reaction, is it possible for the movement to be repeated in the form of a voluntary act. In that inexpressible and complex structure that determines our thinking about or conception of various objects, the decisive role is played by kinesthetic experiences, which are not localized very accurately, as if internal states unlike all other states, since they actually possess an entirely distinctive nerve character and an entirely distinctive perceptual substance.

The presence of these kinesthetic components in every conscious movement is confirmed by Baier's experiments. Baier trained his subjects to move their ears and to perform other usually involuntary movements by inducing the organ to move by mechanical means, after which a kinesthetic reaction was created that enabled the subjects to perform the particular action thereafter whenever they wished to and at their own initiative.

Finally, the third group of these phenomena belongs to the realm of thinking and conceptions of those objects, things, and relations that, at first glance, seem to be difficult to set in motion. In other words, the difficulty lies in establishing the motor nature of those thoughts that are oriented not towards movement, but, for example, towards a high, four-sided tower, towards a blue light, or towards a heavy weight. However, it is not hard to see that, in these instances as well, we are dealing with a series of rudimentary movements that, though difficult to discover, do exist without a doubt. For the most part, we are dealing with movements of perceptual organs that had once been accompanied by the perception of a particular object. For example, when thinking of something loud or quiet, we carry out in rudimentary fashion the very same movements that are needed to adapt our ears and our head to the perception of similar sounds in real life. When thinking of something round, whether large or small, we realize through the movements of our eye muscles the very same adaptive movements, the very same focusing on objects which we had once perceived in actuality.

Even the most abstract thoughts of relations that are difficult to convey in the language of movement, like various mathematical formulas, philosophical maxims, or abstract logical laws, even they are related ultimately to particular residues of former movements now reproduced anew. Imagine that all your muscles were to become utterly paralyzed, then the total cessation of all thinking would be the natural conclusion. Those internal movements in which thoughts become manifest and that are of the greatest importance in man's behavior form a group of their own. This is the group of the so-called *motor speech reactions*, i.e., suppressed, undisclosed movements of the motor speech mechanism that consist in complex elements of respiratory, muscular, and vocal reactions that collectively form the basis of every thought of the educated person, and which it would be entirely correct to refer to as the *system of internal speech* or *silent speech*.

It is curious that prehistoric man and people at the first stages of civilization identify thought and speech in complete agreement with scientific data, defining thinking as "conversation in one's belly" or, as the Bible puts it, "conversation with one's heart." That thought is a form of conversation, except for being concealed in some internal organ and not brought to fruition, not directed towards anyone, but only intended for oneself, is a definition which is subscribed to by both the savage and the modern scientist equally. This is precisely what Sechenov had in mind when he defined thought as the first two-thirds of a mental reflex, or as a reflex that has been broken down up into two-thirds, having in mind a reflex that is not brought to fruition, that is inhibited in its external aspect.

That this is in fact so is shown by the simplest of everyday observation. Try hard to recall some tune, and you will see that you are singing it to yourself. Try hard to recall the words of some poem, and you will notice that you are saying these words silently, to yourself. This retention of speech in an internal mechanism, this restraint against its complete expression, has acquired an especially extensive and important meaning in human society thanks to the extraordinary complexity of the interrelations that arise there, even at the first stages of culture.

Initially, every reflex manifests itself in utter completeness, in all its constituent parts. There is a complete schema of movement here, with the child first speaking, and then thinking. It is extraordinarily important for the teacher to know that what is, in fact, happening is not what usually seems to be happening, i.e., that the child seems to begin to think, and then learns words in order to express his own thoughts by means of these words. The child's first act of thinking is related to his first, as yet inarticulate, sounds. His thinking has a secondary origin. It arises only when, having suppressed all sound, the child learns to cut short the reflex before the final third and to keep it to himself.

It is extraordinarily important to bear in mind those essential psychological consequences that follow from this observation. It would be a simple matter to distinguish a reflex that seems to have been broken into two-thirds from a complete reflex simply quantitatively, by the fact that it has not been brought to fruition. However, the psychological nature also changes in a radical way, and with it, its biological and social purpose.

If it is true that every thought is speech, it is no less true that inner speech differs from outer speech by its very psychological nature. This difference may be reduced to two fundamental points, first, that in every reflex there seems to be three reference points on which the reflex arc rests and at which there occurs an intense discharge and expenditure of nervous energy. This discharge usually begins in some peripheral organ, due to an external impetus or sensation, a beam of light, a gust of air, etc. It is then processed in the central nervous system and in a peripheral responding effector organ.

Psychologists have succeeded in establishing that the expenditure of energy in the central nervous system and in the working organ are in inverse relation. The more intense and the greater the expenditure of central nervous energy, the less intense and weaker is its external manifestation and, conversely, the more intense the external effect of the reaction, the weaker the central component. The organism seems to have available to it a certain reserve of nervous energy, and every reaction seems to be performed within a given energy budget. Every effort and every complication of the central component is compensated by an attenuation of a corresponding movement of some working organ. The principle has been termed by Kornilov the *principle of unipolar expenditure of energy*; it was arrived at on the basis of rigorous experiments performed on various types of reactions.

Kornilov's experiments basically involved measuring the quantity of energy expended in a reaction as the principal mental act was made gradually more complicated. The subject was asked to respond to the ringing of a bell by pressing a button; he was then asked not to respond until he recognized a ringing that he had been asked to listen to previously, before the start of the experiment. Next he was asked to respond to one bell with his right hand, and to another bell with his left hand. In other words, a mental process of recognition, discrimination, and choice was interposed in the reaction between the moment the sensation was perceived and the moment the working organ was to produce a responding motion. As has been demonstrated by Wundt's studies, this mental process manifests itself in an increase in the duration of the reaction and, as has been shown by more recent studies, in a drop in its intensity.

In other words, if we are to perform some movement only after we have succeeded in gaining a thorough understanding of the signal or after we have succeeded in choosing between one signal versus another, in these instances our movement will prove to be weaker and less vigorous than whenever we respond immediately after the signal has been given.

The investigation also demonstrated that this decrease in the expenditure of peripheral energy is connected by a rigorous mathematical relation to the overall quantity of energy consumed in the reaction and, thus, may serve as a measure of the energy consumed in a particular mental process. If it is assumed that a subject expended **A** units of energy in response to a simple signal, and **B** units in the reaction of choosing between two signals, then

$$\frac{A - B}{A}$$

will denote that measure of mental energy which, in this instance, is consumed in the act of choosing between two signals.

Even the simplest observations show how difficult it is to combine any sort of intense physical effort with complex mental operations; it is impossible to solve complex problems while running rapidly through a room; it is impossible to concentrate on some thought and, at the same time, to chop wood. Every thought seems to induce a stupor, a numbness, and, by its very nature, paralyzes and halts all movement. This is why a person who is deep in thought always has the appearance of someone who is pausing, and if something startles us, we will inevitably delay our movement. Thus, it has been established that though thought is also a movement, it is also, strangely enough, just as much a delay of movement, i.e., a form of movement in which the complication of the central components of the reaction have attenuated and are inclined to extinguish every external manifestation of movement.

Hence, psychologists have arrived at a conclusion that is, incidentally, extraordinarily important for pedagogics, that the link between mental and physical labor which is assumed as the basis of occupational education can in no way be understood as a simultaneous synthesis of the two. To dig vegetables and, at the same time, listen to a lesson on botany, to plane a board in a woodworking shop and, at the same time, review the law of addition and multiplication of forces -- this, according to Kornilov, means equally distorting the law of the parallelogram of forces and ruining the board. From the psychological point of view, the connection of theory and practice in education should mean nothing less than an orderly and appropriate alternation of the two forms of labor that realizes in harmonious fashion a rhythmic expenditure of energy, first by one pole of our organism, and then by the other.

Rhythm, because it also denotes a higher form of organic activity and life, constitutes, for all intents and purposes, a kind of alternation of movement and rest, and, therefore, ensures that movement will continue unceasingly and will be flawless. From the psychological point of view, rhythm is nothing less than the most ideal form of the synthesis of movement and rest. This is why the tireless muscles of our heart can accomplish their unparalleled and remarkable work simply by virtue of the rhythmic character of the heart beats. It is only because it beats in bursts, resting after each stroke, that the heart can beat unceasingly throughout life. Thus does the rhythm of the educational process become a psychologically essential principle for the theory and practice of the labor school.

As regards the psychological explanation of thinking, this principle of a unipolar expenditure of energy explains that the subdivision of a reflex into two thirds is compensated for by the amplification and complication of its central part, i.e., the processing that every outgoing sensation is subjected to in the central nervous system. Thus, because of the subdivision and suppression of a reflex, i.e., the transformation of an entire reaction into thought, our reaction gains in terms of the flexibility, subtlety, and complexity of its interrelations with the elements of the world, and all our actions may be realized in infinitely higher and subtler forms.

A further difference between thought and a complete reaction is that, since it manifests itself as internal movement exclusively, the reaction forfeits the meaning of reaction in general, i.e., as a given movement directed outwardly, and assumes an entirely new meaning, becoming an internal guide of our behavior. In fact, a loudly uttered word, like every movement of our organism, is always directed towards something outside us and always strives to create or lead to a distinctive shift in the elements of the environment. A reaction that is not fully disclosed, that is resolved within the organism itself, naturally can have no such purpose—either it must become entirely unnecessary, biologically speaking, and atrophy and be obliterated in the course of development together with mental detritus, or it must obtain an entirely new value and new meaning. It is precisely because this reaction is resolved entirely within the organism that it assumes the value and role of an inner guide of our new reactions. The aggregate of our thoughts seem to organize our behavior ahead of time, and if I think first and only then do something, this means nothing less than a duplication and complication of behavior in which the internal reactions of thought initially prepare and adapt the organism, and then the external reactions carry out what had been established and prepared in thought ahead of time. Thought plays the part of an advance guide of our behavior.

Conscious Behavior and Will

Now that the motor and reflexive nature of our thought processes has been established, it becomes readily apparent, that all distinction between the deliberate or conscious type of behavior and the reflexive or instinctive type vanishes. Quite effortlessly, the thought arises that, in this understanding, the human mind and human behavior become subject to a mechanistic interpretation, that the human organism becomes viewed as a robot that responds by means of various actions to various sensations from the environment. And just as Descartes was able to define animals as mobile machines and to deny them any degree of animation or a psyche, so are modern psychologists inclined to understand and interpret man. However, the entire vast difference between human and animal experience provides a vivid refutation of such a view.

In establishing the distinctive features of man's labor, Marx emphasized the extraordinarily important psychological difference between man's labor and the labor of the animal.

From his reasoning, it is quite a simple matter to then move on to an analysis of conscious or deliberate behavior. "The spider," writes Marx, "performs operations that are similar to those of a human weaver, though the cells of wax constructed by the bee would be the shame of any architect. However, there is something that distinguishes the labor of the most skillful bee from the labor of the most least experienced architect. Were a person to construct a cell out of wax, he would first construct it in his mind. At the end of a process of labor, a result is obtained that, even before the start of this process, existed ideally, i.e., in the imagination of the worker". The structure of the spider's web or the cells of a beehive still pertain wholly to forms of instinctive behavior, i.e., the passive adaption of the organism to the environment, which in no way differs from exactly the same mechanism of digestion in the human stomach or intestine. Man's behavior, in fact, encompasses an essentially new component, the preliminary presence in the mind of the results of work, a guiding stimulus of all reactions. Our concern here, quite obviously, has to do with nothing less than a kind of duplication of our experience.

Man's structures differ from those of the spider only by the fact that man builds as if twice, first in his thoughts, and then in real life. Hence the illusion of the conscious and free will. The active person, in fact, has the impression that his deeds seem to have a dual character, first he desires, and then he acts. The illusion is reinforced by the fact that the first component may be broken off from the second and realized independently of it. There is the impression that wishes and desires, free voluntary effort, seem to be entirely independent and are not subordinated to physical movement. I may wish to raise my hand and, at the same time, I may be aware that it is tied down and, consequently, the movement cannot be accomplished. In all these instances, we are dealing with a manifest illusion, the psychological nature of which may be attributed wholly and without exception to the inner role in which our thoughts manifest themselves.

That every one of our reactions may, in its responding part, become the stimulus part of a new reaction is a fact we have encountered repeatedly, for example, in the chain-like mechanism of the instincts. A dog responding to the sensation of meat will produce saliva, though, under the influence of a stimulus that reappears at this site, it will either expectorate or swallow the saliva and, thus, the responding part of the one reflex (production of saliva) becomes the stimulus of a succeeding reflex.

This transfer of reflexes from certain systems to other systems is also the fundamental mechanism that underlies what is known as *conscious will*. A volitional act inevitably presupposes the presence in our consciousness of certain wishes, desires, and strivings associated, first, with the representation of the ultimate goal we are striving towards and, second, with the representation of those deeds and actions that will be needed by us in order to realize our goal. Thus, duality is at the very foundation of the volitional act, and this duality becomes especially prominent and vivid whenever several motives, several opposing strivings, clash in our consciousness.

It is precisely these components of the struggle of motives that, to our self-observation, appear to be the most persuasive direct proofs for the existence of free will. Man never senses himself as free to act on his own as when he confronts several possibilities and actions simultaneously and, as if in a free act of will, makes a choice between them. But in an objective analysis, no act of our psyche helps in disclosing the genuine determinacy and genuine absence of freedom as does the act of the struggle between motives. It is rather easy to see that, from the objective point of view, the presence of a volitional motive constitutes nothing less than a certain inner sensation that stimulates us to undertake a particular action. The simultaneous clash of several motives denotes the emergence of several inner sensations that struggle over the general motor field with the elemental force of nerve processes. The outcome of the struggle is always determined in advance, on the one hand, by the relative strengths of all the combatant sides, and on the other, by the setting of the struggle, which is generated out of the overall balance of all the forces within the organism.

The ancient philosophical anecdote of Buridan's ass, who perished from the cold while lying between two bales of hay, only because he could not decide which of the two bales held the greater interest for him, is full of psychological import. Of course, it is, in fact, utterly impossible for this to happen, since two stimuli could hardly be completely balanced in reality; furthermore, the previous experience of the ass, which had been accustomed to finding his fodder either on its left or on its right, would have had the decisive effect in this case. But, speaking theoretically, this case expresses a genuine psychological thought, that where all motives with opposing directions are balanced completely and ideally, the result is complete inertia of the will, and in this case the psychic mechanism will function according to all the laws of exact mechanics, according to which a body affected by two identical forces with opposing directions remains at rest.

Thus, the complete volitional act must be understood as a system of behavior that arises on the basis of the organism's instinctive and emotional attractions and is wholly determined by them. In fact, the very appearance of a particular wish or desire in consciousness always has as its cause a particular change in the organism. What we tend to refer to as desires ex nihilo are only such simply because their cause is concealed from us or is buried in the sphere of the unconscious. Moreover, these attractions are usually refracted in complex mental processes; they strive to take possession of our thoughts, so that thought becomes the harbinger of behavior, and he who possesses these harbingers, possesses strength. Thus, thinking is a kind of rudimentary mechanism between attractions and behavior and serves to guide the latter, as a function of those inner urges and promptings that issue from the deep foundations of our psyche. This is why the utter determinacy of our will is, for the psychologist, an entirely well-defined and radical presupposition for the scientific analysis of all the processes of the will; motiveless and nondeterministic phenomena cannot be the subject of scientific study and assertions.

Psychology of Language

It is easiest and simplest to disclose the mechanisms of thinking and will described above using the special example of language, which is the fundamental element realized by our thinking, as a system of inner organization of experience. From the point of view of psychology, language, both personal and social, passes through three distinct stages in its development.

Initially, language arises out of a reflexive shout that is entirely inseparable from all other emotional and instinctive manifestations of behavior. It may be easily shown that in the heightened emotional states of fear, rage, and others, language seems to be a constituent element of the overall biological complex of adaptive movements that execute, in particular, the function of expression, on the one hand, and serve to coordinate behavior, on the other. The expressive shout is associated directly with expressive breathing, i.e., we shout so that we may breathe.

But in the very earliest stages of development, the shout is more than that. In the animal's behavior in the herd, it is a means of summoning help, serving as the leader's signal to the herd, and so on.

It is at this stage, the stage of the reflexive shout, that voice appears in man for the first time. The newborn child cries because a current of air causes its vocal cords to vibrate. In the very first days of life, the reflexive character of the child's cry forms and is developed. It is most likely that language is frozen at this stage in the lower animals. But in the very first months of life in the human infant, a different stage of language arises, constructed in accordance with all the laws of education of the conditioned reflex. The child perceives his own shout and the series of sensations that follow upon it, say, its mother rushing over to it, feeding, a change in swaddling, and so on. Because the two events nearly overlap each other in terms of time, a new conditioned relation is formed in the child, and he now begins to demand the appearance of his mother expressly for this purpose by reproducing the shout. Language as such, in its psychological sense, arises here for the first time, as a relation between a particular act of the organism and a contingent meaning. The child's shout now possesses a meaning, since it expresses something that is understood by the child himself and by his mother.

But at this stage language is as yet extraordinarily limited. It is understandable only to the person who is speaking, i.e., it is fully contingent upon, and limited to, the conditioned relation that was given in man's personal experience. This is the language of animals. That an animal learns to understand the meaning of words and to relate certain sounds with his own actions or with the actions of others, say, sitting down, getting up, obeying its master's bidding, and so on, is an entirely well-known fact. However, this language differs from human language in that it is necessary to repeatedly conduct the conditioned relation that has to be formed between sound and action through the particular animal's individual experience in order to develop an understanding of its meaning. In other words, the understanding of this language is limited exclusively to whatever is part of the individual's consciousness.

Psychological linguistics has demonstrated that all existing languages have gone through this stage and that, in the beginning, every word that has appeared in language was constructed in precisely this way. It is not very hard to see that there are two types of words in modern language. There are words that relate given signs with a given meaning in a perfectly graphic way for us, while others, by contrast, produce such a connection in a way that, for us, is quite incomprehensible. If we consider such words as "pigeon" [*golub'*] and "raven" [*voron*], on the one hand, and "blue" [*goluboi*] and "jet black" [*voronoi*], on the other, it is not hard to see that, in the first group, it is entirely unclear to us why the sounds of *golub'* refer precisely to pigeons, and we can easily imagine that, under certain conditions, we might denote a raven by the word "pigeon," and conversely. On the contrary, when we speak of pigeons and ravens, we are not only hearing sounds, we are not only understanding their meaning, but are also understanding the causal connection according to which these sounds denote precisely this color. It would be absurd for us to refer to a black [*chernaya*] horse as being blue [*golubaya*], or to say that a blue [*goluboe*] sky was jet black [*voronoi*], because *goluboi* recalls the color of a pigeon, the color of a pigeon's wing, whereas *voronoi* recalls the color of a raven's wings.

Thus, psychologists specializing in linguistics distinguish three elements in the word: sound, meaning, and image, the latter understood as relation between the two, as a kind of explanation why a given word is associated with a given sound. In a language words may even be distinguished by the presence or absence of this third element. Etymological investigations have repeatedly demonstrated that even if a word has lost its image, it always possessed an image in its preceding meaning, consequently, no word arises haphazardly, the relation between meaning and sound is nowhere arbitrary, but is always rooted in the confluence of two similar phenomena, which may be easily seen in the origin of such words as *golub* and *voron*. The new word denotes, in this instance, a relation that may be established between one object and another, and such a relation, which is given in experience, turns out to always be present in the origin of absolutely every word.

In other words, at the very moment it appears, every word possesses an image, i.e., a visual motivation of its meaning that is comprehensible to everyone. A word does not only denote, but also shows why it denotes. Gradually, in the course of the growth and development of language, the image fades away, and the word retains only a meaning and a sound. This means that the difference between the two types of words reduces wholly to the growth of a distinction between words, with words that are a bit younger possessing an image, and those that are a bit older having half-forgotten it, though even in these words an image may still be easily found if we try to think hard about them. Very old words disclose their image only after careful historical gleanings of the primitive meanings and forms of words.

To demonstrate how this process of extinction takes place means demonstrating how, starting from the primitive stage of a language, which exists only for those who have created the language, the word enters colloquial language. The image fades away, which is why a word is employed in far broader relationships than those that have served as the reason for its appearance. If we think of such words as "ink" [*chernila*] and "horse-driven carriage" [*konka*], it is not hard to find the image that underlies these words. Meanwhile, we are now perfectly free, without doing any violence to the thought, to speak of red, blue, and green ink, and of so-called steam-driven, horse-driven carriages [*parovaya konka*], though from the standpoint of etymology, such combinations are not possible.[1] Whoever refers to a fluid used in writing as ink would pause at the first feature of this object, at its black color, and, approaching the new phenomenon with the previously cognized feature in mind, would denote the entire object by this feature. But this feature is not so much the most essential feature, in fact the point is that it is its only feature in the object, as happens nearly always. It proves to be fortuitous and sinks into the ensemble of all the other features that collectively serve for the development of the general concept of ink. When ink denoted something that was invariably black, this constituted a relationship that had been established in the individual experience of a particular person; but once this connotation had been added to the ensemble of other experiences, people forgot that ink denoted something that was invariably black, and from one person's conditional relation, the word became a general, social term; put differently, thought pushed aside the image, dissolved the image in itself, and only on the basis of acoustic analogy can anyone readily ascertain the origin of the word.

Hence, it is not hard to see that every process of understanding, including the understanding of language, denotes, speaking psychologically, a relationship. To understand French means to have the ability to establish a relationship between perceived sounds and the meanings of words. This relationship may be either narrowly personal in character (as in the language of animals) or broadly social (as in human language).

But the most remarkable fact for the psychology of language is that language would seem to implement two entirely distinct functions. On the one hand, it serves as a means for the social coordination of the experience of individual people, and on the other, it is the most important tool of our thought.

We always think in some language, that is, we speak to ourselves and organize our behavior within ourselves just as we organize our behavior as a function of the behavior of other people. In other words, thinking readily discloses its social character and demonstrates that our personality is organized according to the same model as is social intercourse, and that the primitive representation of the psyche as a double living inside man is the notion that is closest to our concepts.

Traditional psychological science has looked upon the understanding of the mind of another person as an insoluble conjecture, since none of my mental experiences is accessible to the perception of another person, and each of my mental experiences is disclosed to me only in introspection. I can only get to know my own joy through my own experiences, so how could I ever get to know another person's joy. In all psychological theories, despite all the differences in their construction, the question is always resolved on the basis of the thesis that we can get to know other people insofar as we can get to know ourselves. Whether we interpret the movements of other people by analogy with our own movements, whether we create a sense of empathy, i.e., induce in ourselves emotions appropriate to someone else's facial expression, we are always, as the psychologists put it, translating someone else's mind into the language of our own mind and getting to know another person through ourselves.

In fact, from the genetic standpoint of the development of the child's consciousness and from the standpoint of psychological knowledge of volitional acts, it would be more correct to think of this thesis as a contradictory assertion altogether. We have seen that the very understanding or awareness of our deeds arises as a relation between inner sensations and, like every conditioned-type relation, it arises out of experience in the simultaneity of different stimuli. Thus, before learning to understand other people, and only then on the basis of this model, the child learns to understand himself. It would be more correct to say that we know ourselves insofar as we know other people, or, more precisely, that we are conscious of ourselves only to the extent we are other for ourselves, i.e., somehow alien to ourselves. This is why language, this tool of social intercourse, is, in addition, also a tool of innercommunication between man and himself. The very consciousness of our thoughts and deeds must be understood as the very same mechanism responsible for the transmission of our reflexes to other systems or, speaking in terms of traditional psychology, as a feedback reaction.

Id and Ego

The time when psychologists could think of the human personality as something simple and unified is long gone. Psychological analysis has now discovered in the structure of our personality such highly heterogeneous strata that we can no longer conceive of personality as a kind of unified substance. Instead, a more appropriate representation of personality is achieved if we attempt to represent it in the form of a dialectical clashing of the most diverse tendencies and forces.

Even everyday language very readily draws a distinction between such assertions as, "I wish" [*ya khochy*] or "I do," and the assertion that "It is desired to [i.e., by] me that...." [*mne khochetsya*] establishing thereby an apparent distinction between the two fundamental axes of our personality, those which are denoted provisionally in the new psychology by the terms "id" and "ego."[2] The dual character of our thinking, as a permanent clash between id and ego, discloses itself with absolute exactitude. Freud declares that the ego is like a horseman, and the id like a horse. Now if the horseman does not wish to be thrown by the horse, he will often have to lead it where it wishes to go. In precisely the same way, very often our ego also has to follow inclinations that are embedded in the deepest strata of personality, else there arises considerable outright conflict, resulting in temporary ailments or more prolonged illness. Studies have shown that psychoses and neuroses are exactly the forms assumed by such illnesses, which arise out of the ground of an inner conflict between separate layers of the personality. The ego is also that conscious core of personality which guides behavior, what we always denote as thinking. The ego is the thinking side of our personality; but that dependence in which thinking precipitates from the more radical and more fundamental strivings of the organism then becomes perfectly clear.

We can begin to understand that thinking itself arises only on an instinctive and emotional foundation and is directed precisely by the forces of the latter. Virtually the most important achievement of the psychology of the past several decades has been the determination of the emotional and purposeful character of thinking.

In this sense, thought must always be understood as a special, newly solved problem of behavior or orientation in new circumstances. Thinking always arises out of difficulty. Where everything flows smoothly and where there are no obstacles, there thought does not yet have a reason to emerge. Thought arises wherever behavior encounters a barrier. It is this difficulty, which we may understand as the basic source of thinking, that provide a rationale for all those psychological analyses which establish that our thought is subordinated to a deterministic propensity, i.e., to a foreordained problem which has to be solved right away. Hence, also, all those elements of striving, of searching, of orientation, and of all the other undeveloped and incoherent residues of adaptive activity that arise in thinking.

Pedagogical Conclusions

The first and most important pedagogical conclusion that one naturally asks oneself, given such an understanding of thinking, may be found in the new view of the fundamental nature of education, which is characterized by frank and outright hostility towards visual teaching aids. The pedagogics of the recent past was permeated through and through with this propensity to make all of education easy, it sought to banish every difficulty and to make of it something entirely simple, carefree, and normal. This was an entirely healthy reaction against those back-breaking and superhuman exertions that had been the lot of the student in the preceding epoch.

But together with healthy social propensities, a sizeable proportion of psychological error also crept in. The demand that all of education be graphic, which we may think of as the highest expression of this pedagogics of facilitation, at the same time discloses all its weak points better than anything else. To make everything graphic means, above all, banishing every difficulty of thought beyond the child's reach. It means that everything the child is presented with has to be presented to him, first, in his personal experience, and second, in such an accessible, graphic, and facilitated form that the child has nothing left to guess at, nothing left to conclude, and only has to look and touch.

It's no use pointing out that such a requirement, above all, limits experience to the formation of personal relationships exclusively, which is insufficient even in the most well-appointed school and even with the best of external advantages. Man's experience is always broader than his personal experience; we know far more than we have seen, and if it was someone's desire that we know only as much as we see, by this device he would be restricting us inordinately and narrowing the sphere of our experience.

But it is far more important that such a propensity towards ease is in fundamental contradiction with the educational principles of psychology. It is virtually the same thing as insisting we not make it difficult for children in kindergarten to chew their food, and instead give them everything in half-digested and liquid form. For us, it is far more important to teach the child how to eat than to feed them. In just the same way, in education it is far more important to teach the child how to think than to communicate various bits of knowledge to him. By constructing the easiest and most comfortable path towards the acquisition of various bits of knowledge, graphic approaches, moreover, not only basically paralyze the habit of independent thinking at its very roots, but also take away from the child this concern and deliberately eliminate from education all elements of complex processing of experience, requiring that everything necessary be presented to the child in disconnected, half-digested, and over-done form. Meanwhile, it is necessary to take care to create as many difficulties as possible in the child's education, as starting points for his thoughts.

The child's social environment and all of the child's behavior must be so organized that every day brings with it ever newer connections and unforeseen examples of behavior for which there would not be any pre-set habits or ready answers in the child's store of experience with which he could respond, but which would instead forever require on his part ever newer connections between thoughts. Thinking, you see, denotes nothing less than the participation of all of our previous experience in the resolution of a current problem, and the distinctive feature of this form of behavior is simply that it introduces a creative element into our behavior through the construction of every possible connection between elements in a preliminary experience, which is what thinking is essentially. By this very fact, it multiplies the limitless possibilities of all those connections that may be produced out of human reactions, and makes man's behavior inexhaustibly multifaceted and exceptionally complicated.

Creative labor differs from the labor of the slave precisely by the fact that, in the case of slave labor, the component of preliminary organization of experience is kept apart from the component of execution. Physical labor and mental labor may be distinguished out of the overall unified process of labor simply because they were distributed between different social groups, due to social necessity. To certain groups fell the responsibility for one part—the inner preliminary organization of experience—while to other groups fell the responsibility for the physical implementation of experience. Psychologically speaking, the overall process of labor inevitably presupposes a contradiction, i.e., a unification in each individual act of two elements, a preliminary element and an executive element.

Thus, what is pedagogically correct is not a striving for what is representational, but the absolute inverse striving to let the child himself investigate the most complex and the most involved circumstances. If you would like a child to learn something well, take care to place obstacles in his path.

It goes without saying that it is not a matter of constructing deliberately hopeless situations for the child, which would only lead to fruitless and unsystematic expenditure of the child's efforts. We are only concerned with organizing the child's life, and teaching, so that the child confront the two necessary elements for the development of thinking, as the highest forms of behavior. These two elements are, first, the difficulty or, put differently, the *problem* which is to be solved, and, second, those elements and tools by means of which this problem may be solved.

The very solution of the problem, nine-tenths of which had previously been the responsibility of the teacher, now falls entirely on the student's shoulders. In this sense, the Dalton program of education, which shifts the responsibility for finding and formulating scientific laws from the teacher to the student, which replaces the classroom with laboratories, which reduces the role of the teacher to nothing, to the extent that he can be replaced by books, manuals, pictures, and other instructional material, and which reserves for the teacher only the function of conductor and guide of the student's own experience—this program is, from the psychological point of view, the one that most accords with the nature of the process of educating thinking.

Here the student is forever being given a kind of contract, i.e., a problem that is subdivided and measured out in terms of time. In the laboratory he receives all the necessary materials and tools he might need to solve this problem, and his task is to so organize his work, to so subdivide and allocate his time, that the contract may be fulfilled successfully and on time. This program teaches each student to think independently, to think for himself, whereas the old system of teaching entrusted the responsibility for the entire class to a single teacher. This system of teaching places the student repeatedly in the position of an investigator who is out to establish a particular truth and whom the teacher only guides. Thus is the psychologically complete process of labor preserved, a process that presupposes an inevitably preliminary stage of planning, and the reaction that is executed subsequently receives its full expression precisely within the framework of this plan.

Finally, the very last point, which underscores the advantages of this system of teaching over the previous system, lies in the exclusively concrete character which thinking assumes in this system of education. Wholly abstract thinking is entirely incomprehensible to the student, and, in the Tsarist school, produced a naked and dry literalism, i.e., an infinite propensity for verbal formulations and for verbal definitions without any effort to penetrate into essentials, and instead of a knowledge of subject matter, there was knowledge of words.

Nekrasov, in speaking of one of his heroines, tells how, with all the skills she had gotten out of education, it came to her one day that she felt inadequate in only one area—in the ability to think. She had learned much and was even a superb horseback rider, but she could never think simply because she could not recall even a single minute in her entire life when she had had any difficulty.

It must be said that when students were taught how to think as a routine part of education in the Tsarist school, this always happened despite all the intentions of the school, because the difficulties that it put forward always aroused thought to flow in a direction other than the one which was needed in the course of the pedagogical process.

In the process of developing the ability to think, it is extraordinarily important to establish in the student's consciousness that general relation, that ultimate goal, which is the governing propensity of the entire process of thinking. What is the reason for my thinking—to this question an exact and satisfactory answer has to be given from the very start. Meanwhile, the entire collection of all of our old textbooks was constructed without such a guiding relation, and in passing from one particular to another, students would understand the relation between the individual parts of a subject like a horse understands the relation between each tug on the reins and each individual turn, though the meaning of the entire path as a whole, from its starting point to its last point—the meaning all the individual turns are subordinate to—this was just as much of a secret for the student as it is for the horse.

Analysis and Synthesis

The analytic and synthetic activity of the mind, i.e., the activity that first decomposes the perceptible world into individual elements, and then builds new structures out of these elements, helping us gain a better understanding of our surroundings, is the basic logical form in which our thought becomes manifest. In this regard, it is extraordinarily important to discern the psychological mechanism responsible for the formation of concepts, i.e., those general and cognate reactions that relate not to individual objects, but to an entire class or an entire group of objects simultaneously. In this sense, every reaction constitutes an extraordinarily valuable accumulation of experience, and is essentially already a complete theory. When I say the word, "lamp," having in mind an entire class of homogeneous objects, I am thereby making use of the results of a vast amount of analytic work that has already been completed, i.e., the work of decomposing all the objects already in my experience into their constituent components, into assimilations, i.e., the collocation of similar elements, the rejection of random elements, and the synthesis of the remaining elements into an integral concept.

This analytic activity seemed at one time to be highly conjectural and complex until it was established that an analogous activity always occurs in language when we are dealing even with isolated objects. Even when I speak not of lamps in general, but of a given lamp, I am essentially operating not with naked, sensient experience, but with experience that has undergone substantial reworking. In fact, in my ordinary experience, even this lamp presents itself somewhat differently every time, in other words, experience is always changeable. The lamp is now lit, now it is out, now it is illuminated, now it is not, now it is part of one ensemble of objects, now another, now it is turned towards one corner, now towards another, and now, when I speak about the lamp, I overlook all these partial variants of experience and establish a certain neutral and general meaning of this object.

The natural pedagogical conclusion, therefore, is that students must be allowed to experience as many objects and phenomena as possible that could serve as a means for the acquisition of an appropriate piece of information. Moreover, these objects and phenomena should be selected in such a way as to facilitate the very choice of the objects and seem to suggest analytic and synthetic effort to the student. The pedagogical technique of developing the concept of shape and color in a child may serve as an elementary example. We select objects of varying geometric shape, though of the same color, and then proceed at once in reverse order, and, as a result, the general attribute of shape and color manifests itself especially vividly and distinctly against the background of variable surroundings, as if separated from the objects containing it and, because of its partial repetition, begins to dominate our consciousness and lead a seemingly independent existence there. Thus does analytic work help us group material together, so that the attribute that is subject to discrimination is encountered in the most varied combinations.

And conversely, the synthetic work of adding attributes helps us group material together, so that elements that are to be bound together become as clear and as distinct as might be desired, and, most important, become entirely purified of all alien relation. Bear in mind in this connection the law of inverse proportional dependence between the volume and content of a concept, a law which is of the greatest importance for the teacher. By the *volume* of a concept we understand the quantity of objects or phenomena that may be subsumed under the concept. The *content* of a concept refers to the quantity of attributes that may be conceived in this concept. The broader the volume of some concept, incidentally, the narrower is its content, and conversely.

Thus, the teacher must always be cognizant of the fact that by expanding the volume of some concept, he is contracting its content, and conversely; by filling up content with an infinite quantity of particular details and particulars, he is contracting and restricting its volume.

If we take as an example the concept of man and that of Negro, we may easily explain the meaning of this law. In terms of volume, man the concept is broader than the concept of Negro, though the concept of Negro is just as broader in terms of content, i.e., in terms of the quantity of attributes occurring in it, since all the attributes of the concept man are inherent to that of Negro, though, in addition, specific features may be conceived in this concept that do not occur in the concept man, but are introduced by restricting this concept, which becomes contracted by virtue of apparent distinction.

One psychologist has referred to this law quite correctly as the tragic law of teaching. In fact, here the teacher confronts irreconcilable extremes, in that every expansion of denotation entails just as great a unification of connotation and content associated with the denotation; every enrichment of content contracts its volume. Finding the correct relationship between the two is always a difficult problem for pedagogical tact, which is still unable to achieve a solution in general form until pedagogics has become an exact science.

Value of Thinking for Inner Education

The study of all the various forms of psychopathology and mental defect has demonstrated that an overall low level of development is almost always associated with a low level of development in the intellectual sphere. In other words, pathology discloses the very same relation between thinking and the inner aspect of personality as does psychology.

This is why the teacher must bear in mind that thinking is not only a mechanism that complicates and refines our interaction with the external world, but also guides the inner aspect of our behavior. The reader surely knows how powerless thinking is in the struggle against emotional and instinctive drives. No moral prescription can compel us to act in spite of our drives. To understand how one should act still does not mean acting the way one should.

That the moral health of our behavior must begin with its preliminary forms, that the health of our deeds must begin with the health of our thoughts, this, however, is self-evident and without any doubt for present-day psychology. This is why it is not so much the outer direction of our thoughts as its inner purposefulness, that interior function which is its lot, that has assumed a leading role in educational psychology in recent times. To learn how to think correctly about the world means making certain that the correct relationships between the elements of the world and the student's reactions are set up in his experience. To teach the student how to think correctly about himself means setting up in the student's experience the correct relationships between his thoughts and deeds, i.e., between his preliminary and executive reactions.

Modern psychologists are inclined to see in this *internal* character of mental processes a specific distinctiveness of these processes, by means of which thinking may be set apart in a class of reactions of its own, and thus represents an entirely new form of behavior. From this standpoint, three classes of reactions should be distinguished in man's behavior: (1) instinct (unconditioned reflexes, stereotypical, inherited, pre-set modes of behavior forming the foundation for absolutely all reactions of the two higher classes); (2) training (conditioned or orienting reflexes by means of association and practice, and new mechanisms involving the acquisition of personal experience and built upon the instincts); (3) intelligence (thinking).

The essential distinction of this third form of behavior consists in the fact that these reactions appear all of a sudden. Köhler established the presence of similar sudden guesswork and solutions, i.e., the rudiments of intelligence, in chimpanzees; Thorndike is also of the belief that the suddenness with which such reactions appear, and the fact that they are consolidated "once and for all," so distinguishes these reactions from the ordinary education of the conditioned reflexes, which requires lengthy practice and a gradual approach to their reinforcement, that these new qualities emphasize that there is "nothing greater" than ordinary training.

"Invention," writes Bühler, "constitutes, in the real sense of the word, also the biological work of intelligence." Thinking may thus be defined as "purposeful behavior in new situations, without any tests on the object itself." The absence of external tests and their replacement by internal probing, is also an essential distinguishing feature of thinking. A hen rushing about haphazardly in front of a garden fence who is trying out each hole in order to, ultimately, find the one it can get through is not an example of thinking. In thinking tests are carried out inside. Thinking is characterized by a delay, a cessation of all external movement (reflection), an intensification of the internal stress of nerve currents, and the sudden appearance of a solution, usually accompanied by the exclamation, "Aha!" which is why Bühler referred to it as the "aha experience" or the "aha reaction."

From the physico-chemical standpoint, it turns out that "there are processes which are possible in the nervous system whose initial point of departure is a reaction that arises initially at centers in the brain and which, because of this fact, yields a sense of volition, of spontaneity." Lazarev also allows for the existence of "spontaneous centers of excitation in the brain caused by radioactive processes created by potash salts." Here we are dealing not with conditioned reflexes, but with a new type of reaction, one that is "generated in the cerebral cortex as a voluntary process."

---

[1]Apparently, writing ink was only of one color, so that referring to red, blue, or green ink constituted a misnomer; likewise, *konka* refers to a carriage that is pulled by horses, so it is a misnomer to give it the attribute of *parovaya*, which has the meaning of steam-driven. In both cases, however, the terms are correct grammatically (or, as Vygotsky puts it, in terms of thought) (trans.).

[2]Vygotsky seems be saying that the two expressions, which have basically the same meaning in Russian, (differing only in the fact that the first is a personal and the second an impersonal construction), express, in this grammatical distinction, what we might think of today as a Whorfian distinction between ego and id.

Chapter 10

PSYCHOLOGICAL UNDERSTANDING OF OCCUPATIONAL EDUCATION

Types of Trade Schools

In terms of historical development and psychological potential, there exist three basic forms of labor education. The first type is what is known as vocational or manual training trade schools, where work is made the subject of teaching, in that the task of this type of school is to prepare the student for a particular occupation. To train a technician or craftsman, to foster in him the skills and technical knowledge of his craft—it is this which constitutes the task of this form of education.

With this understanding, occupational education is absolutely no different from any other form of education, since pedagogics likewise always strives to establish a certain new system of behavior, whatever the form assumed by this system. Whether it is an academic school that prepares the future debater, attorney, or advocate, or a manual training school that prepares metal workers and shoe-makers—the preparation for future activity are everywhere the subject of teaching.

Work occupies an entirely different position in the instructional system of such a school. Here it occurs not as a subject of teaching, but as a new method, i.e., as a tool for the study of other subjects. Even if labor is introduced into such a school, the particular labor techniques do not possess any independent value whatsoever. Though the child learns how to saw or how to hammer in nails, the teacher's concern is least of all directed towards teaching him how to do this as best and as plainly as possible.

Whereas in the manual training school habits of work constitute an end in itself, in the prototype (pilot) school they are only a tool to help students master certain other subjects. Speaking historically as well as psychologically, here labor manifests itself as the ultimate triumph of the graphic method, as the ultimate of "facilitative" pedagogics, since making a subject graphic means not only to demonstrate something visually, but also to draw into the process of perception as many organs as possible; to bring the subject to the child not only through the eyes, but also through touch and through movement.

The very system and goals of instruction may remain entirely unchanged, since this form of teaching presupposes that it be realized only *through* the hands, even though it is a matter of teaching *everything whatsoever*. In this system, therefore, labor appears only as exemplar, as the best way of assimilating, understanding, and recalling something. In other words, labor assumes an auxiliary, secondary, and subordinate role.

Suppose history is being studied in such a school. Then the teacher's responsibility, is, as usual, to develop in the students as distinct and as accurate a store of knowledge of historical facts, conditions, and laws as possible. But just to achieve this goal of abstract knowledge, it is useful to lead students into drawing maps, building models of ancient structures, and recreating uniforms and weapons. Hence the highly complex labor activity that becomes the lot of students, though the direction of education and its fundamental striving is forever outside labor.

Finally, the third advantage of the trade school and of occupational education lies in an entirely new view of labor, understood as the very foundation of the educational process. In such a purely trade school, labor is introduced not as a subject of teaching, nor as a method or tool of teaching, but as the very substance of education. In the felicitous phrase of one educator, not only is labor introduced into the school, but the school is introduced into labor.

It is precisely this last understanding of the trade school that, in the proper sense of the term, underlies the Soviet system of education, and it is this, more than anything else, which is in need of psychological evaluation.

That manual training type trade schools possess only negligible educational value should be perfectly obvious to the reader. Bear in mind, above all, that the handicrafts nature of labor had its origin in the workshop system of medieval society, when the actual processes of production were extremely primitive, and when the bulk of the store of skills was concentrated not in the tool, but in the hands of the craftsman. Production was specialized to an infinite degree, required an enormous amount of complicated training and technical workmanship, was confined to the limited scope of the workshop, often passed from father to son and from father-in-law to son-in-law, as a family and inherited treasure, and accordingly, became narrow and closed.

Like every form of labor, of course, there has been built up around handicrafts the creative experience and skill of past generations, but this experience and skill have been narrowly defined, even if the subtlety and elegance of the results have attained a degree of perfection that is not exceeded even today. It is precisely because the master craftsman fashioned everything by hand that it acquired a fully distinctive character, and it is for this reason that there can be no boundary between handicrafts and art. The artist is a craftsman. And the craftsman is an artist in his own work. He creates not products, but individual works whose degree of individual perfection leaves every mass-produced article far behind.

It is, therefore, entirely understandable that the educational value of handicraft labor is quite negligible. The volume of theoretical knowledge the craftsman works with is extremely small, and the range of materials that is amenable to fashioning by a craftsman is insignificant. What might be thought of as his "technical dictionary," i.e., the sum total of techniques and movements he makes use of, is often confined to several dozen stereotypical patterns. In this sense, handicrafts constitutes thankless pedagogical substance requiring an enormous expenditure of effort for the development of subtlety and precision in the movements involved in labor and for making the human hand more capable of functioning automatically, until it begins to approximate the perfection of a tool, though this in no way means replacing the human hand nor does it involve any evolutionary or broadly educational elements.

It is entirely understandable that the psychological character of manual training is bound up with the social character of the manual training school. Manual training schools, in fact, arise in the bourgeois state in response to the demand for a lower-middle class of good sources of craftsmen, and it is just as understandable that such a school takes upon itself the limited role of a supplementary school within the context of a system of universal public education. Understandably, all the other pedagogical constraints of such a school are fully in accord with the narrow character of handicraft work.

Kerschensteiner is the most brilliant proponent of this type of schooling, pointing out quite frankly that the education of respectable citizens and craftsmen trained to maintain the proper attitude towards the existing social, political, and cultural order is the ideal of such occupational education. Thus, this form of education exhibits a far greater concern for the social system than for the student's character.

The second type of trade school, called the *prototype* or *pilot school*, has a far broader mission in this regard, though it, too, proves to be mistaken in conception, speaking psychologically, for a whole number of reasons. First, bear in mind that simply seeking after real-life representation and striving to facilitate the educational process must be considered a long-past stage in pedagogics. The principles of occupational education are far more accord with the demands of pedagogics than are representational teaching methods. And it is also clear that the labor method, understood as the most complete expression of representational teaching, comprises all the defects and all the shortcomings of this principle in its most extreme form.

Here we again see the utter incompatibility of those skills that are needed expressly for a particular form of labor and those that are needed for the particular subject matter in which this form of labor is called upon to serve as prototype. To construct a good model or a good tool is a task that, in and of itself, requires so much attention, so much skill, so much work of the mind and of the hand, that the purely historical value of the subjects that have been developed seem to fade into the background, and, in the expression of one American educator, in such a school the labor time periods become times when the educational process is at a standstill. The study of history seems to cease once students are involved in model building, and labor itself acquires the character not of forward movement, but of stagnant repetition, reinforcement, the assimilation of results already attained, of running in place.

Work on historical models does not move the child forward in the study of history, rather it holds him wholly in the power of what he has already gone over. Even here, however, labor assumes broadened psychological importance by comparison with its status in manual training trade schools. Now it is no longer brought down to the level of professional industry, and, consequently, does not place such a great burden on the student. Now it is no longer withdrawn into the narrow sphere of some one single activity, and instead causes the student's abilities to be scattered about from one activity to another. Now it is already a great teacher of motor skills, giving the student training in mobility and dexterity, and teaching him how to carry himself, how to hold his hands, feet, and trunk. Now it is already assuming the role of a powerful educator of general behavior, accustoming the student to self-control, to monitoring his own behavior and to planning his movements, to the possibility of self-appraisal by means of the graphic results obtained.

But in spite of everything, labor continues to play the role of a *calligrapher of behavior*, i.e., for all that, a fruitless and, in and of itself, unnecessary expenditure of effort, which becomes more fruitless and seems to become even more burdensome simply because here labor is only called upon to repeat and duplicate what has been gone over in the classroom. The student works on what he knows very well, and the point of such labor is clear to the teacher, but is hidden from the student himself.

The vocational trade school is free of this shortcoming. Its own shortcoming has nothing whatsoever to do with what the prototype school suffers from. In this school, labor assumes the appropriate status of seriousness that it possesses in real life. In acquiring these work skills, children who are taught in such a school enter immediately into the workday routine. However, the problem is that such a school inculcates forms of labor that belong more to the past than to the future; everything faces backward, rather than forward. And what it imparts to its students is not of any great value for modern life.

Handicraft labor has virtually no educational value, since it comprises such narrowly accumulated experience as to make it impossible to go beyond the restricted limitations of handicraft itself. Handicraft has long since lost the sense of an artistic craft that was inherent to it in the middle ages, when the title of expert craftsman was applied equally to a painter and to a furniture maker, and when leather, and furniture, and other goods actually bore the impress of individual perfection, and by its very nature, in fact belonged to the realm of artistic manufacture. Every object was engendered out of a particular conception, and the process of manufacturing an object was governed and guided also by the individual constraints involved in the execution of just this conception.

These times have receded far into the past, and in present-day industry the pointless and uninteresting role of side function, the role of patching over the gaps in the larger industry, is now the lot of handicrafts. Handicrafts continue to exist only insofar as the medieval way of life has yet to vanish totally from modern culture. But with each new machine in the factory, with each new improvement in technology, the value of handicrafts is becoming less and less, and, in every sense of the term, handicrafts have become peripheral in real life.

The very division of labor into the different occupations focuses workers' attention on the final, active moment of work, and not its overall preconditions. In other words, handicraft labor emphasizes, in every act of manufacture, not those general elements which are inherent to all forms of human labor, but only those which distinguish a given form of labor from all other forms of labor.

In contrast to this narrow form of professional labor, modern industrial labor is distinguished by "polytechnism", the psychological and pedagogical value of which compels us to see in it a fundamental method of occupational education. Modern industry is polytechnical in nature in terms of the economic and technological aspects of labor, but, more important, in terms of the psychological aspects of labor. To understand the economic reasons for this circumstance, we need look no further than those vast tides and displacements of great masses of working people that are the inevitable accompaniment of the building of capitalism. Marx himself pointed to the economic mechanism which, because of industrial crises and the associated contractions and expansions of production, makes it necessary that there exist a reserve army of the unemployed, with large numbers of workers moving from one form of production, and one factory, to another. The worker who today is working at a bottling plant tomorrow will settle down to producing galoshes, and the day after tomorrow will go to work at an automobile plant, and in every transition from one factory to another the only requirement imposed on the worker is the possession of a minimal general technical development, i.e., the ability to work with machines; no specialized or professional knowledge is required.

Therefore, the economic conditions themselves impose on workers the demand to be a kind of multi-specialized technician, i.e., in any form of production not to have any more profound knowledge than the simple fundamentals, or to perish during the next business crisis. And this in fact is what happens. Nine-tenths of the army of European and American workers have absolutely no sense of professionalism that might lead the worker to become interested in some definite type of production. This brings to mind that great strike in America, when everyone working at some very large factory went on strike. It took only two days for this factory to resume operation at its previous rate with an entirely new staff of workers.

The technical reasons which have also led to the development of multi-specialized technicians are the consequence of mechanical progress, which evens out all the differences between the various types of mechanisms, and leads to more or less uniform types of the most economic and the most suitable machines that also happen to be the least expensive. Competitive conditions are such that the most suitable machines are inevitably introduced in the shortest possible time into all factories of a given type, for otherwise the owners run the risk of their factories being left behind and overwhelmed in the commercial struggle for the market. Never before, in fact, has there been such a triumphant procession of every type of new improvement imaginable with such thundering speed as in the past several decades.

It is in this which defines the very superstructure of every form of machine production, in the sense of fundamental constituents, and these constituent parts prove to be extraordinarily similar in the most diverse enterprises. The most critical parts of the mechanical equipment of absolutely every form of production comprise motors of absolutely the same type for use in the most diverse factories. The driving gears, which are again all of the same type, are next, and differentiation sets in only in the active or working part of the machine, as a function of the ultimate operations it has to carry out in order to place some finished good into the market.

Thus, two-thirds of all of modern production has become entirely uniform, and only in the final third is any variation permitted, and even this is increasingly leveling off with the further development of technology. This is happening for the following simple reason. All the possible types of movement involved in the different labor processes are being resolved into the simplest elementary forms. As a result, it has become possible to ultimately reduce all these movements to 12 fundamental types of elementary movements. It is these elementary movements which are implemented in absolutely all the different forms of complex labor that industry the world over makes use of in all their various combinations and permutations.

This should not surprise us just as we should not be surprised, as Münsterberg puts it, that the 22 [sic] letters of the English alphabet suffice to accommodate all the plays of Shakespeare. From this standpoint, it becomes entirely understandable that the third, or performance component of a machine reduces ultimately to a kind of technical alphabet that is the same in every mode of production. And just as with a real alphabet, it is sufficient to learn this alphabet in order to read any "book" inscribed in this system.

Thus, it is quite probable that we are experiencing the greatest epoch in the consolidation of labor in all of history, and that the concept of professionalism is in its death throes right before our very eyes.

Finally, the most essential point are the psychological prerequisites that polytechnism imposes. These may be summarized as follows. Every process of human labor constitutes a dual process, inasmuch as man constitutes, on the one hand, a direct source of physical energy, and on the other, the director of the labor process. In the most primitive forms of labor, the working man assumes a dual role. On the one hand, he is constituent component of his own machine, the direct source of physical energy, a role in which he may be replaced by draft animals, steam engines, electric motors, and so on, and on the other, he plays the role of director and foreman of his own tools and of his own movements, and in this role there is nothing that can replace him.

The division of labor into mental labor and physical labor occurred in that epoch when these two psychological functions, which had been merged together inseparably into a single act of labor, were distributed among different members of the community because of social differentiation. To some members fell the exclusive responsibility for the directive and supervisory functions, while to others, the responsibility for the function of performance.

Things changed somewhat when machines were introduced, and the role of the worker got stuck somewhere in the middle between the two functions. Once the worker was reduced to operating a machine, he was forced into the role of a mere appendage to the machine, usually responsible for performing some extraordinarily insignificant operation that could not be entrusted to the machine. The expenditure of physical energy was extremely limited, though the mental aspect of labor did not require great effort on the worker's part.

To imagine how stupefying is this form of labor, just recall how, in the most ordinary factories, the raw materials pass through several dozen operations, and over the past several decades it has been the worker's lot to repeat one and same movement with entirely mechanical precision. Those who declare that, before the advent of the machine, labor still possessed, from the psychological point of view, more of a human aspect, than does labor in the age of the machine are, therefore, correct.

However, with the development of technology things changed radically. The component of control and direction of the production process began to increasingly dominate the dual structure of labor, and the component of performance became increasingly negligible. Human energy is now being increasingly replaced by machines, and the worker of today is assuming the role of supervisor and guide of the production process, the ruler of the machine, the monitor and regulator of its action.

In the most highly perfected mode of production, this process reaches such heights that the worker is not even responsible for controlling the machinery directly, instead relying on mechanical controllers which, in turn, regulate the machines. Thus, in factories of this type the worker is a regulator of regulators, i.e., he performs the highest and most complex directive functions. Whoever is familiar with the duties of a stoker under Russian conditions would probably be surprised, once he had become acquainted with the duties of the chief stoker at the largest American factories, to learn that there these duties are carried out with the hands kept absolutely clean. This becomes understandable once it is noted that the actual dirty work of throwing coal into the furnace, unloading residues, removing fused pieces, fanning the flames, opening the flues, cleaning away soot, and so on are performed by automatic machines, metal arms, that report on their own operation and their own status by means of several dozen mechanical attachments placed on a table, moreover that these machines are controlled by means of levers from this table.

The stoker himself, who has the responsibility of heating the largest imaginable factories and, in this sense, performs the very same functions as does our stoker, plays the part of a commander-in-chief of a veritable army of machines, with his work table recalling a field headquarters where dispatches from all sectors are received, requests gathered together, instructions issued, actions coordinated—and all this is accomplished through the agency of the subtlest and most complex of technical devices, demanding on the worker's part considerable mental grasp as well as an alert eye and advanced technical skill in order to control these instruments. The development of labor is increasingly coming to assume just these forms, and the residue of physical labor that is found in these factories is increasingly being confined to negligible movements of small levers that recall the hands of a clock, to depressing electrical switches and buttons, and to slight rotary movements of the handles of a barrel.

Under these conditions, it is natural that labor, understood as a particular expenditure of physical energy, as compulsive deliberate activity, is carried out by a machine, and that the human being has become responsible for the increasingly critical and intellectual work involved in controlling these machines. The contemporary worker's need for polytechnical education, hence, becomes entirely understandable. Recall, too, that despite the exact meaning of the term, polytechnism of this kind should not be taken to refer to any sort of "multi-craftsmanship," i.e., the combination of several specialties in a single individual, but rather a familiarity with the general foundations of human labor, with the "alphabet" from which all its various forms derive, or, figuratively speaking, the extraction of a common factor consisting of all these forms outside a pair of brackets. It goes without saying that the educational value of this form of labor is infinitely great, since it signifies the highest flowering of technology, which itself is realized in step with the highest flowering of science. Technology is also science in action, or science applied to production, and the transition from the one to the other is performed every minute, in entirely imperceptible and elusive forms.

Strange as it may seem, the worker, even the rank-and-file worker in a large enterprise, must keep up with science. An expression of one American industrialist is instructive in this regard: "The worker who is 10 years behind the contemporary development of science cannot count on a position in my factory."

In these forms, labor is transformed into crystallized scientific knowledge, and in order that skills be acquired for such labor, it is actually necessary to possess that entire vast capital of accumulated knowledge of nature that is utilized in every technical improvement. For the first time in all of mankind's history, polytechnical labor is turning into an intersection of all the most important lines of human culture, a result that would have been unthinkable in any earlier epoch. The educational value of this form of labor is without limit, since its complete mastery requires the most complete mastery of everything that science has accumulated through the ages.

Finally, the most important point is that purely instructive effect which labor exerts here. Labor is transformed into deliberate work for the most part and requires that its participants exert all the forces of the mind and their attention as strenuously as possible , with the result that the labor of the rank-and-file worker is lifted up, attaining the highest stages of creative human labor. This is why the introduction of the spirit of the production process [*industrialism*] into the school will get students accustomed to the standards of industry the world over; the ascent to the heights of modern technology constitutes the fundamental demand of the trade school.

It is not hard to see how far off from the above are those types of trade schools that conceive the entire spirit of work as reducing to the conception that the child's lot consists in humiliating and dirty work in the kitchen, bathroom, and lavatory, and in washing the floor, and that have discerned the rudiments of work habits in this gloomy and regressive form of labor. Labor has been revealed to children in the form of extraordinary physical effort and thereby has justified its etymological meaning, which in Russian makes this word synonymous with the words *bolezn'* [illness] and *pechal'* [suffering].

Those forms of labor which can be introduced into the school if, that is, we are guided in our design of the curriculum not by primitive and long-gone forms of domestic physical labor, but by forms of industrial and technically advanced forms of labor, which are of extraordinary interest. Thus, without any effort whatsoever on our part, the child can be directly accustomed to those two realms among which all educational influence on the child is divided—on the one hand, modern natural science, and on the other, modern social life, which through its threads encompasses the entire world.

In the modern factory, the pulse of life and of science the world over beats, and the child who is placed in the factory himself learns to feel this pulse of the contemporary age. It is extremely important to arrange the various forms of the child's active working life and his labor activity in such a way that he enters into entirely deliberate and creative relationships to all those processes he has to deal with. This is achieved not by gradual vocational instruction of the child in the various skills involved in working with machines, but by introducing the child all at once into the overall scheme of a workshop. In this way he is taught to find the place and meaning of different technical instruments, understood as individual necessary constituents of an entire whole.

Cognition of Nature Through Labor

In industrial labor, the child is brought into contact from the very start with the higher forms of processing natural materials, and he is taught to follow those lengthy paths along which raw materials travel from the moment they arrive at a factory to the moment they leave, in the form of treated and finished output. Meanwhile, throughout this lengthy path the material must disclose nearly all its most important and essential properties; it is compelled, in fact, to show that it obeys all the laws of physics and chemistry, that is, the process of treating any raw material seems to represent a demonstration of these laws organized expressly for the student.

Meanwhile, the very properties of one material that distinguish it from all other materials do not play any sort of essential role. The material manifests itself mainly as material as such, as the bearer of certain general properties which vary quantitatively as a function of the mode of production, though not qualitatively. Whether we are dealing with the processing of wood or of some metal, wool or cotton, rock or bone, in all these instances we are dealing with a certain quantity, density, elasticity, deformation of material, and of other general properties of some substance. Thus, the very character of modern production leads us to identify common elements of the most diverse materials whatsoever and to generalize the common properties of materials graphically, right before the student's eyes.

Physical matter in modern production manifests itself—and this is its essential feature—not as such, with all its particular and specific properties, but as a physical body or as a chemical compound, and in this sense, discloses right before the student's eyes—and not just in the pages of a textbook, but also in the pages of life—those general features that are inherent equally, though in different quantities, to the finest threads of cotton and to the most hardened forms of steel. Thus, the general laws of the physics and chemistry of earthly matter march past the student in the process of industrial labor with an entirely graphic and impressive force.

No less important is the fact that in the course of this production all the most important laws governing the processing of this material, laws which are constructed by taking into account scientific mechanics in as precise a fashion as possible, likewise "march" past the students. These laws disclose to the students not statistical natural science, but practical and dynamic science. Familiarity with all three parts of the modern factory presupposes that the student possess the most rigorous knowledge of mechanics, and the ability to control these machines is based ultimately on this knowledge.

At a factory, every workday is a living examination, and there is not the slightest need for specially designed tests in order to discover and evaluate how firmly and how thoroughly this knowledge has taken root.

There is a third aspect related to this that we wish to emphasize as a novel advantage of industrial labor. Here, the student's own movements are restored to him in the form of the finished product of work. This permits him to monitor his own activity and to evaluate his own labor on the basis of the indubitable and objective results of work, and, what is most important, to create the opportunity for realizing a concluding moment of satisfaction, of exultation, of conquest in some sense, thanks to which our strivings and all forms of activity are aroused in essential ways.

Psychologists have long emphasized the psychological value of grades, which William James, for example, considered so significant as to thrust into the background all the obvious harm brought about by grading systems. He insisted not only on preserving grading systems in the school, but also that students be made aware of their grades, since marks introduce a useful element that gives meaning to all the student's labor and allows him to come to a decision as to whether or not his efforts are bearing fruit. Of course, James also agrees that psychological conclusions must give way to the arguments of experience, and admits that, despite the psychological rule, there are times when the teacher has to refrain from announcing grades. This, however, does not solve the psychological problem, and in James' conception there is a wonderful truth here, basically the demand that all work be brought to some crowning point and that this moment of success or failure be reported to the student and lead him to see the meaning of all his labors. The greatest value of occupational education is found here, i.e., that this ultimate moment is nothing foreign and estranged from the entire process of labor, as has been the case, for example, with school marks, and that, consequently, there is absolutely no danger that the student's striving will assume an entirely false direction, as always occurred when the student would get to work only to obtain a good grade. The more the student's strivings and interests are bound up with this ultimate point of his labor efforts, the more powerful and the more effective will be the coordinating and connective effect of these efforts within the overall system of his reactions.

Thus, the distinctive feature of human labor, which requires preliminary knowledge of ultimate results, and the fact that these results coincide with what is presupposed from the very start, finds its most complete and purest expression precisely in the forms of industrial labor. This is just what psychologists are essentially saying when they speak of the overall healthy effect that industrial labor exerts on the individual person. Within the mass of workers, psychologists declare that each individual discovers what seem like enormous mirrors in which he learns to discern the least of his movements and, thus, it is here that he attains the highest level of mastery over his own body and behavior. This via the reflected impression of the group to the student himself, and, in this case, a group of workers plays the role of a vast resonator which amplifies and transmits, though on a vast scale, the very same emotions that are possible in a small group of people. It is in this sense that we can say that emotion grows as a function of the audience that experiences it. Shame experienced in front of a crowd of thousands is thousands of times more powerful than shame experienced in front of a single person. The same may be said of the emotion of satisfaction, which directs all our reactions to an ultimate goal, and which grows and increases in magnitude the larger is the group in whose channel it travels.

Coordination of Labor Efforts

Even in the most primitive forms, labor manifests itself not only as a process between man and nature, but also as a process between people, since even the most primitive forms of labor require, of necessity, a certain degree of coordination of effort, a certain degree of skill in reconciling one's behavior with the behavior of other people, and in coordinating and monitoring one's reaction so that they can become a constituent component of the general fabric of collective behavior. This is why labor, especially in its higher and industrial forms, always signifies the greatest school of social experience. One psychologist has said that nowhere does man learn genuine courtesy and foresight as in the modern factory, since it teaches everyone to coordinate his own movements with the movements of others in as meticulous a fashion as possible.

The most important feature of this learning is that it teaches subordination and mastery simultaneously, eliminating absolutely all the moral drawbacks of both. In this sense, the educational effect of industrial labor fully recalls the educational effect of games, where the child senses himself forever linked to a whole network of complex rules and where, in addition, he is taught not only to obey these rules, but also to subordinate the behavior of others to these rules and to act within the strict guidelines established by the conditions of the game.

Ultimately, both games and industrial labor represent, in this regard, only the purest model of every form of behavior in real life, in that however we relate to these forms of behavior, we will always be dealing with these two elements, i.e., the necessity to first submit to certain rules in order to subordinate ourselves to something else. Thus, the fundamental forms of deliberate behavior and will are also formulated and develop in the process of technical labor, inasmuch as they are determined by these two components.

It is also extraordinarily important that the full complexity of human relations, whether we consider them in geographic, political or cultural contexts, finds its purest expression also in the modern factory. A student who is working in a modern factory always seems to be standing on the chessboard of the modern social struggle and begins to take part in it with each of his steps in entirely practical ways, whether or not he wishes to. In other words, all those problems of public education that would seem to require absolutely special approaches and forms of organization of the school population are resolved painlessly in occupational education.

Finally, the last danger that represents a threat in this regard, i.e., the well-known narrowness of those social relations and connections that arise between people out of the soil of labor, also exist only for the lowest forms of labor and disappears in the higher technical forms of labor. There are many who have declared that labor develops only narrow and one-sided social skills; it trains us to see in another person only a colleague, whether an assistant or a superior, and these aspects of human relations are practiced and polished to artistic perfection. In modern large-scale industry, there are created whole groups of people with interdependent responsibilities who work together as different constituents of one and the same mechanism, fully adjusted and fitted one to the other. However, this accommodation of human relations in large-scale labor must not be understood as an exceptional degree of harmoniousness in their rate and skill in work. In genuine forms of work, one requires from one's colleague not just the ability to pass along a work piece, but also genuine understanding and a degree of intimacy. In advanced forms of technological endeavor, a certain degree of mutual occupational faith, requiring a kind of unified discipline on the part of both sides, becomes the psychological condition for working together. Nowhere in occupational activity do two people come into such close contact as in the modern factory when they speak to each other over the telephone using curt and brief remarks.

To understand the pedagogical value of this circumstance, recall that occupational education presents entirely novel didactic techniques of teaching. Neither the old method of simple transmission of knowledge from teacher to student, in which teacher and student work together to discover knowledge by means of questions, or the heuristic method, in which students themselves search for knowledge succeeds, in general, in capturing the didactic essence of occupational education. All these methods presuppose the presence of an ultimate meaning for knowledge not in the student himself, but in the instructor who is guiding him, and, for this reason, differ in essential respects from occupational education, where the meaning of knowledge and the ultimate point it is to attain, is given to the student himself in the form of a process of production in which he sets about to work.

It is in this sense quite correct to liken the psychological path of occupational education to a circle, since this form of education actually describes a circle and, in its very functioning, returns to the actual starting point from which its movement begins. But this return only occurs when the student has entered a new state, seeing with new eyes the very same things, enriched by new experiences; in other words, he approaches the very same point from a different standpoint, and this particularly assists the student himself in examining all at once, and in a single glance, the entire road he has traversed and, what is most important, to get an idea of the purpose he achieved by traversing this road. All the components of the psychological process: the problem the student confronts, his awareness of ways and means of solving the particular problem, the concern over the assimilation and consolidation of this knowledge, monitoring and testing students, and the final assessment of all the work accomplished in the Tsarist pedagogical system—all of this was put together quite mechanically out of different and entirely unrelated pedagogical techniques. We need only recall all those examinations, grades, explanations of lessons, memorization, and so on in order to convince ourselves that these components of the pedagogical process all lacked organic interconnection and were put together only mechanically into a common process simply because they followed one after the other.

On the contrary, in occupational education there occurs a fusion and integration of the entire pedagogical process, an organic unification of all its components into a single whole, and this cyclic character of occupational education emphasizes even more clearly that all the successive stages of this process form and close a complete circle.

Value of Effort in Labor

The psychological value of the efforts made in work manifests itself in the fact that it points to a complete and entirely finished process of a reaction. A sensation that had begun with stimulation of external organs travels through the central nerve pathways and makes it's appearance in the form of an responding act of an active or working organ. Nothing remains stuck inside the organism, there are no residues of mental effort left there, all the sensations of the organism are completely and fairly responded to.

This resembles what happens when a diversion channel designed to direct the flow of a liquid diverts absolutely all the liquid entering it without retaining even the slightest quantity of dregs, residue, or impurities from the flow. Thus, the very presence of effort demonstrates that the organism is functioning entirely, properly and without error, since it is precisely effort of this sort that turns into a switch guiding every sensation and every reaction whatsoever into assuming the correct direction.

The most important result which is achieved thereby is that labor becomes meaningful, and the student who is involved in labor does not have the slightest question as to what might be the meaning of his work. Meaning is given in advance, even before effort itself is induced, and the presence of effort is already an indication that meaning is present.

Meanwhile, every pedagogical science that has treated knowledge in isolation from praxis has virtually always produced entirely unwarranted efforts and, from the psychological point of view, has acquired the character of fruitless Sisyphean labor, like pouring water into a bottomless pit. The common perplexity of gymnasts underscores quite eloquently the meaninglessness of the labor that falls to the lot of students. What could be the purpose of solving problems in arithmetic if all the solutions were given to them long ago and if the answers are printed at the backs of the book? What could be the purpose of translating Latin tests when the word-for-word translations were given to them long ago and are right there in between the lines—this is something my students could not understand at all.

Come to think of it, every exercise in school is so designed that it's as if the student were being asked to work on something for awhile but is first told that this work is quite pointless, is not needed for anything, and is, for all intents and purposes, worthless. Every imaginable way of straying off from this labor has, therefore, become a universal tool in the struggle of students against their teacher's effort to champion the intelligibility and worth of their labor. An educational system lacking all orientation has, accordingly, been created that has never been able to answer the question as to what might be the point of studying this or that subject.

Psychologists have always pointed to the value of what is termed *formal discipline*, asserting that, regardless of the immediate knowledge the student acquires in the study of a particular subject, the educational value of every subject is nevertheless still a matter of perfecting our capacities, of a developmental effect, which these subjects exert on our mind. For example, it is believed that the study of Latin words not only gives the student the ability to read books written in Latin, but also somehow develops and improves his memory. The study of arithmetic and geometry not only teaches him how to multiply and how to prove theorems, but, it is believed, also contributes to the development of the ability to think logically and of a sense of precision when working with quantities. In other words, it is believed that the educational effect of every subject transcends its immediate effect and in some fashion assumes an expanded interpretation and expanded value.

Quite frankly, it was from this point of view that the entire system of classical education was constructed in pre-revolutionary Russia insofar as it found its reflection in the *gymnasia*. Everyone understood perfectly well that nine-tenths of the subjects our gymnasia were burdened with had absolutely no independent pedagogical significance, and that the value of these subjects was limited exclusively to the formal discipline, the "developmental effect" on our mind, which they were supposed to exert. Recall that natural science subjects were introduced into the gymnasium only very recently, and all of them had to undergo quite a struggle before they could attain a position in the curriculum.

From our standpoint, such a pedagogical theory represents, historically speaking, a successor of the medieval scholastic academy, where unending verbal exercises, constructions, and operations constituted the only material and subject of knowledge, and where it was believed that the mind could be developed in the same way that the body could be developed by means of physical exercises. But underlying the pedagogics that was constructed on the basis of such a "gymnastics" of educational subjects was the belief that, just as was maintained by the science of gymnastics proper, all attention had to be focused not on this or that movement in and of itself, but on the developmental force of a particular movement for some group of muscles and organs.

Instruction in Old Church Slavonic could be, in and of itself, just as pointless in the form it was taught in the Tsarist school as is the lifting of weights in Swedish gymnastics, and in the future life of the student the grammar of Old Church Slavonic the student learns by rote has just as little use for him as do the various techniques of Swedish gymnastics in the life of most of us. But it was believed that learning the grammar of Old Church Slavonic is just as healthy and bracing an exercise for the mind as is Swedish exercise for the arm muscles. From the standpoint of psychology, in fact, this theory is based wholly on the old "psychology of capacities," which divided up the entire apparatus of the mind into a whole series of individual mental abilities, found a place for each of them in the brain, and supposed that human psychology could be put together out of the coordinated action of these capacities in the same way that man's body is put together out of individual organs.

Quite frankly, neither the psychological nor the pedagogical basis of this theory has undergone any sort of criticism, and, both in theory as well as in practical applications, views of this sort smack of medieval obscurantism, from the standpoint of modern knowledge. Pedagogical experience has discovered, first, that the formal discipline supplied by a particular subject is quite negligible. It would be more correct to say that it does, indeed, assume an enormous scale, though only in a very narrow range. The memorization of Latin verbs or of irregular conjugations can have a powerful effect on the development of habits of recall, but only for Latin verbs. General processes of recall either do not manifest any sort of improvement whatsoever or only an extremely insignificant improvement. Thus, the formal discipline produced by every subject turns out to be associated only with negligible improvements as regards the accumulation of specialized skills and, consequently, its educational value is confined exclusively to vocational training.

Thus, prolonged acquaintance with the "cuisine" of Latin grammar will improve a pharmacist's memory for prescriptions, and, similarly, a librarian will learn to recognize tens of thousands of books from their tickets and recall where each of them belongs on the shelf, but neither the memory of a pharmacist and his knowledge of foreign languages, nor the memory of a librarian for something else entirely, is improved through vocational practice. On the contrary, there is every reason for supposing that such a specialization of our capacities is always purchased at the expense of a certain limitation of these capacities in other areas and is paid for quite dearly.

Nowadays, psychologists are more inclined to emphasize instead the harm of such early specialization rather than its utility. In particular, as regards memory, they say quite frankly that the real goal of pedagogics is to find out how to teach children to forget what is unnecessary, and not how to force them to remember what is necessary. To properly understand questions in the psychology of memory one might refer to the words of Themistocles, who, in response to the suggestion to learn, is recalled as having said, "Teach me rather to forget."

As in the investigation of memory, the investigation of other abilities has led to the same results, i.e., it has been shown that the formal discipline supplied by each subject affects the development of specialized habits to a certain degree. In other words, our capacity seems to become specialized, and assumes a certain one-sided and extraordinarily narrow character. Of course, whatever is lost in breadth because of this one-sidedness is compensated by the appreciable gain both in overall productivity and in the flexibility of this capacity, though, paradoxical as it may seem, on the whole the formal discipline supplied by individual subjects tends to have a stupefying and restrictive effect rather than a developmental and expansive influence.

In a saying from the French, every definition is already a restriction, and in no other realm is this as true as in the development of our abilities. In present-day psychology, therefore, most researchers are inclined to be most suspicious of those subjects that have become part of the curriculum for their formal value alone. That is, the utility of any subject and its relevance in a pedagogical system is determined, above all and primarily, by the immediate benefit and immediate value that may be ascribed to the knowledge this subject imparts.

Finally, the very psychological conception of man's labors, understood as having been formed out of a multiplicity of individual capacities, does not stand up to rigorous criticism. Every one of our "abilities," in fact, functions in such a complex unity that, taken in and of itself, no one ability can give us even an approximate idea of the real potentiality of its effect. If we study a person with a poor memory in isolation, he may turn out to remember better than someone with a good memory, simply by virtue of the fact that memory never manifests itself in and of itself, but only in close collaboration with attention, overall orientation, thinking, and so on, and it may even prove to be the case that the aggregate effect of these different abilities is always entirely independent of the absolute magnitude of each of the constituents.

It goes without saying, therefore, that the principle of practical instruction assumes the foreground in pedagogics. If knowledge has an extraordinarily slight effect on the development of our mental capacities, value can even be conferred on knowledge only insofar as it is necessary, in and of itself, and only to an extremely limited extent, insofar as it is needed for the development of certain general skills. The formal aspect of the development of these skills is, thus, confined to those elementary and very primitive movements to which the particular school subject, in the course of which these movements may be acquired, becomes nearly neutral.

Consequently, the only criterion of knowledge is its vital value, its need in the real world, i.e., the principle of practicality. The fundamental law of education is, thus, the law of education of conditional reflexes, which says the same thing. If, later on in our life, we wish to discover some relation between various events or facts, on the one hand, and a person's particular reaction, on the other, we must connect the two together in the course of education, not once, but repeatedly, and only then may we be certain that the new relation we require has, in fact, been formed. Thus, the school—the greatest mechanism for the formation of new relations—indeed, all of school, must be geared to life, since only with such striving can the techniques employed there obtain their justification and meaning.

Synthetic Knowledge

Until now, our schools have suffered from a profound dualism, which it inherited from the Tsarist school. Whatever standpoint we assume in relation to our school system, we cannot but note that our school curriculum may still be broken down into two large and incompatible groups. On the one hand, the natural sciences, the sciences that deal with nature, and on the other, the humanities, the sciences of the mind, between which there is no bridge in the edifice of the educational system. Students learn and are brought up seemingly with the unconscious conviction that there are, in fact, two distinct worlds, the world of nature and the world of man, and that they are separated from each other by an impassable gulf.

Not a word connects one realm of entities with the other, and if students acquire other views and another understanding of the world, this occurs despite the school. The school proves to have no effect here, and its exertions are directed toward imparting and emphasizing this duality of our knowledge and of experience. When the student moves from the world of physics to the world of political economy and literature, it's as if he becomes transported to an entirely new world, a world which obeys laws all of its own, where there is not a single point that recalls the world just left, the world of the natural sciences.

And this is not an unintended vice of the Russian school, but rather is the historically inevitable culmination of the entire course of development of European science and of the European system of education. In this case, the school reflects only what had been instituted in the course of the very development of philosophy and science. Only labor, understood as a subject of study, can make it possible to unify the two psychologically, simply because, on the one hand, as a process that occurs between man and nature, labor is wholly dependent upon natural science, and on the other, as a process involved with bringing together social forces, labor is a foundation of the humanities and the social sciences.[1]

Labor, which we may conceive as having been fashioned on the basis of a system of conscious reactions, is also a bridge thrown across the gulf separating the world of the natural sciences and the world of the humanities. It is the only "subject" that is the object of study of both.

In fact, when man is studied in the natural sciences in school, it is only that part of man which is part of anatomy and physiology which is studied and only insofar as he is a mammal; the world of nature from which man is excluded proves to be infinitely ill-fated and infinitely impoverished by comparison with the wealth of real life. And conversely, the world of human actions and deeds seems to hang in thin air, like a rainbow suspended over nature without having sunk any roots into the earth.

Only in its historical meaning and in its psychological essence does labor become the point of encounter in man of the biological and the supra-biological foundation, in which the animal and man are knotted together, and the natural sciences and the humanities become interwoven.

Praxis

"Occupational education" writes Blonskii, "constitutes the education of the ruler of nature", [2] because technology is nothing less than the genuine and materialized dominance of man over nature, a dominance that obeys the laws of nature for the benefit of man.

In this sense, labor reveals itself in what is very nearly its most valuable psychological aspect, that which it exposes to praxis. It is extraordinarily instructive that, in European philosophy of the last several decades, the principle of praxis, in one form or another, has been advanced by the most diverse schools of thought as constituting the only possibility for the construction of scientific knowledge. Come to think of it, praxis constitutes the ultimate test that any scientific discipline may be subjected to, and Marx's expression, that philosophers have done enough in explaining the world, now it is time to think about remaking it, wholly covers the true history of science.

All knowledge ultimately, has arisen, and will arise always, out of some sort of practical need or necessity, and if, in the course of the development of knowledge, it loses touch with the practical problems that gave rise to it, at its final points of its development it will again be oriented towards praxis and find in praxis its ultimate justification, confirmation, and verification.

In particular, the fact that knowledge was presented as entirely abstract and lifeless was the greatest psychological sin of the entire scholastic and classical system of education. Knowledge was assimilated as if a prepared dish, and absolutely no one knew what to do with it. The very nature of knowledge, and likewise the very nature of science, was forgotten, the fact that knowledge is not a kind of prepared dish or pre-set capital reserve, but is always a process of activity, mankind's battle for the mastery of nature.

Scientific truth is mortal, it lives tens, perhaps hundreds of years, and then passes away, since in its struggle to become master of nature, mankind is always moving forward. Science as studied in our schools has been utterly at variance with this standpoint wherever it distorted those truths the student had to learn into dogmatic forms. No psychological conception of truth has been so falsified as that which our students draw out of their textbooks in school.

Truth is presented to them as something finished and all done with, as the result of some kind of process that was finally discovered and is unconditionally certain. It is curious how the greatest disrespect for scientific truth was fostered in students as a result of their learning the scientific truths from the pages of Kraevich and Savodnik, where truth seemed to have been broken down into sections, and where the student could not distinguish in any way what was a scientific fact versus what were the didactic techniques adopted by the compilers of the textbook.

The very process of disclosing truth was hidden, and it was presented not in the dynamic context of its appearance, but in the static of an already discovered rule. And since everything was learned by heart and on faith, it is entirely natural that our student' attitude towards science and towards scientific truth did not differ too much from the attitude of a savage towards his beliefs; and it is just as natural that superstitious and blind devotion to the letter of the facts taught in the school, which, in the Tsarist school, had been the ultimate of pedagogic wisdom, was really capable only of training civilized savages.

Moreover, truth was presented in the school always in the form of an abstract theoretical rule, attained not in the course of a search and of labor, but as if in purely mental work. It was never related to the vital needs that gave rise to it, nor to the vital conclusions that flowed from it. Meanwhile, the very nature of scientific truth, whether it has to do with some minor rule of health or the theory of relativity, nevertheless is practical in nature, or, in other words, truth is always concrete.

Finally, even the most experienced philosopher of teaching methods could not make sense of that infinite melange of scientific truths which was presented to the student without arriving at the most inappropriate conclusions. In any course of studies, all scientific truths were lumped together, in the full sense of this word, and not even the most resourceful educator could explain what might the relationship between Latin declensions, the Napoleonic wars, and the laws of electrolysis.

Because of the uncoordinated and patchwork nature of school learning, the student's perception was weighted down with an infinite number of isolated facts, preventing him from attaining a unifying and connected point of view on the object. It is for this reason that, in the realm of philosophy and general outlook, there has dominated among educated people in Russia the most embarrassing superficiality, a propensity for the use of the most flippant phraseology, and the most incredible degree of ignorance as regards the most elementary of questions. These three sins of the Tsarist school are all easily overcome in occupational education, which, first, synthesizes and unifies all subjects, second, confers on all subjects a practical bent by providing them with applications, and, third, discloses the very process involved in uncovering truths, and the progress of truth that has been discovered.

Vocation and Polytechnism

Though the trend of modern industry is towards the utter multi-specialization of labor, nevertheless this process cannot be considered complete in the slightest degree, even in such a highly developed capitalist country as America, and even less so here in Russia.

Thus, polytechnism is a truth for some future day towards which the school must be oriented in its own efforts, but this truth has still not been realized today, and the school confronts the task not only to implement a program of polytechnical education, but to also satisfy the immediate everyday needs which are presented to it. We have to understand the sense of vocational career that has to be fostered by our schools as a concession to the real world, as a bridge from public education to everyday experience.

This means that, in its bias in favor of vocations, the school does not in any way lose its polytechnical character, and the polytechnical spirit remains as its principal and fundamental core, though polytechnical education of this sort is concentrated at one end, as if sharpened so that it may more easily enter directly into the world from this end. In this regard, the relationship between general and special education, now expressed in a new light, however, is fully encompassed by that old formula that has long been advanced by psychology, which asserts that *everyone should know something about everything, and everything about something*. That everyone should know something about everything simply means that the most elementary and the most general ideas of the most important elements of the whole world must be the foundation of every person's general education. And for us to know everything about something, our educational system has to gather together absolutely every piece of knowledge about some one realm directly related to our work.

It is not hard to see that this old formula is fully applicable to occupational education if by "knowing everything about something," we understand the demands of professional career, and if by "knowing something about every-thing," we understand polytechnism.

None of the pedagogical principles that are now put forward threatens such adverse consequences, if not understood correctly, as does the principle of the trade school. Quite frankly, the Russian experience with trade schools has been a vivid example of such misinterpretation. Blonskii, in his book on trade schools [*Trudovaya shkola*], declares that there is not a single page nor a single principle that could not be converted into the most malicious parody of the labor principle:

> I have seen communal schools that have completely revived the spirit of orphanages. I have seen teachers who have developed a 'child's day' for an entire district down to an accuracy of 15 minutes. I have watched girls too young for school teach five-year-old children to cook in a smelly kitchen. Children have rushed over even to me, hoping to escape from having to work in vegetable gardens that had brought them to the point of utter exhaustion. I have seen teachers who thought that trade schools consist in hauling heavy and dirty loads of firewood, cleaning up bathrooms, and sweeping up, though to me this seems like unhealthy labor, and reminiscent of hard labor even for grown-ups. I have seen woodworking shops where I, a grown-up, was forced to gasp for breath, and where children worked on their feet, forced to stand in incredible positions. I have seen children working in metal shops after which, it would seem to me, they would all end up with a case of pneumonia. I have watched people chatter away who thought that their lengthy conversations on every imaginable daily trifle meant that they were conducting a trade school. I have discovered departments responsible for speaking with teachers on how to run school lunch rooms. I am certain that a number of instructors lead children into the hell of factories, put teenagers into the din and heat of workshops, place them right next to dangerous machinery, fill their lungs with lungs with coal and dust, and then go around confident they are teaching using 'Blonskii's method'. [3]

[1] These remarks seem to prefigure the work of C.P. Snow by 30 years, in which Snow describes how education becomes possible in the trade school.

[2] Original source not known.

[3] Original source not known.

Chapter 11

SOCIAL BEHAVIOR AND THE CHILD'S DEVELOPMENT

The Concept of Adaptation

Contemporary biology sees in the concept of adaptation a fundamental principle governing the development of organic life on earth. In pedagogics, we also say that adapting the child to the environment in which he will have to live and function is the ultimate goal of every form of education.

But there are two things to keep in mind here. First, the process of adapting to the environment may display the most diverse features imaginable. A cunning career-seeker, a sharp operator, or a swindler who possesses a magnificent sense for the slightest disturbance in his surroundings, who knows how to respond to it with the appropriate reaction, and who succeeds in satisfying all his own vital needs and thereby experiences the greatest sense of self-satisfaction, as expressed in positive emotional affect, giving him the opportunity to always be in the dominant position—these people, too, are adapted to the environment.

One might ask whether such a person is, from the pedagogical standpoint, the ultimate of the educated personality. And, conversely, is a revolutionary who cannot get on in any social group at all, who rises up in rebellion against society and is always in conflict with his surroundings, thus exhibiting his maladjustment—do we say that such a person is badly or incorrectly educated?

The other problem is that, because of the very features of his development, every child adapts himself to his surroundings in different ways.

Thus, we have to consider the problem of adaptation to the environment also as a function of the child's behavior as he grows up. Let us consider both questions in turn.

To start with, we have to say that adaptation has to be considered in no other way than from the social point of view. One must never proceed from the given and existing environment as if from something constant and unchanging. The social environment comprises an inexhaustible collection of the most diverse aspects and elements, which are always in the most outright contradiction with each other and always engaged in the most brutal struggle against each other. We should not think of the environment as a whole as a static, elemental, and stable system of elements, but rather as a dialectically developing dynamic process.

From the point of view of society, therefore, the revolutionary may prove to be more adapted to the highest tendencies of the environment than the career-seeker, simply because he is adapted to the social dynamic, and not to the social static.

Man's relationship to his surroundings must always bear the character of purposefulness, of activity, and not simple dependence. Adaptation to the environment may, therefore, denote the most brutal struggle with individual elements of the environment, and always denotes certain purposeful inter-relations with it. Consequently, the individual may assume entirely different social orientations in different social environments. It's all a matter of the direction in which this purposefulness is guided.

The other question is solved if we note the following. A child actually passes through many stages of adaptation to the social environment, and the functions of his social behavior are highly variable, depending on particular developmental stages. The child's social behavior, therefore, must be thought of as behavior that has been refracted innumerable times as a function of the biological development of the organism.

The Child and the Environment

Zalkind conveys the objective and materialist meaning of Freud's teachings in the following, rough form:

Freud, according to Zalkind, establishes two principles to which man's activity is subordinated, the pleasure principle and the reality principle. Man's deeply embedded conscious and unconscious desires in interaction with the environment are the source of man's psyche. "All of emotional life is guided by the desire for pleasure and the aversion to suffering." These desires for pleasure guide the entire orientation of the personality, filling attention, memory, and thought with actual content. "The aggregate of man's psychological world is nothing but the sum total of his desires and experience in the struggle for their fulfillment." But the desire for pleasure comes into conflict with the demands of the real world, which the individual must adapt himself to, and, thus, the pleasure principle is in conflict with the reality principle. There are many desires the organism must deny itself. Any such unfulfilled desire is exiled to the realm of the unconscious, and there continues to exist in concealed form, "breaking through into mental life, attempting in its own way to subordinate to its influence these unconscious and exiled desires. The pleasure principle, where it has not achieved a compromise with the reality principle, avenges itself by creating in place of, or in addition to, the real world, another world of its own—a world of unrealized, exiled, unconscious desires. Two realities that would seem to be incompatible are created in man, an external reality that man can become aware of, that comprises elements of adaptation to the surrounding environment, and a mental reality that is alien and hostile to the external environment, which is driven underground into the unconscious by the external environment, but remaining hungry and unsatisfied, and forcing its way upward. All of mental life is permeated by a furious struggle between these two realities." This struggle expresses itself in what is known as a *censor*, which distorts the suppressed desires that are forced upward whenever the conscious state is in a weakened position, whether in sleep or when distracted.

The highest form of this conflict, this disharmony with the environment, is expressed in what is referred to as the escape into illness, a process that must be understood as an unhealthy attitude towards reality, a special form of behavior, in which the exiled and unsatisfied desires that have been isolated in a kind of "complex," or group of representations associated with some effective experience, gain the upper hand.

Even our thinking seems to be guided along the lines set out by these exiled desires or complexes, to say nothing of the fact that all other mental forces are subordinated to this law. "Man, it turns out, directs to the environment around him only part of his creative wealth, the rest being preserved for internal use, use that is alien to the obligations made by this environment. The sum total of attention, memory, the substance of mental processes, those qualities of general and special abilities, that quantity of stamina and versatility that an individual manifests in acts of his real adaptation, frequently constitute a negligible scrap of his creative potentiality. The overwhelming mass of this potentiality remains hidden from our eyes, shut in, and directed towards isolated, internal processes, nourishing extraneous, unreal, and uncreative sensations. This occurs not only in so-called pathological ill personalities, but also in entirely normal people, bearing in mind the extraordinary relativity of the very concept of mental health, what with the insanity characteristic of the contemporary social environment. The innate structure of personality and the habits that personality accumulates from early natural childhood prove to be in inevitable conflict with the demands of the surrounding reality in the course of the individual's subsequent growth. Inner disarray, utter disruption, and a sharp personality split that returns to the environment only that which personality has been forced to renounce grows, while the bulk of the reserves of personality is left in a state of hungry potential tension."

Freud believes that the bulk of these suppressed desires are of sexual origin, and he ascribes the development of the sex instinct to very early childhood. Of course, he does not mean there is any sort of fully developed and outright sex instinct in the child. Rather, he sees more of a matter of embryonic, incomplete elements, isolated sensations, that emanate from the mucous membranes, from the functioning of individual organs, constituting the rudiments of future sexual feelings, the so-called "libido."

It turns out that the child's primitive instinctive experience, like the earliest habits of childhood, what we call "infantile behavior," occurs chiefly under the influence of the pleasure principle. Adaptation to the environment is the concern of the grown-up. It is the grown-up who helps the child establish the first inter-relations with the environment. This also imposes a special imprint on infantile behavior in the early period of childhood, which is formed, first, out of unconditional innate reactions and, second, out of those first-degree conditional reflexes which are closest to them.

This also explains the tragic contradiction "between the innate reserves, early childhood experience, and the much later acquisitions of experience." It is because there exists the greatest incompatibility imaginable between this early childhood experience, which has grown up on the foundations of biological habits, and the environment with all its objective demands, that man's biological disarray arises, and the transition from infantile behavior to adult behavior always constitute a tragedy, which Freud has referred to as the struggle between the pleasure principle and the reality principle.

Zalkind points out that these conclusions are fully in agreement with results learned from experiments performed in Pavlov's laboratory. Here can be seen in experimental form the reproduction of the *definition* of childhood experience as it manifests itself in life. A dog is presented with scented powdered meat, and responds to it with prehensile and salivary reflexes. The dog, however, is given powder only if there has already been some sort of preceding signal, whether light or sound. Otherwise, the dog is not given any food. The dog at first picks at the powder every time, produces saliva, and so on. But as a result of persistent repetitions of the experiment, it begins to inhibit its fundamental reflex. Without obtaining any resolution, without a conditional signal, it is, biochemically speaking, simply not capable of eating (no saliva or other gastric juices are produced), does not have any appetite, and does want to eat.

The Contemporary Environment and Education

Because of its own chaotic system of influences, the contemporary social environment, i.e., the environment of capitalist society, creates a radical contradiction between the child's early experience and its subsequent forms of adaptation. The organism must, therefore, master certain forms of inhibition, certain ways of reining in its own desires, and these desires manifest themselves and find an outlet in sleep, though not completely, but only in masked form, since they are hindered by the censor. A decisive contradiction between the environment and personality is created as a result. This is how Zalkind paints the picture which thereby arises: All unfulfilled desires are pointed in an incorrect direction, and flow back to the sex instinct, which feeds off them, like a parasite feeding off a host.

The chaotic agglomeration of contemporary social stimulations creates a crude incompatibility between the inherited reserves, the experience of early childhood, and the later, more mature psychological build-up. Hence, the vast proportion of man's biological and emotional forces are restrained, and hence the perverted employment of these forces and the fact that only a negligible proportion of this energy is made use of by the social environment. Powerful reserves that anticipate appropriate social sensations and which possess an extraordinary degree of plasticity are found at the very base of man's psychophysiology. Raising these reserves up from the depths, undertaking the social liberation of this energy, means realizing a process we may describe in the following way. Masses of energy are embedded in man in the form of conscious and unconscious desires and strivings; part of this energy does not obtain any satisfaction, because of the reality principle, and is exiled to the unconscious. For the remainder, there are now three outlets possible. It may enter into a struggle with the conscious forms of behavior, conquer them, and avenge itself on the reality principle; it is this which constitutes the flight into illness or psychoneurosis. Second, the struggle may end in a draw, or, more properly, it may not end at all, and the individual, while retaining normal forms of behavior, lives in a constant, prolonged conflict between the environment and himself, and within himself. Finally, the third outlet: energy that has been driven off into the subconscious and exiled from reality is again liberated, again assumes the status of reality, though now it is guided in socially useful, creative directions. Here the environment is fully triumphant, since it has not only banished forces that are in contradiction to it, but has once again taken possession of them, though in altered form.

Thus, this process, or sublimation, also constitutes the greatest realization imaginable of all our desires, but only in socially useful directions. Consequently, this is also the road that education must travel. Sublimation understood this way has much in common with the ordinary forms of disinhibition of reflexes, even those that have not been banished to the subconscious. To explain the mechanism by which sublimation functions, we will use an everyday illustration given by Zalkind:

A minor official has been roughly insulted by his superior. Previously, "irritations" of this sort had always induced in the official a typical inhibition, rather than an aggressive reflex, which in this case would usually not obtain the required nourishment, since the bureaucratic environment in the Tsarist system, of course, did not create a favorable soil for the development of nascent aggressive reflexes. The sum total of this inhibited arousal could manifest itself externally in either of two directions:

(1) The official is at home, sitting down to dinner, and some trifle, perhaps a little mishap, occurs at the table, 'irritates' him, and the irritation ends up within the field of the inhibited arousal, and suddenly there is a sharp, rough outburst, and with the enormous force of an aggressive reflex the dishes are thrown at the wife, at the children, the official begins to pound the table and there is shouting throughout the apartment (the Freudian catharsis is an explosion, an impetuous outpouring of an inhibited arousal). This is one path.

(2) Another path is possible. Inhibition remains in force, and all the superior's subsequent insults sustain, nourish, and condense it. But, in addition, there appear new sensations as well, for example, a revolutionary uprising through-out the city, underground proclamations that call for a struggle against 'superiors' in general, give instructions as to what methods should be followed in such a struggle, which becomes a prolonged, persistent, and disciplined struggle. The aggressive reflex is liberated, but not impetuously, but instead in a disciplined form that unfolds over a lengthy period of time, turning into a persistent, underground revolutionary effort. The aggressive reflex is disciplined and sublimated; a lower-order reflex is transformed by means of the encrustation or accumulation of sensations all about it, through its prolonged inhibition and its slow liberation, into a higher-order reflex, into a *creative process.* [1]

Hence, it is clear that education which is ideally practicable is possible only on the basis of an appropriately guided social environment and, consequently, the crucial questions of education can be solved in no other way than through the resolution of the social question in all its entirety. But the conclusion follows, therefore, that man's substance possesses infinite plasticity in a properly guided social environment. Everything that is found in man may be educated and re-educated if the appropriate societal influence is applied. Even personality must be understood in this regard not as some finished form, but as a constantly coursing dynamic form of interaction between the organism and the environment.

Recall that if absolutely everything in the human organism is potentially capable of being educated, under the genuine conditions of our century, education as we are understanding it, runs up against a whole series of obstacles. Let us consider the genuine forms of the child's social behavior.

Genuine Forms of Social Behavior

In real life, people sustain their existence by adapting nature to their needs in the course of labor. Human industry is collective in nature, and always requires a certain degree of organization of social forces, as a preliminary moment for its appearance.

In life, in general, there exists a close relationship between organisms of the same form. The forms of human society, however, differ from the forms of animal communities. Any animal community always arises on the basis of the instincts of feeding, protection, aggression, and reproduction, all of which require the combined cooperation of different individuals. In mankind, these instincts led to the formation and appearance of economic activity, which underlies all of historical development. Marx says in this regard that,

> ...in the form of social production characteristic of their times, people enter into definite and necessary relations that are independent of their will, that is, production relations, which correspond to a definite stage of development of the material production forces of the community. The aggregate of these production relations constitutes the economic structure of society, which is the genuine foundation of the legal and political superstructure and which corresponds to a particular form of social consciousness. As the economic foundation changes, there occurs, sooner or later, an upheaval throughout the entire vast superstructure. In considering such upheavals, we always have to distinguish between the material upheaval in the economic conditions of production, which may be ascertained with the precision of the natural sciences, and the legal, political, religious, artistic, or philosophical upheavals, in brief, the ideological forms in which people are aware of this upheaval and struggle among themselves on the soil of this upheaval. (*Das Capital*).

Thus, from the standpoint of historical materialism, the fundamental causes of all social changes and all political upheavals must be sought not in peoples' minds, Engels said, and not in their views of eternal truths and justice, but in changes in the means of production and distribution. They must be sought not in philosophy, but in the economics of each epoch. Thus, in mankind the production process assumes the broadest possible social character, which at the present time encompasses the entire world. Accordingly, there arise the most complex forms of organization of human social behavior with which the child encounters before he directly confronts nature.

The nature of man's education, therefore, is wholly determined by the social environment in which he grows and develops. But this environment does not always affect man directly and straightforwardly, but also indirectly, through his ideology. By ideology, we will understand all the social stimuli that have been established in the course of historical development and have become hardened in the form of legal statutes, moral precepts, artistic tastes, and so on. These standards are permeated through and through with the class structure of society that generated them and serve as the class organization of production. They are responsible for all of human behavior, and in this sense we are justified in speaking of man's class behavior.

We know that absolutely every one of man's conditional reflexes is determined by those environmental influences that reach him from outside. This social environment is class-based in its very structure insofar as, obviously, all new relations are imprinted by the class basis of the environment. This is why certain investigators have decided to speak not only of class psychology, but also of class physiology. The boldest minds have decided to speak of the "total social immersion" [*vsepropitannost'*] of the organism, and have pointed out that the most intimate of our functions are, ultimately, expressions of this social nature. We breathe and carry out the most important functions of our organism always in accordance with those stimuli which affect us. If we were to analyze the psychology of modern man, we would find such a mass of other people's views, words, and thoughts that there would be absolutely no way we could tell where the individual personality begins and the social personality ends. In modern society, every person, therefore, whether he likes it or not, is inevitably a spokesman of a particular class.

Since we know that each person's individual experience is conditioned by the role he plays in his environment, and that it is the class membership which also defines this role, it is clear that class membership defines man's psychology and man's behavior. "Thus", writes Blonskii, "there are no invariant and obligatory laws of human behavior in society whatsoever. In class society the concept, 'man,' is generally an empty and abstract concept. Man's social behavior is determined by the behavior of his class, and each person is inevitably a person from a particular class". [2] In this regard, we must be profoundly historical and must always present man's behavior in relation to the class situation at the given moment. This must be the fundamental psychological technique for every social psychologist. Recall that the class structure of society defines the standpoint which man occupies in organized social labor. Consequently, class membership defines at one fell swoop both the cultural and the natural orientation of personality in the environment. "Hence", Blonskii continued, "every person is a kind of exemplar (intermediate, most common, best, worst, and so on) of a particular social class. It follows that the behavior of the individual is a derivative of the behavior of the corresponding class". [3]

In fact, human labor, i.e., the struggle for existence, assumes, by necessity, forms of the social struggle and, accordingly, places whole masses of people under the same conditions, forcing them to develop identical forms of behavior. These identical forms of behavior are made up of all those widespread religious beliefs, ceremonies, and customs within which a given society lives. Thus, whether we like it or not, education is, either consciously or unconsciously, always guided along class lines.

For the psychologist this means that the aggregate of stimuli that forms the aggregate of the child's behavior comprises class stimuli.

This should be kept in mind whenever present-day pedagogics confronts the old question as to what constitutes the ideal of education, whether an international type that would be suitable for all mankind, or a national type. It is essential to keep in mind the class nature of all ideals, and recall that the ideals of nationalism, patriotism, and so on are only masked forms of the class trend of education. This is why neither can serve as a genuine solution for our pedagogics. On the contrary, since present-day education adapts itself to the international working class out in the historical arena, to that extent the ideals of international development and of class solidarity have to overcome the ideal of national education and the ideal of education "appropriate for all mankind."

This does not at all mean, however, that contemporary pedagogics requires that we not attend to national forms of development. In fact, national forms of development constitute a great and undoubted historical fact. It goes without saying, therefore, that these forms of development occur as an indispensable psychological condition in our schools. Everything we teach the child must be adapted to those special forms of behavior, language, customs, morals and manners, and habits which the child perceives.

Meanwhile, it is important to avoid the fundamental errors that pedagogics usually makes in this understanding. First is the extraordinary cult of ethnicity [*narodnost'*], which intensifies the national element in behavior beyond all reasonable limits, and fosters nationalism in students in place of a sense of nationality. This is usually associated with a whole series of adverse phenomena, such as negative attitudes towards other ethnic groups and "rabid patriotism," i.e., the propensity for external, ostentatious signs of one's ethnic origin. Like all cultural acquisitions, the ethnic complexion of human behavior constitutes the greatest of all human values, though only when it is not a matter of pulling the wool over one's eyes, like a snail crawling into its shell, and not when it screens the individual off from all external influence.

The collision between different cultures has often brought with it mixed and false forms of language, art, and so on, though, in addition, it has produced brilliant results through the development of novel forms of cultural creativity. Loyalty to one's ethnic group is loyalty to one's individuality, and is also the only healthy and nonartificial path of behavior.

The extraordinary degree of concern around these questions represents a further danger of nationalism. In fact, national forms of culture are acquired seemingly spontaneously and occur as an unconscious constituent in the structure of our behavior. In this sense, speaking both psychologically and pedagogically, nationality is not in contradiction with class, and instead both possess their own extremely important psychological function.

Variations in the Development of Children

Child development constitutes the fundamental principle of psychology. The child is not a finished being, but a developing organism and, consequently, his behavior is formed not only under the exclusive impact of the systematic influence of the environment, but also as a function of certain cycles or periods in the development of the child's own organism, which, in turn, defines the relationship of man to the environment. The child does not develop in uniform or gradual fashion, through the accumulation of slight variations, but by fits and starts, harmonically, so that periods during which the child's growth is on the rise follow periods of stagnation and abatement.

This irregularity of rhythmic oscillations constitutes the fundamental law of the child's behavior and manifests itself even in daily and annual oscillations. Meumann, for example, has suggested that the child's psyche expresses itself with greatest intensity in autumn and winter; mental forces experience the greatest tension from October to February, beginning to fall in March and vanishing entirely by summer. Alongside the annual oscillations, there are also daily oscillations; because of these oscillations, pedagogical science has been led to propose that student lessons be distributed in such a way that the most difficult lessons are presented at times when energy is at its peak. The harm produced by lessons held at night or in the evening, at times when energy has dropped the most, as well as after supper, when there occurs an appreciable outflow of blood from the brain and inflow into the stomach because of the intensification of digestive activity, has been particularly noted.

In the present context, this principle of periodicity may be termed the *dialectical principle of the child's development*, since it manifests itself not by slow and gradual changes, but by fits and starts at particular critical points, where quantity turns into quality all of a sudden; and we have every right to distinguish different qualitative periods of child development. Precisely the same thing happens when water subjected to uniform cooling suddenly begins to turn into ice at the freezing point, or, when subjected to uniform heating, begins to be transformed into a vapor all at once as it passes through the boiling point. In other words, in the course of child development, just as with everything else in nature, there occurs a dialectical path of development composed of contradictions and a transition of quantity into quality.

Aristotle long ago demonstrated in rough outline the transition from one stage to another stage that, in general, coincides with those divisions everyone is more or less in agreement about. Now we tend to distinguish four basic stages in the development of the child, each of which has its own special biological meaning and, consequently, its own relationship to the environment.

The first period may be termed the *period of early childhood*, when the child's activity is virtually nil. His biological functions are principally determined by feeding; the child eats and sleeps, grows and breathes, and his behavior is wholly determined by these very important functions. Those forms of his behavior, therefore, develop which help him carry on these functions. Nearly all the child's reactions of this period are directed towards making even the slightest acquaintance with the environment. Even at this time, the child exhibits a number of reactions associated with play. At this stage, the child plays, is oriented towards the environment, and exercises his most important organs of perception and movement. It is right at this time that the greatest event in the life of the child occurs: he learns to direct his movements, coordinating for the first time the activity of his eyes and hands, and learns how to reach out to an object that is in front of him. At this time, he is shut off from the environment by grown-ups, who carry out on his behalf the most important functions involved in adapting to the environment. By this time, however, the child has fallen under the influence of those around him, his situation, and, principally, the role his surroundings play with respect to him.

His mother, therefore, assumes the primary role and, as one psychologist has correctly put it, it is she who is the primary social environment for the child. A turning point occurs at this time with the eruption of baby teeth, when the child, in the course of switching over to other food, also changes its relationship to the environment. In general, the entire period of early childhood is rich in events in which the child learns how to walk, speak, and move about, and first begins to gain a sense of direction in the environment. This period lasts, thus, for six or seven years, constituting the early period of childhood.

At this time of continuous growth, the child finally becomes proficient in all his movements, and his relationships to the environment are governed by the fact that the environment reaches him through adults. This entire period is called by some psychologists the *play period.*

A kind of crisis sets in at this point, a lag in growth, which would appear to represent what we may think of as a boiling or freezing point, after which the new, qualitatively distinctive period of late childhood begins, which lasts from the age of seven through 13 or 14. In this period, the child finds himself in an unmediated relation with the environment, acquiring all those skills that an adult requires. The forms of his behavior become complicated, and he enters into new relationships with the environment. It seems like a new, second wave immerses him ever more deeply into the world, into a more intimate relationship with the world. This period concludes with puberty, which psychologists are all in agreement in referring to as a tragic period in the life of the child. Absolutely everyone notices a sudden change, whether in the voice or in the appearance and structure of the body, "when all its parts," in Rubinshtein's expression, "seem to be as if at a cross-roads, having abandoned the stage of childhood wholeness but still not having succeeded in establishing the solidly cohesive harmony of the adult body.

This period is characterized by the greatest discord with the environment. It is accompanied by internal and external shocks, and is often a source of subsequent illnesses and disturbances in the organism that last for the individual's entire lifetime. This is because a powerful and impetuous instinct that suddenly manifests itself in the body is condemned to inaction, as a consequence of which there arises a grave conflict between the child and the environment and within the child himself. The period is also characterized by an extraordinarily heightened sensitivity and awkwardness, as if the child were constantly aware of his maladjustment to the environment. Thus, it is, in every sense of the word, a critical age.

It is also a decisive stage for education in the sense that it is at this time that the basic forms of sublimation are established in the child, by virtue of the outflow of sexual energy that sublimation receives under the influence of education.

After this delay there follows the period of adolescence, lasting from age 13 to 18, which is characterized by the ultimate formation of the individual's relation to the environment. This is clear if only from the fact that, during puberty, the brain gains the third of its full weight; the first third is present in the newborn infant, while the second third builds up throughout childhood up through the age of 14. The period of youth, the time when the individual becomes finally accustomed to the environment, follows this period and lasts until the age of 18. All these divisions must be looked upon as conventional lacking absolutely exact points of division. They are accompanied by a whole series of transitional mental features that are, to a enormous extent, distinctive of each period.

One example is the time of childhood negativism, which is typical of children in the pre-school period. A love for arguments, denial, and deeds of defiance represent its clearest manifestation. Some psychologists ascribe this period to the age of 3 to 5, though, for various reasons, it would appear to occur at a later age, and is often encountered the most in subtle forms in seven- and eight-year old children.

The psychological meaning of this behavior would appear to consist in a sudden change in the child's activity in relation to the environment, which grows as he gets older. To everything, such a child says, "Let me do it myself," suffering all the time from an "itch to negate." One has only to approach a child at this age and say to her over and over, "yes," in order to hear in response a sharp and decisive "no." A moment after your "no" the child answers "yes," speaking in a flat tone. One has only to approach a child at this age, dressed all in white, and say to her, "Today you'll wear your white dress," in order to hear the response, "No, my black dress." In this period, according to Rubinshtein, children often respond both to requests and to injunctions, and even to a simple summons, by expressing themselves in the form of a negation: "Not Volodya," "Not Mama," and so on. One mother who was quite confused by the following example, which represents only an intensified form of this argumentative period, once turned to me for advice. Her four-year boy, who responded to everything with a "no," whether it was the right or wrong thing to say, at the same time often did not refuse to do what he was asked. Once, while getting ready to go to sleep, his mother asked him to read a common prayer with her, and he responded by performing the request in an entirely unexpected form: 'No to father, no to us, no to them, no to the heavens. . .

Such instances are often encountered, though perhaps in less aggravated form. The present author once had to observe how a girl, having reached the age of negativism, copied out her lessons on the blackboard in reverse order, from right to left. Her example was contagious, with the entire class following suit, and the teacher, who was generally on good terms with the class, was entirely unable to cope with this fit of negativism. But what was most curious was that this instance was painlessly overcome once, at the suggestion of the present author, the teacher herself began to write on the blackboard from right to left. That day the children resumed the normal style of writing.

Negativism of this sort is only a special instance of the manifestation of that general maladjustment which is the basic feature of childhood. From the time it is born and throughout its childhood, the child is an organism which is maladjusted and uncertain in its relationship to the environment to the greatest degree imaginable. This is why a child is always in need of grown-ups to steady him, even if unnaturally. This is why a child, that most emotional of all beings, will laugh or cry, but will rarely be indifferent. You see, emotions are also points of imbalance in our behavior, points when we feel either weighed down by our surroundings or triumphant over them.

The tragic aspect cannot, therefore, be effaced from the processes of childhood development and education, and the child's entry into the world was and always will be a process involving a painful break and the creation of ruptures in tissues and in their birth. Buhler was entirely correct when he referred to "the transformation of our children into grown-ups [as] the greatest of all the dramas of development." Like a tooth that breaks through the gums, the child, with difficulty and great effort, enters the world.

---

[1] Original source not known.
[2] Original source not known.
[3] Original source not known.

Chapter 12

ETHICAL BEHAVIOR

The Nature of Ethics from the Psychological Point of View

The problem of moral education is among those questions that are now undergoing a reassessment in psychology and in culture in the most decisive and most thorough-going fashion. The thousand-year link between morality and religion has been broken, and, under the force of analysis, morality is beginning to acquire an increasingly temporal character. It is now possible to establish beyond all reasonable doubt the experiential, temporal character of morality, and its dependence on historical and social conditions, and its class character.

Every nationality and every epoch, and likewise every class, possesses its own morality, which is always a product of social psychology. There is the morality of the Hottentot, who, it is said, responds when asked the question, "What do you consider to be good, and what do you consider to be bad?" by declaring, "Good is when I steal a wife; bad is when I'm robbed."

Moral concepts and ideas vary depending upon the social environment, and what is considered bad at one time and in one place, elsewhere might be considered the greatest of all virtues. And if there are any common feature in all these different manifestations of moral consciousness that can be identified, this is only because certain common elements shared by every human society were once part of the social order.

Thus, from the standpoint of social psychology, ethics must be looked upon as a certain form of social behavior that was established and evolved in the interests of the ruling class, and is different for different classes. This is why there has always existed a morality of the ruler and a morality of slaves, and this is why epochs characterized by crises have represented the greatest crises of morality.

It is said that in the schools of ancient Sparta, children were forced to wait upon a common table while the adults had their meals. A child had to steal something from the table, and he would be punished only if he couldn't do this, or only if he were caught red-handed. The moral lesson of this experiment was to steal and not get caught. Such an ideal was entirely conditioned by the

Communist order of the closed aristocratic society of Sparta, in which concern for property did not constitute the standard of morality, in which stealing, therefore, was not considered a sin, but where force, craftiness, cunning, and composure constituted the ideal of all citizens of Sparta, and where the greatest sin was the inability to deceive someone else and to control one's emotions.

As in every school of thought, moral education here coincides entirely with the class morality which guides the school. In France, where special classes in ethics have been introduced and where there are textbooks of morality in use, the educational ideal consists in those bourgeois virtues which permeate the mind and soul of the French middle-class. In one French textbook on morality, for example, there are hardly any "ethical standards," according to M.M. Rubinshtein, and in their place thriftiness is exalted and bank books turned into the criterion of morality.

Such class ideals are inherent to all other systems of education. This was also the case in the pre-revolutionary secondary schools, which were constructed on authoritarian foundations, in which obedience was considered the ideal for the student, and the general goals of moral education were to educate a loyal subject or a hard-working official.

Now that the world has experienced the cleansing threat of social revolution, the very foundations of bourgeois morality are trembling, and it is very possible that in no other realm do we meet up with such shapeless and tenuous ideas as in the domain of ethical standards. All those rules of bourgeois morality, which were fully laden with hypocrisy and mendacity, have lost their meaning. Bourgeois morality was compelled to be hypocritical, because it taught one thing and did another, because it was constructed at the juncture of class interests and, preaching the kingdom of God after death, implanted a kingdom of enslavers in the world. Lies and hypocrisy were the natural source of such a form of morality, and sanctimoniousness was its inevitable accompaniment. The child saw one thing out in the world and was told something else altogether, and all the school's endeavor was oriented towards reconciling this divergence between real life and morality in the child as effortlessly as possible.

The child either was unable to reconcile the two, or, if he was taught how to do so, he would become accustomed to viewing morality as a kind of social decorum that everyone had to observe, though this always entailed great effort, in fact, it was only through such effort that he could assume this point of view. The child's moral consciousness could be reduced to the convictions of Griboedov's chambermaid, i.e., that "There's nothing wrong with sinning, just don't spread rumors."

The fear of moral retribution supplied the compulsory sanction for morality, in addition to public opinion, and, in his moral behavior, man was easily guided psychologically by the very same custodial rules—this you should not do, but that you may do—and usually guided himself in all his behavior in precisely this way. One Russian philosopher was right, in this sense, to refer to these moral concepts as embodying a kind of "moral policeman," since the force of moral precepts was rooted in the compulsory and humiliating power of fear in the face of moral punishment and the pangs of conscience. There was a special morality of the strong and the weak, and just as in regard to external laws, so in regard to the laws of conscience, the weak would submit to them, and the strong would rebel against them and break these laws. In its revolt against bourgeois morality, European philosophy proclaimed the immorality of its own basic laws, and speaking through Nietsche's lips, declared itself to be beyond good and evil.

Shestov says that man's relation to the categorical imperative is just like the attitude of the Russian peasant towards that forest of tall trees which Peter the Great had forbidden to cut down. In both cases, there is the attraction of an entirely arbitrary deed, though the individual still confronts the fear of retribution and punishment, in the one case external and in the other case internal. The moral commandment, "do not kill," has always been understood in just this sense; that is, "do not kill, not because that's the wrong road to take, but because you yourself will die from the pangs of conscience." This, the internal contradiction of bourgeois morality, was exposed by Dostoyevskii in *Crime and Punishment*. In Nietzsche's revolt, the overall negative critical work of his thinking, in its attack on bourgeois morality, had the force of a stick of dynamite, exploding the very foundations of Christian morality from within.

A new morality will be created once a new human society will have been created, but at that point it is likely that moral behavior will have been entirely dissolved into general forms of behavior. All of behavior in general will be moral, because there will be no basis whatsoever for any conflict between the behavior of one person and the behavior of society in general.

Here it is possible to take note only of several points that the pedagogics of moral behavior must deal with.

Note, first, the negation of the absolute, supra-empirical roots of morality, or of any innate morality of feelings. From the psychological point of view, moral behavior, like everything else, arises *on the foundation* of innate and instinctive reactions, and evolves under the influence of the methodical effects of the environment. Without question, the foundation of moral feelings have to be sought in the instinctive sense of sympathy for another person, in social instincts, and in much else besides. As it comes into contact with every imaginable datum, concept, and phenomenon in the process of growth, these innate reactions turn into those conditional forms of behavior we refer to collectively as moral behavior.

Hence the general conclusion that moral behavior is a form of behavior which is amenable to education through the social environment in exactly the same way as is everything else.

We should also bear in mind the uncertainty that now pervades morality. On the one hand, revolutionary boldness is needed, not a narrow-minded view of things, in order to discern what is happening, what is its genuine meaning, and to know how to reject all those prejudices which only recently everyone believed to be unshakeable moral tenets. All that is left of bourgeois morality, like the corrupt legacy of a previous life, all this must be swept clear out of our schools. On the other hand, however, there is a certain risk concealed in this impermanence of present-day morality, the risk that all moral restraint will be lifted and the child's behavior become entirely arbitrary.

Bear in mind that such utter amoralism, the complete absence of all restraining principles, will return us to those naive ideals where our natural instincts are pursued, ideals which we have left far behind and which modern man can in no way agree with. We cannot agree to the blind pursuit of the demands of our instincts, because we know in advance that these demands were begotten by previous epochs, and are the residue of the long-past experience of adaptation to vanished environmental conditions, and, consequently, pull us back, rather than carry us forward. Moreover, that the instincts must inevitably be restricted to, and adapt to new conditions in the world, constitutes the essential condition of education.

Consequently, within that uncertain chaos which the present-day state of morality presents, there are a number of such moral standards which have been the basis of man's social behavior and which nevertheless have to be recognized. It is not the responsibility of educational psychology to arrive at exact definitions of the form and content of these moral standards. This is the something for social ethics, while the business of psychology is simply to find out whether it is even conceivable to put this into practice in the real world.

Bear in mind that all those revolutionary epochs when the old order breaks down and falls apart often represent such an improbable combination of the most diverse moral cultures that the child may sometimes find it utterly impossible to make any sense of this confusion. Moral crises, therefore, lie in wait for the child at every step of the way, and, consequently, the teacher and educator can in no way ignore questions of moral education. No other epoch creates such magnificent opportunities for moral heroism, and in no other epoch is there such a risk of moral degradation.

Getting accustomed to the spirit of the epoch, to those great currents which permeate the world, is the only criterion here. The purely aesthetic and passive perception of the clarion call of revolution, to which Blok passionately summoned the Russian intelligentsia, writing that, "With all your body, with all your heart, with all your consciousness, heed the call of revolution"—this cannot serve as a foundation of moral education, inasmuch as heeding the call of revolution once upon a time will not lead to active involvement in revolution, and if the poet's summons is to be applied to our actions, it has to so resonate that its meaning express the demand not simply to listen to, but to himself create the music of revolution.

The third basic feature of moral education in our epoch is found in that aspect of truth that distinguishes the ethical outlook which is being created right before our eyes. Truth and the unflinching capacity to face reality squarely in the eye in all the most difficult and all the most confusing circumstances in life—this is the first demand of revolutionary morality. Never before could moral education have reached such an inexorable and absolute truth as now, when absolutely every undisclosed moral "value" has been put on the map and revealed in its true form.

In this as in all other realms, a revolutionary epoch is scarcely able to suggest consummate systems of morality, whatever the previous epochs might have boasted of. Though on the other hand, we may impose on our moral education various individual demands that go well beyond the demands imposed in preceding epochs. We can require that Soviet education train fighters and revolutionaries in the realm of morality, as in all other realms. We should not set out with the abstract ideal of creating an entire personality, since such a personality does not exist and since such an education would neglect contemporary goals and turn into a game of verbal gymnastics. We confront the concrete goals of training the adults of the next epoch, the adults of the next generation, in full accord with the historical role which will be their lot. Hence the extraordinary degree of specificity and integrity which have become the foundation of moral education in our epoch.

Principles of Moral Education

The first question which comes up is to decide on the relationship between moral education and the general education of the personality. In this area, Tolstoy leaned to a negation of all culture, and found that wherever the higher forms of culture flourished, there the higher forms of immorality flourished too. Hence, his conclusions were in the spirit of Rousseau, that the moral ideal lies not in the future, but in the past, that it consists in the negation of civilization and in a return to nature.

That such a view is in radical contradiction to the revolutionary ideology of consciousness of class, an ideology by virtue of which mankind will, in the long run, come to believe in the vigor and dominance of the culturally armed man over nature—this is something no one can deny. There is, however, in Tolstoy's critique of culture an entirely healthy aspect, and this critique may be adopted, though with some corrective, if we take into account the fact that here it is not a matter of culture in general, but of capitalist culture, in particular. There can be no doubt that the moral contradictions reach their zenith at the highest stages of human culture, and that a tribal village represents a healthier moral climate than a European city. But from this one can only conclude that European culture has outlived itself, not that culture in general is antagonistic to morality. On the contrary, since the time of Socrates, the contrary view has been put forward, one which identifies moral behavior with moral consciousness.

"Morality," says Socrates, "is knowledge, and immorality is the fruit of ignorance." Here there is a real psychological problem which is in need of analysis. According to William James "The hackneyed example of moral deliberation is the case of an habitual drunkard under temptation. He has made a resolve to reform, but he is now solicited again by the bottle. His moral triumph or failure literally consists in his finding the right *name* for the case. If he says that it is a case of not wasting good liquor already poured out, or a case of not being churlish and unsociable when in the midst of friends, or a case of learning something at last about a brand of whiskey which he never met before, or a case of celebrating a public holiday, or a case of stimulating himself to a more energetic resolve in favor of abstinence than any he has ever yet made, then he is lost; his choice of the wrong name seals his doom. But if, in spite of all the plausible good names with which his thirsty fancy so copiously furnishes him, he unwaveringly clings to the truer bad name, and apperceives the case as that of `being a drunkard, being a drunkard, being a drunkard,' his feet are planted on the road to salvation; he saves himself by thinking rightly."[1] Thus, it's as if there was a complete identity established between moral behavior and moral consciousness. "Our moral effort, properly so called, terminates in our holding fast to the appropriate idea. If, then, you are asked, *in what does a moral act consist* when reduced to its simplest and most elementary form? you can make only one reply. You can say that *it consists in the effort of attention by which we hold fast to an idea* which but for that effort of attention would be driven out of the mind by the other psychological tendencies that are there. *To think*, in short, is the secret of will, just as it is the secret of memory".[2]

To find a way out of this awkward situation, we should add that there are facts which at once point to the reverse relationship between consciousness and moral behavior. The reader surely knows that it is one thing to know how to act, and an entirely different thing to act correctly. One can understand perfectly well that alcohol is harmful and nevertheless not have the willpower to give up being an alcoholic. Obviously, here it is essential to bear in mind that consciousness, of course, plays a kind of role, though not the decisive one, and that it is only one of several components and, quite often, inferior to other, more powerful instinctive drives. Consequently, it is still not enough to provoke the awareness that some good deed is necessary, rather it is far more important to make certain that this idea dominate consciousness, and this means disciplining the child's consciousness so as to assist him in gaining the upper hand over all his conscious and unconscious desires.

Once again, it is not a matter of reducing consciousness to just one thing. In his analysis of the mental state of the alcoholic, James is right to point out that the alcoholic's moral victory or defeat depends wholly on whether he gives the correct name to his state. But one must also ask what this state depends on, and this question, of course, may be answered only in the sense that the very appearance of this or that idea in consciousness depends, in turn, on the different stimuli which have preceded it, and these are usually powerful emotional drives. Consequently, we can speak of conscious influence only when we understand this as something connected with the nervous system, as a system formed by precisely those reactions which all of behavior consists in, though we are speaking only of those reactions which inhibit and regulate the rest of behavior. In other words, only an understanding of consciousness as involving preparatory forms of organization of behavior can supply us with an explanation of the role of consciousness in ensuring proper behavior.

Hence follow several conclusions. There can be no doubt that consciousness exerts a decisive influence on our moral behavior, though there is no direct dependence whatsoever which can be established between the two. It was for this reason that Meumann was able to show that moral development and the general level of education go hand in hand, while Witheft established the rule that success in school has fundamental importance for the student's entire moral existence. The question has to be asked in such a way as to disclose the relationship between success in school and behavior, though this does not mean also explaining this relationship.

We can see this if we take a look at morally backward children. We know that intellectual development may be associated with the greatest immorality, and, consequently, intellectual development, in and of itself, is hardly a guarantee of moral behavior. We also know of the converse, that one may be blessed with luminous moral behavior even though one's intellect is greatly retarded, that retarded children may display a genuinely keen and understanding heart, and, consequently, mental development cannot be taken as even a necessary condition of moral giftedness. Nevertheless, we are still justified in claiming that there exists a profound relationship between the two, and that mental development is a propitious condition for moral education.

Such a relationship denotes a finer life, more complex and more diverse forms of behavior, and, consequently, allows for far greater opportunities and possibilities for educational intervention. In the mentally underdeveloped child, the process of behavior is far simpler and, consequently, there is no opportunity for all those infinitely involved schemes children have to be drawn into in order to influence their behavior.

However, only that form of consciousness proves to be decisive for morality which is directly associated with behavior and realized directly in activity, for otherwise a correct consciousness may lead to incorrect deeds.

All attempts at moral education, at moral sermonizing, must, for these reasons, have to be seen as quite futile. Morality has to constitute an inseparable part of education as a whole at its very roots, and he is acting morally who does not notice that he is acting morally. Just like health, which we notice only when it is disturbed, like the air which we breathe, so does the way we behave in terms of morality arouse in us a whole series of concerns only when there is something seriously wrong with it. Herbart's rule, "not to teach too much," is nowhere as applicable to this extent as in moral education.

It is for this reason that we feel it is pointless to teach morality. Moral precepts, in and of themselves, will, in the student's mind, seem like a collection of purely verbal responses that have absolutely nothing to do with behavior. At its best, such a system is like a motor that has not started up some device and which is doomed to remain idle. At its best, therefore, it may cause some conflict between the child's behavior and the moral precepts. There can be no doubt whatsoever that, for example, the struggle of Tsarist pedagogics against certain childish vices associated with sexual behavior not only did not lead to useful results, but, on the contrary, turned out to have harmful effects, in that it created complex and agonizing feelings in the child's soul. The child who did not feel capable of dealing with his own desires, who did not know how to counter them, suffered from the consciousness of his own guilt, his own fears, and his own shame, and, as a result, things that were, in and of themselves, not so terrible, were transformed into severe mental and nervous shocks under the influence of such unwise education.

Not only does education in morality seem pointless and harmful, but every form of moral education already seems to attest to a degree of abnormality in this realm. Moral education should be dissolved entirely imperceptibly into all those general modes of behavior that may be established and regulated by the social environment. Neither student nor teacher should think special instruction in morality is called for. Our understanding of moral behavior becomes enlarged, inasmuch as we are then justified in speaking not only of moral behavior in the narrow sense of the term, but also of a moral relationship to things, to oneself, to one's body, and so on.

Moral behavior will always be that which is associated with the free choice of social forms of behavior. Spinoza writes that if a person runs away from something on the grounds that it is bad, he is acting like a slave. Only that person is free, in Spinoza's view, who runs away from something because something else is better. With this as a ground rule, William James gives a perfectly rigorous technique for moral education, on the basis of the principle that one must always proceed not from evil, but from good. "See to it now, I beg you, that you make freemen of your pupils by habituating them to act, whenever possible, under the notion of a good. Get them habitually to tell the truth, not so much through showing them the wickedness of lying as by arousing their enthusiasm for honor and veracity ... And in the lessons which you may be legally obliged to conduct upon the bad effects of alcohol, lay less stress than the books do on the drunkard's stomach, kidneys, nerves, and social miseries, and more on the blessings of having an organism kept in lifelong possession of its full youthful elasticity by a sweet, sound blood, to which stimulants and narcotics are unknown, and to which the morning sun and air and dew will daily come as sufficiently powerful intoxicants".[3]

In other words, we should not proceed in moral education the same way we proceed in thinking of laws in the criminal code, when we refrain from some deed simply because we fear the punishment that would ensue. Do not, in other words, turn morality into the internal policeman of the soul. To avoid something out of fear still does not mean you are performing a good deed. In this sense, Rousseau was profoundly in error when, wishing to keep his hero Emile away from dangerous and sordid affairs, placed him as a child in a clinic for venereal diseases in the hope that ulcers, stench, shame, and the abasement of the human body would frighten the youth. From the psychological point of view, chastity purchased at the price of fear sullies the soul worse than outright debauchery, inasmuch as it does not destroy all base wishes and desires in the child's mind, but only creates in his mind a petty and mean struggle between these desires and the no less humiliating and no less servile feelings of fear. Only that chastity has any value which is procured by a positive attitude towards action and by an understanding of its true essence. Not to do something out of a fear of dire consequences is just as immoral as to do it. Every unfree attitude towards things, all fear and dependence, already denotes the absence of any moral sensibility. In its psychological sense, the moral is always free.

In this sense, present-day pedagogics is in radical contradiction with religious and, in particular, Christian morality, whose principle tool has been intimidation, threats, and the like. "He whose life is based upon the word 'no,' who tells the truth because a lie is wicked, and who has constantly to grapple with his envious and cowardly and mean propensities, is in an inferior situation in every respect to what he would be if the love of truth and magnanimity positively possessed him from the outset, and he felt no inferior temptations. Your born gentleman is certainly, for this world's purposes, a more valuable being than your 'Crump,' with his grunting resistance to his native devils,' even though in God's sight the latter may, as the Catholic theologians say, be rolling up great stores of 'merit'".[4]

There are three irrefutable drawbacks of this type of pedagogics. First is the fact that it can never be certain of success. It frightens the weak, but arouses resistance in the strong and imparts a special charm of strength, boldness, and challenge to the breaking of rules. It is profoundly remarkable for moral psychology that rebels and those who break the rules of moral psychology are always portrayed in man's imagination in an attractive light simply because they represent strength, unyielding pride, and insubordination to rules. From Byron's passionate heroes to the most commonplace school wit—everything that is insolent and which refuses to surrender to intimidation quite naturally draws the child's sympathies. In such instances, the child seems to respond with the words of the Apostle: "I see what is better and approve of it, but instead I follow what is worse."

The second drawback of this form of moral education, which is always based on the absence of freedom, is that it creates an entirely false picture of moral values, assigning to moral virtue a kind of wealth, arousing self-esteem and a contemptuous attitude towards everything which is wrong. Everyone is forced to experience the sort of agonizing moral conflict that Andreev described in his story, "Darkness," sooner or later, and the time comes for everyone when he recognizes that it is sometimes shameful to be good, just as it is shameful to be rich when it is combined with the terrible darkness of the unenlightened human soul. And then the honest and morally pure person who has been totally consumed in the enthusiasm to perform good deeds discovers the degradation and insignificance of his own moral purity when confronted by a vulgar prostitute and decides that if we are powerless to illuminate the darkness with our pitiful lanterns, then it is better to extinguish them and start to crawl about on all fours in this darkness.

Finally, the third danger is that every description of misdeeds, by creating a succession of images in the child's mind, creates, at the same time, the impulse and inclination to perform these deeds. Recall that every act of consciousness is a nascent activity, and that, consequently, by cautioning our pupils against what they should not do, we are, at the same time, focusing their attention on these deeds, and thereby encouraging them to perform them. The common expression, that the forbidden fruit is sweetest, contains a great psychological truth, and communicates some of what we have been speaking of here. There is no better way of compelling a child who has picked up a glass to break it than by repeatedly cautioning him. "Now look, don't break it," or "you're going to break it. I'm sure of that." In the same way, there is no surer method of leading a child into carrying out some immoral deed than by describing it in great detail.

This is why Thorndike is quite correct to emphasize the harm brought about by discussing with children in painstaking detail and at great length the motives, methods, and opportunities for committing suicide, as is done in certain French textbooks on morality. To do this means creating in the student's mind propitious conditions and material that might take hold of the child's mind at some point in the future and guide his behavior not away from suicide, but towards it. Explains Thorndike, do not speak to children by telling them, "You must not cut a cat open in order to see what is inside." Every consciousness of some phenomenon contains a certain motor impulse, and this impulse is especially strong in children. All of us know how much power is exerted over a child's behavior by a book he has just finished reading, in the same way that children who have begun to read James Fenimore Cooper and Captain Mayne-Reade will run off to America to become Indians. Consequently, there is nothing more dangerous in childhood than such teaching of morality, in which, by virtue of natural psychological consequences, the teaching of morality turns into the teaching of immorality. Here we can say, without fear of falling into error, that whereas knowledge of a good deed is far from any guarantee that it will be performed, knowledge of bad deeds will always serve as encouragement.

Moral Transgressions in Childhood

Every teacher is forced to deal with moral misdeeds committed by children. These misdeeds may range over an extraordinarily lengthy scale, from slight and insignificant faults to genuine and serious offences, in the form of murder, arson, and so on. Quite analogously, the steps taken by teachers against such children begin with slight and simple verbal reproofs and end in penal colonies for young offenders, where children are kept behind bars and subjected to prison conditions.

How should we view these moral misdeeds in children from the psychological point of view? Until the true nature of morality was discovered, moral behavior seemed to be just as objectively necessary for behavior as are the rules of logic for thinking. Both the adult and the child who has transgressed moral precepts seem to be abnormal, and ill. In such instances, pedagogics spoke of a moral deficiency in the child, as if speaking of an illness, in the same sense one usually speaks of a mental or physical impairment. It is supposed, moreover, that a moral deficiency is an inborn defect attributable to biological causes, to heredity, or to physiological causes of some defect in the structure of the organism, like congenital blindness or deafness. Thus, it is claimed that there are people who, from the time they are born, are moral and others who, from the time they are born, are immoral, and that, consequently, there are children who, by their very nature, are condemned to sit behind bars, because they are born criminals, just as a blind person is fated never to see light, since he is born without vision.

It goes without saying that, from the point of view of physiology and psychology, such ideas are nonsense. No physiologist has ever had to deal with any sort of special organs of morality in the human body which, if injured, would lead to an absolute love for criminal behavior and for practical jokes. No psychologist in analyzing the forms of human behavior and in explaining the laws governing their development has ever had to confront the existence of such innate reactions that might govern moral or immoral behavior. Thus, the concept of moral imperfection is not a biological concept, but a social concept. It is not innate, but acquired, and arises not from biological factors that guide the development of the organism and its behavior, but from social factors that guide and adapt this behavior to the conditions of existence in the particular environment in which the child has to live.

Thus, moral imperfection always derives from experience and always denotes not a defect in innate reactions and instincts, i.e., not a defect of the organism and of behavior, but a defect of conditional relations for adaptation to the conditions of the environment, i.e., a defect in education. It is, therefore, far more correct to speak not of the moral deficiency of a child, but of his social underdevelopment or neglect. Hence a general conclusion becomes perfectly clear, a conclusion which should serve as a starting point in all questions having to do with the education of such children. These children require no special pedagogics, no protective, corrective, or punitive measures whatsoever, only redoubled social attention and quadrupled educational influence from the direction of the environment. In every case of moral misdeeds in children, from the least significant on up to the most serious, we are dealing with a conflict between the child and the environment, and we have to recognize that every child is a congenital moral criminal simply by virtue of the fact that he is born with reactions that are notoriously maladjusted to the environment. Even in the utterly most well-educated families, no child is born with the ready ability to behave properly; on the contrary, in absolutely none of his normal actions and deeds does he obey the rules of good breeding and morality, and in this sense the whole task of education is only to help the child adapt to the conditions of his surroundings.

The educational influence of the environment the child is immersed in is the only tool for the adaptation of these reactions. And since under the conditions of the modern order, the social environment is always is always organized in the most discordant way imaginable, consequently, by virtue of the contradictions it contains, there will inevitably always be people in whom anti-social behavioral patterns will consequently evolve simply because they fell under the influence of inauspicious circumstances. Consequently, in these instances we have to think of social re-education as being the only pedagogical tool for overcoming these evils.

Such a child has to be placed in an environment that would foster in him, in place of the anti-social behavioral patterns already established in him, new ways of interacting with people that would also adapt him to the conditions of his existence. A morally imperfect deed is anti-social above all, and moral education is, above all, social education. In this sense, the rule of scientific pedagogics is quite the reverse of what is often employed as regards those who break laws in society and in government. There, banishment from the social environment is the natural thing to do, whereas here, in contrast, the most involved forms of participation, and of social contact, are appropriate. There, we have an extraordinarily slight concern with the character of the offender himself, and all our concern is directed towards rendering him harmless and safeguarding the environment from his influence. Here, in contrast, our concern must be directed towards preserving and transforming the child's character and, consequently, our goal is the most thoroughgoing re-education of the child. Nowadays, even the state in its punitive policies has begun to assume that point of view towards offenders which views punishment as being intended to serve the purposes of re-education rather than of intimidation and retribution. And just as in the case of serious offences, so does the slightest misdeed committed by a child ultimately always point to a greater or lesser schism in the child's social behavior.

Therefore, like criminal behavior generally, criminal behavior in children does not at all point to a low overall development of the individual. On the contrary, an offence points often to a certain strength, the capacity to rebel, considerable freedom, and the capacity for powerful feelings—and the capacity to desire much and to achieve much. Under the conditions of bourgeois morality and truth, everything that exceeds the bounds of the average man is banished to become the province of criminals, of those who sense a force in themselves and who cannot be reconciled with the established way of life. Dostoyevskii, in speaking of his novel, *The House of the Dead*, remarked that in the prisons for hard labor, one could find the most gifted, the most forceful members of the populace gathered there, except for the fact those forces had been corrupted, perverted, and employed for evil purposes.

Similarly, childhood offenses not only do not indicate any sort of defect in the child's psyche, but, on the contrary, are bound up with and are quite compatible with considerable overall giftedness. Moral offenses not only do not point to an inability in the child for the acquisition of social skills or his incapacity for social relationships, on the contrary, very often such a child will exhibit an extraordinary degree of guile, cunning, ingenuity, true heroism, and, what is most important, the greatest devotion to a special morality of his own, whether of street thieves or pickpockets, who have their own morality, their own professional ethics, their own concept of good and evil.

More often than not, this moral imbalance in a child springs from two fundamental causes. First, there is homelessness, which constitutes a fact of enormous social significance and, in its true sense, is comparable to the absence of all social education, i.e., all concern for the development of adaptive reactions to the environment. On the other hand, there is the problem of children who, though highly gifted, cannot find any outlet for their energy in ordinary patterns of behavior. On the contrary, in terms of morality, obedient children usually represent a vivid example of ungiftedness, simply because they tend very often to suffer from rickets or are anemic or are dull and narrow-minded, follow the line of easiest adaptation to the environment, and either do not need very much, or who, very early in childhood, grasped the secret of a happy life and value it above all other blessings. People with great passions, people who accomplish great deeds, people who possess strong feelings, even people with great minds and a strong personality, rarely come out of good little boys and girls.

There is no one feature of the traditional moral education that attests so eloquently against this system as do these instances. In other words, not only in those instances when moral education has not succeeded, but far more often in those instances when it has succeeded, does moral education reveal its utter impotence. Nowhere has it achieved such degradation as where it achieved everything it wished. It is here that its true nature stands revealed. We have seen that wherever it did not succeed, it testified to its own utter impotence, creating, in theory, a concept of congenital moral deficiency, and, in practice, replacing desks in school by bars in prison and the school routine by forced labor conditions, entrusting prison wardens with the responsibility of completing those duties that teachers had left incomplete.

But this also happened whenever it experienced the triumph of its own force and power, wherever it reaped total success, even where it discovered it was capable only of creating a loyal and cautious child, one who was faint-hearted and inclined to be obedient, timid, and dutiful. This occurred simply because the whole system of moral education was constructed on authoritarian principles, i.e., with the recognition of that special compulsory value of the authority of parents and teachers, which sustained the sanctions of punishments and rewards, deterrence and happiness. "Listen to your elders, and you'll be good, otherwise you'll be bad"—such is the inelegant, though exact formula of this form of pedagogics.

The higher moral value was recognized in an obedience that was motivated by fear, whereas, from the psychological point of view, obedience itself lacks all power of moral instruction, inasmuch as it supposes in advance an unfree and servile attitude towards things and towards deeds. Thus, the fundamental psychological mechanism that served as the foundation of moral education was, in fact, the most profound pedagogical delusion imaginable.

It is extraordinarily important to note in this regard that this mechanism has penetrated so deeply into our flesh and blood that even the most progressive teacher and the most well-educated parent is unable to free himself of this timeworn technique, and when a mother tells her child, "Don't do this, else Mama won't love you," she is making the very same mistake, except in gentler form, as the police do when they put a very young thief behind bars. A child can, in fact, abstain from his misdeeds, but the moral and educational influence of his abstention will either be null, or can even be negative, inasmuch as it is purchased at the price of fear, at the price of humiliation, and not at the price of the child's true rebirth. This is why obedience is, for us, of negligible moral value, and the good behavior purchased at the price of obedience is not, in our eyes, a pedagogical ideal.

All the same, the authoritarian principle in morality from which this authority must have emanated in one way or another must be demolished, and in its place something entirely new must be erected. The closest we can get to a definition of this new principle, which is to become the foundation of moral education, is to view it from general approaches to education, as consisting in the social coordination of one's own behavior with the behavior of the group, and here obedience must be replaced throughout by free social coordination. The rule that originates from everyone, from the group, and which is directed likewise to the entire group and sustained by the actual effective mechanism of the self-discipline and routine of daily life in the school has to itself replace that "pedagogical singsong" which prevails between teacher and student in the authoritarian system.

It is not obedience to someone or obedience to something, but the free adoption of those patterns of behavior which will vouchsafe the consonance of all of behavior. This mechanism is not something alien to the child, something that grips him, on the contrary, it lies within the child's very nature, and play is the natural mechanism which develops and connects these skills together. Nowhere is the child's behavior so regulated by rules as in play, and nowhere does it assume such a free and morally instructive form as in play. Nowhere in play do we find any patterns whatsoever that an adult might have prescribed and which the child only enact.

On the contrary, games are the natural seedlings of future moral behavior. The child obeys the rules of a game not because he is threatened with punishment or, on the other hand, because he is scared of failing in something or of losing something, but only because observing the rules—which is a promise that he renews from one minute to the next—vouchsafes him the inner satisfaction that comes from playing a game, because here he acts as part of the general enterprise that is formed out of a group at play. Breaking a rule does not represent any threat whatsoever other than the fact that, at that moment, the game has not worked out, and the child has lost interest in it, and this is a powerful enough incentive for regulating the child's behavior.

Accordingly, it is clear what steps have to be taken by the teacher to counter the various moral transgressions a child may commit. In the authoritarian system of morality, every moral rule was accompanied by a particular sanction which entailed punishing the child in the event of disobedience, and awarding him when he obeyed. Punishment and rewards assumed the most diverse forms, from corporeal punishment, being sent to bed without supper, or being locked up in a jail cell, and all the various kinds of rewards right up through rather fine and delicate forms, for example, reprimands, censure, and, in the case of rewards, praise. The pedagogical utility, or, more properly, the harm produced by these measures was extremely variable, though they all served as tools for producing commonplace, unthinking reactions and, in the best case, taught only the virtue of obedience, only the single moral rule—avoidance of what is unpleasant.

And if we were to imagine that this sanction were lifted and the child could imagine that his misdeeds would produce not the slightest reaction on the part of those around him, he would not have the slightest reason to refrain from engaging in these deeds. Moral behavior must be based not on external prohibition, but on internal restraint, even more properly, on the fact that man is naturally drawn to the good and the beautiful. Moral behavior must become the individual's true nature and be enacted freely and effortlessly.

The idea that the child's own will is his best teacher is still very much alive in pedagogics. There is the view held by many instructors which teaches not to protect children from danger, but to let them experience the unhealthy consequences of their own deeds as if in an experiment, and to learn to avoid them on their own. Thus, if a child is in the habit of instinctively reaching out to a lit candle or to a hot samovar, it is the opinion of these teachers that he should not be kept from doing so. On the contrary, he should be given the opportunity to burn himself, that this is the best school for the child, it is this which teaches him to beware of fire better than any other measure. In the very psychological mechanism of pain and the striving to avoid it, teachers have found a mighty tool, and the example just presented represents a typical instance of such an education.

In critically examining this approach, we have to bear in mind that, when applied to instances of this type, in which a healthy effect is associated directly with some deed, this type of educational measure could hardly become widespread and assume the status of a general principle. How should a teacher proceed if he wishes to act in accordance with this rule and allow children to have the experience of the adverse consequences of their deeds, and how should he proceed when the adverse consequence of some deed does not manifest itself immediately, but only after a prolonged period of time, or only after many years? Isn't it true that, after all this time, the child could end up becoming accustomed to bad habits, and that all the harm he finds out about afterwards will not be able to save him from it? The harmful consequences of a single cigarette may be negligible and, in fact, imperceptible, but if we allow the child to, in fact, experience the harm of smoking, we run the risk of fostering in him an experienced smoker long before he comes to the realization that he has to renounce the very idea of being a smoker.

Instances in which harmful consequences are associated with just such a connection with some deed are just as likely, which makes the relationship between this deed and its adverse consequences difficult and incomprehensible to the child's understanding. Finally, there are a whole series of deeds that induce such destructive consequences as to make it extremely risky to trust in their educational influence. If a child has a yearning to jump out the window, a teacher would hardly think it reasonable to allow him to do so in order to actually learn the harmful consequences that this would bring about. There is an extraordinarily large number of such instances, with effects that not only involve physical harm, but also moral harm.

Thus, the application of this principle could be limited to insignificant cases of the type presented above, but it cannot be of general pedagogical value, and, in particular, it is entirely inappropriate for the education of moral behavior. It lacks that essential freedom of choice which alone is capable of leading to moral behavior. Natorp says somewhere that we don't in the least think that people without jobs could turn into angels if they were to be given their freedom. We only know that they become devils when they feel they are being oppressed. And in the same sense, it seems entirely clear and self-evident that this principle of pain is not appropriate for justifying punishment. The child learns very quickly to understand that punishment is not at all necessarily related to his misdeeds, but that there is an additional and intermediate component here expressed in the intervention of adults, and he learns to avoid this intervention, to conceal his deeds, to tell lies, and so on.

Besides, every form of punishment places both the teacher and the student in the most painful and difficult of positions. Neither love nor respect nor trust can be preserved between a teacher who is inflicting punishment and the child he is punishing. Every form of punishment, no matter what it involves, always places the student in a humiliating position, and undermines his love and trust. Herbart says in this regard that, "Threats are a poor educational tool; they tempt strong natures and are of little effect in keeping weak natures away from misdeeds, because they do not have the power to combat their negative desires. Desires make mincemeat of the fear of punishment."

In other words, every form of punishment is harmful, from the psychological point of view, and there is no place whatsoever for punishment in Soviet schools. The very idea of a child committing some misdeed always points to a defect in the educational process. An offense committed by a student is, above all, an offense committed by the school, and only the elimination of this defect in the social organization of the school itself is appropriate. In this sense, self-governance in the school and the self-discipline of the children themselves are the best tools for moral education in the school.

One must take care that the forms assumed by such self-governance not turn into a mere replica of adult behavioral patterns, and that interest in artificial formalities does not kill the vital sense of community in the child. Accordingly, organizing the social environment in the school is not simply a matter of creating a constitution of school governance and of summoning children to general assemblies at regular intervals of time, of making choices and maintaining all those forms of communal organization that children are so eager to copy from adults. Rather, it means concern for those genuinely social relations that have to permeate this environment. Beginning with intimate and friendly relations that reach down to the smallest social groups, then moving on to the broadest associations of comrades, and ending in the broadest and largest forms of children's movements, the school has to penetrate and envelop the life of the child with a myriad of social relations that could assist in the development of moral character. In no other realm does the general thesis of education—that to educate means to impart a discipline to life, and in a properly conducted life, it means to raise children properly—possess as much force and validity as here.

Hence, the relation between education and life, and between the school and the social order, becomes understandable, moreover that this relation must serve as a starting point for pedagogics. Questions of education will be fully solved only when questions of social order have been fully solved. Every attempt at constructing educational ideals in a society with social contradictions is a utopian dream, since, as we have seen, the social environment is the only educational factor that can establish new reactions in the child, and so long as it harbors unresolved contradictions, these contradictions will create cracks in the most well thought-out and most inspired educational system.

Accordingly, in the present transitional epoch we will always have to deal with undesirable patterns of behavior in children, and, before anything else, we have to be ready to deal with the complex and difficult work of re-education. Next we have to find out how to retain the positive aspects of the system of rewards and punishment as educational measures for Soviet pedagogics. Though rewards and punishments have to be banished from Soviet schools because of their harmful influence, it is nevertheless beyond question that some portion of their effect will have to be retained, for otherwise the nature of children's drives, which happen to be a powerful motivation of their deeds, will have to be made use of in the realm of moral education. This positive element should be retained, and manifest itself through the reversion, or return, of every one of a child's actions back to him in the form of the impressions of the effect it has on those around him. Nothing so arouses us to act as the satisfaction associated with it.

This is the reason why William James was able to discern a positive element in the system of grades, and even insisted that children be told their grades. It is here that James discovered a realization of that psychological law according to which, through the work cycle, our own deed reverts back to us, in the form of a reflected impression. "We thus receive sensible news of our behavior and its results. We hear the words we have spoken, feel our own blow as we give it, or read in the bystander's eyes the success or failure of our conduct. Now this return wave of impression pertains to the completeness of the whole experience But so far as our psychological deduction goes, it would suggest that the pupil's eagerness to know how well he does is in the line of his normal completeness of function, and should never be balked except for very definite reasons indeed. Acquaint them, therefore, with their marks and standing and prospects, unless in the individual case you have some special practical reason for not so doing."[5]

We have not presented these thoughts of William James not in order to make a defense of the grading systems used in public schools. On the contrary, that grading systems are psychologically inappropriate is entirely self-evident from the reasoning presented above in our discussion of punishment. A grade is a form of assessment so alien to the entire course of school work that it very quickly starts to dominate the natural concerns of teaching, and the student begins to learn for the sake of avoiding bad grades or for the sake of obtaining good grades. Similarly, grades combine all the negative aspects of praise and censure. There is in these remarks of his a great psychological truth, however, that the child should always know the ultimate results of his own deeds, and that this knowledge is a powerful educational tool in the hands of the teacher.

Therefore, a public school should not be understood as simply consisting in a crowd of children who have nothing to do with one other. We all know that bringing together any large group of children who have nothing to do with one other and who do not share any common interests makes each child feel his isolation and loneliness even more acutely. Nowhere does a person feel so alone as when he is in a crowd he has no connection to or when he is in a modern capitalist city, where no one has any feelings for or understanding of another person. Such a system is capable only of stifling the child, and has a profoundly oppressive effect upon him. Obviously, in the Soviet school we have to be concerned with those forms of public education that would induce vital interaction between children so that the child would place a high value on the satisfaction or dissatisfaction of his classmates. With these social structures in place, the environment becomes a powerful mechanism that is forever conveying to the child the reflected impression of his own actions.

In a properly ordered social environment, the child will always think of himself as fully transparent, as if reflected by a vast resonator, and all those reflected impressions of his own deeds he will be discovering all the time will become the most powerful educational tool in the hands of the teacher.

It is thus not hard to see that the child's relationship to his surroundings will not in the least always bear that propitious and idyllic character in which "free" education pictures itself.

The ideals of free education, i.e., the absolutely uninhibited pursuit of the child's deeds, arouses objections from two points of view. First, it is almost never possible to actually realize free education in its entirety, and, consequently, we are always left with only a pedagogical principle possessing a certain degree of relative force within quite narrow limits. The child's desires will always encompass much that is destructive and harmful, and, left to his own devices, a child could cause himself so much harm that no teacher in his right mind would be opposed to discouraging a child from undertaking this or that deed in the name of the principles of free education.

Moreover, complete freedom in education means rejecting all forethought and all social adaptation, i.e., in other words, all educational influence. But, education denotes a restriction and restraint of freedom from the very outset. To the extent that education is an unavoidable process in man's life, to that extent free education denotes not a rejection of constraints in general, rather it means imparting to those constraints the elemental force of the situation in which the child lives. If a person refuses education proper, he begins to be educated by furniture, by the street, and by things in general.

Thus, free education must be understood exclusively as denoting education which is as free as it can be within the constraints of an overall educational program and within the constraints of the social environment. Thus may it always turn out, and, in fact, it often turns out that the child's behavior is far from the same thing as the interests of the group. Then conflict may always arise, which, without forcing the child to do anything in particular, will make him see the value of changing the way he behaves so as to accord with the interests of the group. The school routine should be so organized that the child finds it best to go in step with the group, in the same way as when he is at play; that any departure from the group seem just as meaningless as quitting a game. Just like playing a game, life should demand a constant straining at the leash, a constant joy in concerted activity.

Ultimately, the theory of free education is the other side of the theory of innateness of moral sensibility. Both concede that pedagogical intervention is powerless and of no use in the development and growth of the child, and both suppose that what is most important in the child's moral response is already present at birth. Thus do both come to the conclusion quite naturally that there are children who are good and children who are bad, children who are moral and children who are immoral, from the moment they are born and in their very nature.

In the belief that "moral degradation is inherited," Gaupp presented in confirmation of this thesis testimony given by parents who, in speaking of their own child, declared that "[he] *could not be normal*; he is altogether different from other children; from the very beginning he was not the same as other children; he possessed an ineradicable desire to do evil."

Tolstoy, likewise, supposes that the child possesses an ineradicable drive to do good. There is the very same mistake being made here; faith in the innateness of moral behavior and a lack of understanding of the fact that moral behavior is wholly the product of education.

Education does not know of any "ineradicable drive to do evil"; *these very drives* may be turned towards the good.

---

[1] William James, *Talks to Teachers*, p. 110.
[2] *Ibid.*, pp. 109-110.
[3] *Op. cit.*, pp. 113-114.
[4] *Op. cit.*, p. 113.
[5] *Op. cit.*, p. 32.

Chapter 13

ESTHETIC EDUCATION

Esthetics in the Service of Pedagogics

The nature, ultimate meaning, purpose, and methods of esthetic education are still unresolved questions in the realm of psychology as well as in pedagogical theory. From time immemorial and right up to the present day, extreme and opposing viewpoints have been adopted towards these questions, viewpoints which, with each passing decade, seem to find ever newer confirmation in a whole series of psychological investigations. Thus, the controversy not only has not been resolved and not only is not drawing to a close, but rather is becoming increasingly more complicated, as if marching in step with the forward advance of scientific knowledge.

Many writers are inclined to reject the thesis that esthetic experiences possesses any educational value whatsoever, and the system of pedagogics which is associated with these writers and which has grown up from the very same roots persists in maintaining this idea, granting only a narrow and restricted value to esthetic education. In contrast, psychologists who subscribe to a different system in psychology are inclined to overstate the value of esthetic experience to an extraordinary degree, and to see in these experiences a slightly radical pedagogical tool that can take care of absolutely all the difficult and complex problems of education.

Between these two extreme points there is a whole series of moderate views on the role of esthetics in the life of the child. In most cases, these views are usually inclined to see in esthetics a form of amusement and a way for children to have fun. Where some discover a serious and profound meaning in esthetic experiences, it is nearly everywhere a matter not of esthetic education *as an end in itself*, but only as a tool for attaining pedagogical goals that are *alien* to esthetics. *Esthetics in the service of pedagogics*, as this may be termed, always fulfills exotic purposes and, in the opinion of some educators, should serve as a means and method for the education of cognition, sensibility, or moral will.

That this view is misguided and irrational can now be considered established beyond all reasonable doubt. All three goals, which are alien to yet bound up with esthetics—cognition, feeling, and morality—have played a role in the historical evolution of this problem that has greatly delayed all efforts to understand it correctly.

Morality and Art

It is usually supposed that a work of art possesses a good or bad, though nevertheless direct moral effect, and in evaluating esthetic impressions, particularly among children and teenagers, we are inclined to proceed, above all, on the basis of an evaluation of this moral impulse, which emanates from every object. Children's libraries are set up with the intention of leading children to draw instructive moral examples out of books, while a hortatory tone, tedious copybook maxims, and unctuous preachiness seem to be the essential style of self-conscious children's literature.

The only real lesson the child may draw out of contact with art—so it is said—is a more or less life-like illustration of a particular moral rule. Everything else is declared to be too difficult for children to understand, and outside the realm of morality children's literature is usually limited to nonsense verse and gibberish, as if there was nothing else children are able to grasp.[1] Hence arises that silly sentimentality so natural to children's literature as to be its distinctive feature. An adult who tries to affect children's psychology will, under the impression that real feelings are too difficult for children, present sugarcoated version of events and heroes that are clumsily and unskillfully made up; feelings are replaced by sensitivity and emotions by sentiment. Sentimentality is nothing less than silly feelings.

It is for this reason that, children's literature usually represents a vivid example of bad taste, of the coarse violation of all notion of esthetic style, and of the most dismal misunderstanding of the mind of the child.

We must, above all, reject such an approach, the belief that experiences should possess some kind of direct relationship to moral experience, as if every work of art incorporates a kind of incentive to moral behavior. An extraordinarily curious fact has been reported in the American pedagogical literature regarding the moral influence of that seemingly indisputably humanistic work of Harriet Beecher Stowe's, *Uncle Tom's Cabin*. When asked what were their feelings and thoughts after reading the book, several American students declared that, more than anything else, they were sorry that the time of slavery was gone and that there weren't any slaves in America now. This is even more remarkable in that, in this case, we are dealing not with some kind of exceptional moral obtuseness or misunderstanding, rather that the possibility of such a conclusion lies within the very nature of the child's esthetic experiences, and that we can never be certain ahead of time what will be the moral influence of a particular book.

Chekhov's story of the medieval monk, who, with the skill of a wondrous artist, tells his monastic brothers of the power of the devil, of the debauchery, the horrors, and the temptations he had been led to see in the city, is instructive in this regard. The narrator was inspired by the most sincere indignation, and since he was a true artist and spoke with great enthusiasm, eloquently and resoundingly, he depicted the force of the devil and the mortal temptations of sin so vividly that by morning there was not a single monk left in the monastery, all of them having run off to the city.

The moral effect of art very often recalls the fate of this sermon, and we can never be certain that our well-laid plans will always come out just the way we want them to when dealing with children. Actual observations of the child's life and facts taken from psychology that discuss the way children understand Krylov's stories are extremely instructive in this regard. Whenever children are not trying to guess what sort of response their teacher is expecting, but speak sincerely and on their own, their judgements are so at variance with the moral the teacher may be hoping to impart that some educators have come to think that even indisputably "ethical" works may turn out to exert a morally harmful influence when they are passed through the prism of a child's mind. It is necessary to take account of the laws governing this refractive medium, for otherwise we run the risk of obtaining results along the lines described above.

In his story, *The Fox and the Raven*, for example, all the child's sympathies are directed towards the fox. It arouses the child's admiration, and the child comes to think of the fox as a being who is clever and subtle in his mockery of the dumb raven. The effect which the teacher hopes to obtain—of aversion towards flattery and adulation—is not achieved. Children laugh at the raven, while the fox' deeds appear in the most favorable light. In no way are children led to the thought, "Oh, how wicked and harmful is flattery," from reading the story and instead end up with quite the opposite moral sensibility from what they are taught initially.

In the same way, in Krylov's story, *The Dragon Fly and the Ant*, the child's sympathies are aroused by the carefree and lyrical dragon fly who, all summer long, is always singing, while the morose and tiresome ant seems loathsome, and children come to believe that the entire story is directed against the ant's slow-witted and complacent miserliness. Again, the bite of mockery is pointed in the wrong direction, and instead of instilling children with respect for business-like efficiency and for work, the story suggests the joy and charm of an easy and carefree existence.

And, finally, in Krylov's story, *The Wolf in the Kennel*, children tend to see the wolf as a heroic figure, since they feel he is truly majestic, irreverent, and in splendid defiance towards the hunters and their hounds once he not only does not cry for help, but proudly and arrogantly undertakes to defend and protect himself. The story as a whole discloses its true meaning to children not from the aspect of any moral sense, i.e., the wolf's punishment, but from the aspect of, if one may be so bold, the tragic grandeur of the destruction of a hero.

There are any number of examples and instances that may be taken from these or other stories which confirm the same result. Meanwhile, Russian schools, without any regard whatsoever for the psychological fact that there is always a multitude of possible interpretations and moral conclusions, has forever sought to subsume all artistic experience under a particular moral dogma, and has always been content with imparting a single interpretation of this dogma without suspecting that, often, a literary text not only does not help us when we wish to gain an understanding of the text itself, but, on the contrary, suggests a moral conception which leads altogether in the opposite direction. Blonskii is quite correct in his description of our esthetic education when he writes that poetry as such is absent from literature classes in the Soviet Union, and that all distinction between the text of Krylov's stories and the prosaic presentation of its content has been lost.

The ultimate, a virtual travesty is reached when it is matter of searching for the main theme of a given work of art, for an explanation of "what the author wanted to say" and what might be the moral value of each character individually. Sologub presents just such an interpretation by the teacher Peredonov of a line from one of Pushkin's poems "Together with his hungry mate, the wolf went on its way."[2] Here is an exaggerated, though not distorted picture of all those methodical prosaic renderings [*prozaizirovanie*] of poetry that have served as the basis of esthetic education in general, in which we extracting from a literary work all its nonesthetic elements and make up conjectures regarding this work from the standpoint of certain moral rules.

We have to note that this tends to have a predatory effect on the very possibility of esthetic perception and the esthetic attitude towards the object, not to mention the fact that it is in radical contradiction with the nature of esthetic experience.

Art and the Study of Reality

Another, no less harmful psychological confusion in esthetic education has been the imposition on esthetics of yet other goals and problems that are likewise foreign to it, though these are no longer moral in nature, but rather social and cognitive. Esthetic education is taken to be a tool for expanding students' cognition. All those courses on the history of literature once studied, for example, were constructed on the basis of this principle, and the acquisition of facts about art and the laws governing art, were replaced, quite deliberately, by the study of the social elements found in these works of art. It is of more than slight importance that the most popular textbooks on the history of Russian literature, which all our leading philologists have used in their teaching, bear such titles as *History of the Russian Intelligentsia* (Ovsyanniko-Kulikovskii) and *History of Russian Social Thought* (Ivanov-Razumnik). It is not literary events and facts that are deliberately and intentionally studied, but the history of the intelligentsia and the history of social thought, i.e., subjects that are, in essence, alien and foreign to esthetic education.

All these factors once possessed considerable historical meaning and value in previous epochs, when our schools were like the Great Wall of China, isolated from all social and civil discipline, and when we would receive the true rudiments of civil and social education in lessons in literature. But now that the social disciplines have assumed their proper place, such an exchange of esthetic values for social values is equally harmful for the one realm as for the other. Moreover, such a confusion of different realms of knowledge resembles those marriages where both sides are equally interested in a separation.

Above all, when we study society on the basis of models drawn from literature, we are always learning about it in false and distorted forms, inasmuch as works of art never reflect reality in all its entirety or in all its genuine truth. Works of art always constitute an extremely complicated product achieved through a reworking of the elements of reality, in which a whole series of utterly foreign elements are brought into reality. And, ultimately, whoever knows the history of the Russian intelligentsia only from Pushkin's Eugene Onegin and Chatskii runs the risk of possessing a wholly inaccurate view of this history. Far wiser is he who undertakes to study the history of the Russian intelligentsia on the basis of historical documents, letters, diaries, and all those other materials on which historical study is constructed, where the most modest role, very nearly the last in importance, is that of literary creations. It is just as impossible to study the history of the Russian intelligentsia using works of Russian literature as it is to study geography using the novels of Jules Verne, though, of course, both have left their mark in literature.

This view is based on the false conception that literature constitutes a kind of replica of reality, a kind of model photograph that resembles a group portrait. Such a group portrait, in which any number of people in the same group may be photographed with the same plate superimposes the features of one person on someone else's likeness, as a result of which all those standard features that are frequently encountered in a given group are identified especially vividly, as if in a relief map. Individual and random features, on the other hand, are hidden and, by this simple device, a standard portrait of a family, a group of patients, or a group of criminals may be created. It is believed that a figure taken from literature is something like a group photograph, and that, say, the figure of Eugene Onegin absorbed and accommodated all the typical personalities of the Russian intelligentsia of the 1820s and may, therefore, serve as authentic material for the study of this epoch. Meanwhile, it is not hard to see that, in this as in any other figure drawn from literature, the truth of art and the truth of reality exist in extraordinarily complicated relationships, and that, in any work of art, reality is always so transformed and so altered that there is no way whatsoever that meaning may be transferred directly from phenomena in art to phenomena in real life.

We also run the risk not only of ending up with a false understanding of reality, but also of entirely eliminating all the purely esthetic elements in such teaching. Interest in and regard for the study of the man of the 1820s has, psychologically speaking, nothing in common with interest in and regard for Pushkin's poetry; they manifest themselves in entirely different responses, emotions, and psychological states, and make use only of common matter for entirely different needs. Thus, the roof of an architectural structure may be utilized for protection against the rain, as an observation post, as a restaurant, and for any other purpose whatsoever, but in all these instances the esthetic value of the roof, as a part of an esthetic whole, as a part of an architectural scheme, is entirely lost sight of.

Art as an End in Itself

Finally, it remains for us to consider the third point of confusion where traditional pedagogy sins whenever it reduces esthetics to the sense of the percipient, to the appreciation of works of art, and sees in it an end in itself, in other words, where it reduces the entire meaning of esthetic experience to the unmediated sense of pleasure and joy which it arouses in children. Once again, the work of art is interpreted as a tool for arousing pleasurable reactions and is, practically speaking, placed in the same category as other analogous reactions and sensations that are utterly real. Whoever thinks of planting the field of esthetics in education to serve as a source of pleasure runs the risk of forever encountering the most powerful rivals in the very first tasting and the very first test drive. The special feature of childhood consists precisely in the fact that the immediate force of a real and concrete experience for a child is far greater than the force of an imagined emotion.

Thus, we see that traditional pedagogics is at a dead end when it comes to questions of esthetic education, striving to bound up with it entirely foreign goals that have nothing to do with it, and as a result, first, its proper value is overlooked, and, second, results are often attained that are at variance with what might have been expected.

Passivity and Activity in Esthetic Experience

The opportunity for such psychological confusion is the result not simply of the ignorance of instructors, but of the far more glaring and far more profound error of psychological science itself as regards questions of esthetics. For a long time, psychology viewed esthetic perception as constituting an entirely passive experience, a matter of giving oneself over entirely to one's feelings, the cessation of absolutely every activity of the organism. Psychologists would even explain that disinterestedness, unselfish admiration, the utter suppression of the will, and the absence of all personal relationship to the esthetic object amounted to necessary conditions for the realization of an esthetic reaction. This is all profoundly true, though it is only part of the truth, and thus yields an entirely false impression of the nature of this reaction as a whole.

There can be no doubt that a certain degree of passivity and disinterestedness are indispensable psychological pre-conditions for the esthetic act. The moment the viewer or reader assumes the role of active participant in the work of art he is apprehending, he is beyond the realm of esthetics irrevocably and once and for all. If while looking at apples that happen to be depicted in a painting, the thought of the activity associated with the intention of tasting real apples becomes overwhelmingly powerful in me, what is nevertheless clear is that the picture is now outside my field of apprehension. It is, however, not too difficult to see that this is only the other side of another, incomparably more serious activity, i.e., the activity by means of which the esthetic act is realized. What this is, may actually be easily gauged at least from the fact that a work of art is far from accessible to everyone's grasp, that the apprehension of a work of art involves arduous and difficult mental strain. Obviously, a work of art is not apprehended by an utterly passive individual, and not just by the eyes and the ears, but through unimaginably complex interior activity in which listening and looking are only the first step, the first impetus, the elemental impulse.

If the purpose of a painting were to consist solely in caressing our eyes, and that of music in supplying agreeable experiences to our ears, the apprehension of paintings and of musical compositions would not represent any difficulty, and, except for the blind and deaf, everyone would have a calling in regard to the appreciation of these works of art to the same degree. Meanwhile, the elements of perception of sensations constitute only an essential primary impetus for the arousal of more complex activity and, *in and of itself*, lack all esthetic meaning whatsoever. Christensen says that to amuse our senses, is not the ultimate goal of a work of art. What is important in music is what is inaudible, and in the plastic arts, what is invisible and imperceptible.

This invisible and imperceptible element must be understood as simply consisting in placing emphasis in the esthetic process on the responding elements of the reaction to sense impressions emanating from without. From this point of view, we can say outright that the esthetic experience is constructed from an entirely exact model of an ordinary reaction that presupposes, of necessity, the presence of three components, i.e., sensation, processing, and response. The component of perception of form, i.e., the labor which is performed by the eyes and the ears, amounts to only the first and primitive component of the esthetic experience, and there are two other components to consider. We know that a work of art is, for all intents and purposes, only a collection of external impressions or sensible effects on the individual which are organized in a special way. These sensible effects are, however, organized and constructed in such a way as to arouse a kind of reaction in the individual that differs from the sort of reactions that usually occur, and it is this special activity, associated with esthetic sensations, which happens to constitute the esthetic experience.

We still cannot say precisely what it consists in, since psychological analysis has yet to have the final word on the composition of the esthetic experience, though we already know that it involves the most complex constructive activity imaginable, an activity in which the listener or viewer himself constructs and creates an esthetic object out of the external impressions which are presented to him, and all his subsequent reactions are now referred to this object. Come to think of it, a painting is not really just a rectangular piece of canvas to which a certain quantity of paint has been applied. Once this canvas and these paints are interpreted by a viewer as the portrayal of a person, or of an object, or of an event, this complex work of transformation of painted canvas into picture occurs wholly within the mind of the viewer. Lines have to be connected, and closed up into the outlines of shapes, related to each other, and interpreted in terms of perspective in such a way as to recall the figure of a person or the appearance of a landscape.

Next, a complex effort at recollection, of the formation of associations, is needed in order to apprehend what sort of person or what sort of landscape is depicted in the painting, and what might be the relationship between the different parts of the painting. This essential labor may be referred to collectively as *secondarily creative synthesis*, inasmuch as it entails on the part of the spectator the amassing and synthesis of disparate elements of an esthetic unity. If a melody says anything to our soul, it is because we can ourselves put together sounds that come to us from without. Psychologists have long spoken of the fact that all that content and all those feelings we associate with a work of art involve nothing other than what we ourselves have introduced into it, that we seem to sense them in the esthetic image, and in fact, psychologists have referred to the very act of apprehension as *empathy*. The complex activity of empathy reduces, for all practical purposes, to the reconstitution of a series of internal reactions, to their mutual accommodation, and to a certain degree of creative reworking of the object we confront. This activity also constitutes a fundamental esthetic activity, which, by its very nature, is nevertheless an activity of the organism in response to external sensations.

Biological Value of Esthetic Activity

The biological value of esthetic activity is another troubling and debatable point. Only at the lowest stages of nascent esthetic activity is it possible to grasp the biological meaning of this activity. Initially, art arises to meet the needs of life, and rhythm is the primitive form of organization of labor and of struggle, ornamentation occurs as a component of sexual courting, and art bears an explicitly utilitarian and serviceable character. However, the genuine biological meaning of art in the modern era, of new art, that is, must be sought somewhere else. While a savage might replace martial songs by orders and battle plans, and while he might think that sobbing at a funeral is a means of directly reaching the soul of the departed, there is no way we can ascribe such unmediated and ordinary functions to modern art, and we have to seek its biological value somewhere else entirely.

The most widely accepted view here is that represented by Herbert Spencer's *law of economy of creative forces*, according to which the value of a work of art and the pleasure it provides are fully explainable by an economy of spiritual forces, by the conservation of attention which accompanies every apprehension of a work of art. Esthetic experience is the most efficient and the most profitable of all experiences for an individual, it produces a maximal effect with minimal consumption of energy, and this savings in energy also constitutes a kind of basis of esthetic pleasure. "The virtue of style," writes Aleksandr Veselovskii, "consists precisely in the fact that it supplies the greatest number of thoughts possible in the least number of words possible." One usually points to the facilitative value of symmetry, to the beneficial respite afforded by the interruption in rhythm, as vivid examples of this law.

However, even if it were valid, this law would, for all intents and purposes, have virtually nothing to do with questions of art, since we could find the very same economy of forces essentially wherever human creativity manifests itself; we find no lesser an economy of forces in mathematical formulas or in physical laws, in the classification of plants or in the study of the circulatory system, than in works of art, and if it were claimed that here it is a matter of an economy of esthetic influence, we would be at a loss in explaining how esthetic economy might be distinguished from the overall economy of all of creativity. But apart from that, the law does not express a psychological truth and is at variance with rigorous investigations in the realm of art. The study of esthetic form has shown that, in an esthetic experience, we are dealing not with a facilitative, but with a more demanding reproduction of reality, and some of the more radical students in the field have come to speak of the "condensation" (*ostranenie*) of objects as constituting the fundamental law of art. In any case, it should be clear that poetic speech is a more difficult form of speech by comparison with prose, and that its unusual arrangement of words, its subdivision into verses, and its rhythmic character not only does not relieve our attention from any sort of effort, but, on the contrary, demands ceaseless exertion of attention towards elements which manifest themselves for the first time here and which are utterly lacking in ordinary speech.

For the present-day study of art, it has become a tautology that, in a work of art, the apprehension of any one of its elements gets away from automatism and becomes conscious and tangible. For example, in everyday speech we do not focus our attention on the phonetic aspect of the word. Sounds are perceived automatically and are automatically associated with a particular meaning. William James has pointed out how strange and extraordinary our native language would appear to us if we were to listen to it without understanding it, as if it were a foreign language. Recall that the law of poetic speech simply asserts that when sounds come to the surface in the luminous field of consciousness, the act of focusing our attention on them induces an emotional relation to them. Thus, the apprehension of poetic speech is not only not facilitative, but even more demanding, i.e., it requires additional work by comparison with ordinary speech. Obviously, the biological meaning of esthetic activity does not in the least express the sort of parasitic relationship that would inevitably arise if all esthetic pleasure were to be purchased at the expense of an economizing on spiritual forces which had been achieved thanks to the labor of others.

An understanding of the biological meaning of the esthetic act must be sought along the path followed by modern psychology, in an unraveling of the psychology of the creative work of the artist and in a convergence of our understanding of apprehension and of the process of creation. Before we ask ourselves why it is that we read, we must ask ourselves why it is that people write. The question of creative effort and its psychological sources again presents extraordinary difficulties, so that here we pass from one obstacle to the next. The general thesis, according to which creative effort represents the most profound demand of our psyche in pursuit of the sublimation of certain lower forms of energy is, however, no longer open to question. According to contemporary psychology, the most reasonable interpretation of creative effort is that which views it as sublimation, as the conversion of lower forms of mental energy which have not been consumed and which have not found an outlet in the individual's everyday activity, into higher forms of mental energy. Earlier, we presented on explanation of the concept of sublimation from the standpoint of the study of the instincts and, in particular, discussed the thesis that the creative processes and the sublimation of sexual energy exist in the closest imaginable relationship. In the words of one psychologist, in questions having to do with creative effort, there are people who are "rich" and people who are "poor," people who disburse their entire reserve of energy on the maintenance of everyday life, and people who seem to set aside and save, enlarging the range of needs that have to be satisfied. Here, too, creative effort arises the moment a certain quantity of energy that has not been put to use, that has not been consumed for immediate purposes, has not been apportioned, passes beyond the threshold of consciousness, whence it returns transformed into new forms of activity.

Earlier, we explained at some length that our capacities exceed our activity, that what a person accomplished in life is only a insignificant fraction of all those sensations that arise in the nervous system, and that it is precisely this discrepancy between capacities and realization, between the potential and the real in our life, which is fully encompassed by creative effort. Thus does the identity between acts of creation and acts of apprehension in art become a fundamental psychological presupposition. To be Shakespeare and to read Shakespeare are phenomena that are infinitely disparate in terms of degree, though entirely identical in terms of nature, as Yulii Aikhenval'd correctly explained. The reader must be sympathetic to the poet, and, in our apprehension of any work of art, we seem to be recreating it all over again. Thus, we are entirely justified in defining processes of apprehension as consisting in the reproduction and recapitulation of creative processes. And if that is so, the conclusion is unavoidable that such processes represent the very same biological form of sublimation of certain types of spiritual energy as do creative processes themselves. It is precisely in art that that fraction of our life which occurs, in fact, in the form of excitations in our nervous system becomes manifest to us, though it remains unrealized in activity, as a consequence of the fact that our nervous system apprehends more stimuli than it can respond to.

The fact is that there is always present in man this excess of possibilities over life, this residue of unrealized behavior, as has been demonstrated in the study of the struggle for the total motor field, and this excess must always seek for itself some outlet. If this residue does not find an appropriate outlet, it finds itself in conflict with man's psyche. Abnormal forms of behavior usually arise out of such unrealized behavior, expressed in the form of psychoses and neuroses, which denote nothing other than a collision between unrealized, subconscious desires and the conscious part of our behavior. That which remains unrealized in our life must be sublimated, and there are only two outlets for what remains unrealized in life—either sublimation or neurosis. Thus, from the psychological point of view, art constitutes an imperishable and biologically essential mechanism by means of which excitations that have remained unrealized in life are discarded, and, in one form or another, is an entirely inevitable companion of every human existence.

In artistic creation, such sublimation is realized in extraordinarily vigorous and mighty forms, through esthetic apprehension, in forms that are facilitated and simplified, and prepared in advance by the aggregate of all those stimuli which impinge upon us. That esthetic education, interpreted as the creation of permanent skills for the sublimation of the subconscious possesses an extraordinarily important and autonomous value, is, therefore, entirely understandable. To educate someone in esthetics means creating in that person a permanent and properly functioning channel for the diversion and abstraction of the inner forces of the subconscious into useful skills. Sublimation fulfills in socially useful forms that which sleep and illness fulfill in private and pathological forms.

Psychological Description of Esthetic Reactions

The most cursory glance at esthetic reactions is enough for us to see that their ultimate goal is not to reproduce any genuine reaction, but to transcend it and triumph over it. If the ultimate goal of a poem about melancholy was only to tell us about melancholy, this would be a rather sad state of affairs for art. Obviously, in this case the goal of lyric poetry is not just to afflict us, as Leo Tolstoy puts it, with someone else's feelings, in this case, someone else's melancholy, but to be victorious over it, to transcend melancholy. In this sense, the Bukharinist definition of art as the socialization of feelings, just like the Tolstoyan theme of the affliction of a multitude of people with the feelings of one person are, *speaking psychologically*, not entirely correct.

In this case, the "wonder" of art would recall that dismal miracle from the scriptures when five loaves of bread and two fish were enough to feed five thousand people, except for women and children, and everyone ate and was satisfied; and the remaining pieces of food filled twenty baskets. The "miracle" here lies only in the extraordinary multiplication of experience, though everyone who ate, ate only bread and fish, fish and bread. As in the socialization of feelings in art, there is achieved a multiplication of one person's feelings by a factor of a thousand, though feeling itself nevertheless remains an ordinary psychological type of emotion, and no work of art can incorporate anything that might go beyond the limits of this immeasurably vast emotion. It is entirely understandable that the purpose of art would then be rather puny, inasmuch as every genuine object and every genuine emotion would prove to be many times more powerful, more sharply defined, and more intensive and, consequently, all the pleasure of art would spring from man's hunger and poverty, whereas in fact, it springs from man's wealth, from the fact that every person possesses more wealth than he is able to realize in his own life.

Thus, art is not a means of making up for a lack in life, but issues from what it is in man that exceeds life. The "wonder" of art is far more reminiscent of that time when water was turned into wine, and, therefore, every work of art forever bears some genuine objective theme or some entirely ordinary feeling about the world. But what we understand by form and style refers to the fact that this genuine objective theme or this emotional tinge of things is overcome and transformed into something entirely novel. It is for this reason that the meaning of esthetic activity has been understood since time immemorial as catharsis, i.e., as a liberation and resolution of the spirit from the passions which torment it. In the psychology of ancient times, this concept assumed the purely medicinal and restorative value of a healing of the soul, and there can be no doubt that it was far more in accord with the genuine nature of art than a host of contemporary theories. "Psalms heal a suffering spirit"—these words of the poet express more correctly than anything else that watershed which separates art from illness.

It is not without reason that many psychologists have found it extremely tempting to search for features that might be common to art and illness, to declare that genius is akin to madness, and to view as abnormal both human creation and human folly. It is only in this way that we are able to understand the cognitive, the ethical, the emotional value of art. All these aspects do, undoubtedly, exist, but always as secondary components, as a kind of sequel to the work of art, arising in no other way than as a follow-up to its fully realized esthetic effect.

There can be no doubt that art possesses a moral testament, which manifests itself in nothing less than a certain internal clarification of the spiritual world, in a certain transcendence of one's innermost conflicts and, consequently, in a liberation of certain constrained and exiled forces, particularly the forces of moral behavior. A shining illustration of this principle may be found in Chekhov's short story, *The House*, where the father, a public prosecutor, who all his life has exercised his talents in devising every imaginable from of preventive punishment, in inventing all sorts of warnings and penalties, finds himself in an extremely embarrassing situation when he comes up against the small matter of his own son, a seven-year boy, having committed an offense, as the governess informs him, having grabbed some tobacco off his father's table and smoked it. How many times the father had tried to explain to his son why he must not smoke, why he must not take someone else's tobacco—none of his admonitions had achieved their purpose, since they had encountered insurmountable obstacles in the mind of his very own child, who apprehended and interpreted the world in a very original way entirely his own. When the father explains to him that one should not take someone else's things, the boy responded by pointing out that right over there was his little yellow puppy sitting on the table next to his father, that there was nothing to be said against that, what if his father needed some of his things and felt he was welcome to take it and wouldn't feel ashamed either? When his father tried to explain to him that it was harmful to smoke, that Uncle Grigorii had smoked and, therefore, had passed away, this example turned out to have quite the reverse effect on his son, since the boy associated the image of Uncle Grigorii with a kind of poetic feeling; he remembered that Uncle Grigorii was quite a wonderful violinist, and his uncle's fate not only did not help him avoid doing what his uncle had done, but, quite the opposite, imparted to smoking a new and seductive meaning.

Thus, not having gotten anywhere, the father concluded his conversation with his son, and it was only just before going to sleep, when, as was his wont, he began to tell his son a story, clumsily linking together the first thoughts that came to mind into traditional story models, that his story unexpectedly assumed the form of a naive and silly tale of that old tsar who had a son, the son smoked, fell ill with consumption, and died at an early age; enemies invaded and destroyed the palace, and killed the old man, and "... now there are no longer any sweet cherries in the garden, neither birds nor bells ..." The father himself felt that this story was naive and silly; however, it produced an unexpected effect in his son, who, speaking in a thoughtful and low voice, which his father found quite unexpected, said that he would no longer smoke.

The simple act of telling the story aroused and illuminated new forces in the child's psyche that made it possible for him to sense his father's fear and his father's concern for his health with such renewed vigor that the moral aftereffect of this new force, impelled by his father's initial persistence, had the unexpected effect his father had previously attempted to achieve, but in vain.

But now let us recall the two essential psychological features that distinguish this aftereffect. First, it is realized in the form of the child's own innermost, internal process of attention, it is by no means achieved through a process of rational extraction of some moral or through a sermon taken from a fable or short story. On the contrary, the more powerful is one's agitation and one's passion within whose atmosphere the esthetic impression works its effect, the higher is the emotional lift which accompanies it, the more powerful are the forces that accumulate about the moral aftereffect, and the more faithful is this esthetic impression realized.

Second, from such a vantage point, the moral effect of esthetics may be fortuitous and secondary, so that, at the least, it is an unwise and uncertain proposition to use this moral effect as the basis of the education of moral behavior. There is that story where the father quite properly puts a lot of thought into deciding whether it is really right for "medicine to be sweet and truth beautiful." In drawing its own convictions from novels and poetry, historical knowledge from operas and epic tales, and morality from fables, society, of course, never succeeds in reaching any firm and secure point in any of these realms. Chekhov was entirely correct in calling this a fancy that man has affected ever since the time of Adam, and in this regard it is entirely identical with that form of pedagogics which demands that children receive a stern moral upbringing based on truth.[3]

Psychologists who have studied the visual stimuli that emanate from paintings have all come to the same conclusion, that the principal role in our experience of a painting is played by the kinesthetic senses, i.e., by motor reactions as well, and that we read a picture more with our muscles than with our eyes; its esthetic effect manifests itself in our fingertips as much as in our eyes, since it speaks to our tactile and motor imagination no less than to our visual imagination.

Finally, such an aftereffect may also manifest itself in the hedonistic moment of pleasure or delight in a work of art, and this, too, may exert an educational influence on our senses, though this influence will always be secondary relative to the basic effect of poetry and art. This is not too different from what psychologists have referred to as the "liberating force of the higher emotions." And just as in ancient times, when the incantatory force of the rhythmic word and of poetic speech would banish the spirits and combat them, so too does modern poetry banish and resolve internal forces that possess inimical effects, because in both instances there is a kind of resolution of internal conflict.

It's worth recalling the rather curious fact that the pleasure produced by works of poetry always reveals itself along indirect and contradictory paths, and inevitably originates in a transcendence of the immediate impressions of the object and of the work of art. The tragic and the comic in art are the clearest exemplars of this psychological law, as anyone should be able to recall. Tragedy always speaks of destruction, and induces in us, in Aristotle's definition, fear, awe, and compassion. If we contemplate tragedy not from the vantage point of these lofty feelings, but with a slight smile, then its tragic effect, of course, becomes incomprehensible to us. How agony can, all by itself, become the subject of the experience of the beautiful, and why the contemplation of someone else's downfall can give the audience watching a tragedy such sublime pleasure, was a problem that engaged the attention of philosophers even in ancient times. Then this was attributed naively to a biological antithesis, and philosophers attempted to reduce the enjoyment we experience from tragedy to the feelings of security and pleasure man experiences every time misfortune strikes someone else. In this psychological theory, it is said that the tragedy of Oedipus gives a spectator the greatest pleasure imaginable simply because he learns from it to value his happiness and the fact that he isn't blind. However, even the simplest examples presented by these writers completely refute this thesis, one writer having claimed, for example, that people who happen to be standing along the sea shore and who see a ship sinking into the ocean would, in such cases, have to feel the greatest delight imaginable from their awareness that they themselves are safe.

Even the simplest psychological observation shows us that in the experience of a tragedy, we are inevitably placed by the playwright in an empathetic relationship with a hero, which grows as he approaches his destruction and which feeds into our feelings of fear and rapture. Consequently, the source of this enjoyment must be sought elsewhere, and, of course, we find it only in catharsis, i.e., in the resolution of the passions that are aroused by tragedy, which is the ultimate purpose of art. "Awe," writes Christensen, "is not portrayed for its own sake, but only as an impetus for transcending it."

In precisely the same way, the comic, or that which is, in and of itself, mean and repulsive, also leads, along a path that, at first glance, seems utterly incomprehensible, to great delight. In Gogol's "The Inspector," there is not a single sweetly sounding word, on the contrary, the author has tried to hunt down every word that might sound rusty, tinny, and coarse in the Russian language. There is not a single character in the story who is not repulsive, not a single event that is not trivial, not a single thought which is in any way luminous. Nevertheless, in this piling up of the trivial and the repulsive, a kind of special meaning thrusts itself through and becomes manifest, which Gogol is right to attribute to laughter, i.e., to the psychological reaction which draws the spectator out of himself but which is not within the farce itself. In a farce no one laughs; everyone, on the contrary, is anxious and in earnest, though all this material is arranged in such a way that it inevitably induces in the spectator hearty laughter, which can be ranked with the unfolding of lyric poetry and which Gogol correctly calls the only worthy character of his farce.

German esthetics has long referred to this psychological aspect of art as the esthetic of the grotesque, and through these examples demonstrated with extraordinary persuasiveness the dialectical character of esthetic experience. Contradiction, alienation, transcendence, triumph—these are all essential constituents of the esthetic event. It is necessary to see the grotesque in its full flowering in order to then rise above it in laughter. It is necessary to experience with the hero the absolute consummation of destruction in order to rise above it, together with the chorus. This dialectical, reconstitutive behavior of the emotions always bears within itself art, and, therefore, always points to the most complex of all activities of internal struggle, which is resolved in catharsis.

Education of Creativity, Esthetic Reasoning, and Technical Skills

Carried over to education, this thesis naturally breaks down into three separate problems. Education may have before it the demand to foster the child's creativity, or to give children vocational training in the different technical skills involved in art, or to inculcate in children the capacity of esthetic reasoning, i.e., the skill to apprehend and experience a work of art.

The question of children's creativity is, without a doubt, of extraordinary pedagogical importance, though it has virtually no independent esthetic value. A child's drawing is always an educationally gratifying event, though it is sometimes also esthetically grotesque. It always teaches the child to master the aggregate of his own experiences, to conquer and transcend them, and, as one writer has expressed it rather elegantly, teaches the psyche how to ascend. A child who has drawn a picture of a dog has, thereby, conquered, transcended, and risen above his immediate experience of a dog.

In this sense, too, it becomes pedagogically essential to be able to discern the psychological content of children's drawings, i.e, to examine and take notice of all those experiences that lead to the genesis of a drawing, rather than making objective evaluations of the points and lines themselves. Therefore, any effort at smoothing out or correcting a child's drawing represents only a crude intrusion in the psychological order of his experience and risks becoming an impediment to this experience. While it is true that by changing and correcting the lines a child has drawn, we may very well be introducing a strict order into the sheet of paper in front of us, we will be most certainly introducing conflict into the child's psyche and making him insensitive. Complete freedom for the child's creativity, the renunciation of all effort to place it on a par with adult consciousness, the recognition of its originality and of its distinctive features, constitute a fundamental requirement of psychology.

The boy in Chekhov's story, *The House*, when asked by his father why he was placing a soldier above a house in his drawing, even though he was well aware that a person cannot stand higher than a house, answered in a serious tone that if he were to make the soldier little, then you couldn't see his eyes. It is in this striving to emphasize the main point he is involved in at any moment, the main subject of a drawing, and to subordinate to it all other relationships, that we find the basic feature of children's drawings, and, for all practical purposes, the child's tendency to disregard and remain unencumbered by the true contours of objects springs not from any inability to see objects as such—the way things really are—but from the fact that the child is never indifferent to the object. Every one of his drawings, provided it is not created at the behest of some adult, always originates out of the child's innermost feelings, and this we have to see as the fundamental property of the child's psyche, which, therefore, always distorts the insignificant elements of the object in favor of what is the most important and the most fundamental.

Tolstoy suggests the very same rule in his theory of pedagogy in his insistence that children's compositions not be corrected by adults even orthographically, claiming that any correction of a finished product of an act of creation always distorts the internal motivation which engendered it. In a famous essay, "Who Should Teach Whom to Write: Should we Teach the Children of Peasants or Should the Children of Peasants Teach Us?" Tolstoy defended the thesis, which seems paradoxical at first glance, that a "half-literate peasant boy displays the conscious force of a true author, that not even Goethe, from the lofty heights of his art, can attain." "It seems to me so odd and so insulting," continues Tolstoy, "that, when it comes to art, I, the author of `Childhood,' a work which has achieved a degree of critical acclaim and which has been recognized for its literary talents by the educated public in Russia, was unable to explain or assist 11-year old Semka and Fedka, except in the slightest degree, and then only at the fortuitous moment of excitement, when I was able to grasp what they were getting at, and to understand them." Tolstoy discovered more poetic truth in these children's compositions than in the greatest creations of literature. And if there were some banal moments in their compositions, this was always the fault of Tolstoy himself; whenever the children were left to their own devices, they did not utter a single affected word. Thus was Tolstoy led to conclude that the ideal of esthetic education, like the ideal of moral education, lies not ahead of us, but behind us—not in bringing the soul of the child closer to the soul of the adult, but in preserving the natural properties the child's soul is endowed with from the very start.

"Education corrupts, and does not reform people." In this sense, the concerns of education reduce almost exclusively to not corrupting the child's spiritual wealth, and the precept, "Be like children," seems like the ultimate pedagogical ideal when it comes to aesthetics.

That there is in this view a great and undeniable truth, that in the child's creativity we are dealing with pure examples of poetry at the absolutely elemental level lacking all traces of the adult's trained eye—this is something virtually no one now disputes. But it is also necessary to recognize that such creativity is of an order all its own; it is, so to speak, transient creativity, giving rise to no objective values and needed more by the child himself than by those around him. Like children's games, it has healing powers and is invigorating, but not outside the child himself, but only within him. Tolstoy's Fed'ka and Semka grew up, but did not become great writers, even though at the age of 11 they were given to use language which, as Tolstoy, with all his prestige, was forced to admit, went far beyond that found in novels and was the equal of the most felicitous passages in Goethe.

Hence, the most unquestionable mistake of this view can be found in its extraordinary overestimation and idolizing of the works of children's creative efforts, and in its inability to understand that, though it is capable of realizing works of the greatest emotional tension, here the primordial force of the creative act is, nevertheless, always circumscribed within a narrow range of the most elementary, the most primitive, and, basically, the most impoverished forms.

In this sense, the pedagogical rule as regards the education of children's creativity must always proceed from a purely psychological view of its utility and should never look upon the child who is writing poetry as if he were a future Pushkin, or look upon the child who is drawing pictures as if he were a future artist. A child writes poetry or draws pictures not at all because a future poet or future painter is struggling to burst through him, but because these acts of creation are *now* necessary for him, and even more so because there are certain creative potentialities concealed in each of us. The very processes by which genius and talent are selected are still so dimly understood, so well hidden, and have been so little studied that pedagogics is entirely powerless to say precisely which steps might help preserve and foster future geniuses.

Here we confront the extraordinarily involved question of the very possibility of esthetic education. We have already seen that Tolstoy's views do not draw out the essential difference between artistic creativity in the adult and in the child. Therefore, Tolstoy does not take into account, first, that immeasurably vast importance which, in the realm of art, is subserved by the element of workmanship, an element which, though of course utterly self-evident, is the result of education. Workmanship encompasses not only the technical skills of art, but something far greater, whether in the subtlest knowledge of the laws of one's own art, in the feeling for style, in the talent for creative effort, in taste, and so on. There was a time when the concept of craftsman fully encompassed the concept of artist.

But, in addition, the conception of the mystical nature of inspiration, of spiritual possession, and so on gave way in scholarly discourse to an entirely different view of the nature of acts of creation. And Tolstoy's thesis that, "once he has been born, man constitutes a prototype of harmony, of truth, of beauty, and of goodness," has to be recognized as a legend rather than a scientific truth. It is true that, in childhood, immediate urges and creative impulses are more powerful and more vivid, but, as we showed earlier, the nature of these urges and impulses are not at all the same as in adults. No matter how sublime and how exquisite are those works Semka and Fed'ka produced, their creative impulses were always of a different order than Goethe's or Tolstoy's in their very essence.

The view maintained by Aikhenval'd, Gershenzon, and others, that literature cannot become a subject for instruction in public schools, represents a separate question altogether. But this view originates in an overly narrow view of public schools that forever has in mind those lessons that used to be given in the schools before the revolution. The wealth of educational potentialities in the Soviet school is lost sight of. Esthetic feelings have to become just as much a subject of education as is everything else, but only in special ways.

It is from this point of view that we should approach vocational training in the techniques of this or that realm of art. The instructive value of these techniques is extraordinarily great, in the same way as is every form of labor and every form of complex activity; it becomes even greater still once it is turned into a tool for training children in the apprehension of works of art, inasmuch as it is impossible to fully enter into a work of art if the techniques that are part of its idiom remain utterly foreign. It is for this reason that a certain minimal technical familiarity with the system of every art has to become part of public education.

In this sense, those schools which have made mastery of the techniques of each of the arts an educational requirement are proceeding entirely properly from the standpoint of pedagogy.

Vocational training in art, however, harbors far more pedagogical risks than benefits. To the psychologist, all those grandiose and useless experiments at teaching music to absolutely every child, which became the rule for the middle classes in Europe and pre-revolutionary Russia over the last several decades, seemed to have had only an oppressive effect. If we think of how much energy was spent on mastering the most complex piano techniques imaginable, and if we compare this with the negligible results which were obtained after many years' of practice, we have to admit that this enormous experiment, on experiment that was performed on an entire social class, ended in an utterly embarrassing failure. Not only has the art of musicianship not gained or acquired anything of value from this program, but, as is generally recognized, even the simple musical education of the art of appreciation, apprehension, and experience of music never and nowhere stood so low as in that milieu where learning how to play music became a mandatory rule of good breeding.

In terms of overall pedagogical influence, such instruction was, quite frankly, harmful and destructive, since almost nowhere and almost never was it associated with the child's immediate interests, and wherever this instruction was undertaken, it was always on behalf of outside interests, which, for the most part, subordinated the child to the interests of his surroundings and refracted in the child's psyche the most brutish and the most vulgar everyday thoughts of those around him.

Hence, vocational training in the techniques of each of the various arts, if we understand it as a task of general education and edification, has to be introduced within certain limits and reduced to a minimum, and the main thing is to conform with the other two paths of esthetic education, first, the child's own creative potential, and, second, the cultural level of his esthetic apprehension. Only that instruction in techniques is useful which goes *beyond these techniques* and teaches creative skills, whether those involved in creating or those involved in apprehending.

Finally, until very recently questions as to the cultural level of esthetic apprehension had received the least amount of attention, inasmuch as educators had no idea how truly complex it was, nor did they think there was any problem here. To look at and to listen, to obtain pleasure—this seemed to be the sort of uncomplicated mental effort for which special instruction was absolutely unnecessary, whereas, in fact, it is just this element which constitutes the principal goal and principal task of general education.

The overall structure of public education is oriented towards expanding the scope of finite personal experience as far as possible, towards adjusting the interface between the child's psyche and the broadest possible spheres of the social experience he has accumulated so far, as if to include the child in the broadest possible network in the world. These general goals wholly define the paths of esthetic education. In art mankind has accumulated such an exceptional and vast store of experience that all experience of one's own creativity and one's own personal achievements seem puny and wretched by comparison. Therefore, when we speak of esthetic education within the context of general education, we must always bear in mind, basically, such an orientation of the child towards the esthetic experience of mankind as a means of bringing the child face to face with real art and, through this experience, to include the child's psyche in that general labor mankind throughout the world has been engaged in for thousands of years, sublimating the child's own psyche in art—here is a fundamental task and the fundamental goal.

And it is because efforts at understanding works of art usually resort to impractical techniques involving logical interpretation that specialized training and the development of special skills for the reconstitution of works of art are required, and, in this sense, lessons that consist in looking at paintings, like those lessons in "slow reading" that have been introduced in certain European schools, are true exemplars of esthetic education.

Here is the key to the most important task of esthetic education—the introduction of esthetic reactions into life itself. Art transforms reality not only in the constructions of fantasy, but also in a genuine recreation of things, objects, and situations. Dwellings and dress, conversation and reading, school holidays and strolls, all may serve, in equal measure, as the most gratifying substance for esthetic treatment.

Beauty has to be converted from a rare and festive thing into a demand of everyday existence. And creative effort has to nourish every movement, every utterance, every smile of the child's. Potebnya put it quite elegantly when he said that, just as electricity is present not only where there are thunderstorms, so is poetry present not only where there are great works of art, but wherever man speaks. This is the poetry "of every moment," and it is this which is the most important of all the tasks of esthetic education.

But it is still essential to keep in mind the most serious of all dangers, the risk that an artificiality might be introduced into life which, in children, is something that easily turns into affectation and pretension. There is nothing in worst taste than this "acting cute" [*krasivost'*], those mannerisms some children introduce into games, into their way of walking, and so on. The rule to follow here is not the embellishment of life, but the creative reworking of reality, a processing of things and the movements of things which will illuminate and elevate everyday experience to the level of the creative.

Fables

Fables are usually thought of as the exclusive province of childhood. Two psychological arguments have been advanced in defense of this view.

The first asserts that the child is not yet old enough to have a rational understanding of reality, and therefore has a need for a kind of "surrogate" or mediative explanation of the world. It is for this reason that the child readily accepts the interpretation of reality given in fables, and, second, discovers in fables what adults discover in religion, science, and art, that is, the primary explanation and understanding of the world, the reduction of the discordant chaos of impressions into a unified and integral system. For a child, fables are philosophy, science, and art.

There is another approach which claims that, in accordance with the biogenetic law, the child, in the course of his development, repeats in abbreviated and compressed form the principal stages and epochs that mankind has experienced in its development. Hence that rather popular view which discovers a confluence between the child's psyche and creative urges, on the one hand, and the creative urges of the savage and primitive man, on the other, and the claim that, as he grows up, the child inevitably experiences animism, the sense of all things being alive, and anthropomorphism, just as mankind as a whole has. It is felt necessary, for this reason, to transcend all these primitive attitudes and beliefs at some stage of development, and to introduce into the child's world all those ideas of devils, witches, wizards, and good and evil spirits which were once the companions of human culture. This approach sees in fables a necessary evil, a psychological concession to childhood, in the expression of one psychologist, an esthetic pacifier.

Both these views are profoundly mistaken at their very roots. As regards the first view, pedagogics has long rejected all kinds of mediation, inasmuch as the harm it introduces always outweighs any possible benefit. The point is that any benefit is always temporary, it exists until the child grows up and no longer has any need for such a mediative explanation of the world. The harm, however, remains forever, because in the psyche, as in the real world, nothing happens without leaving a trace, nothing disappears, rather everything creates its own habits, which then remain for all one's life. "Expressed with scientific rigor," William James asserts, "one may say that nothing may be entirely effaced from anything we do." This is especially true in the period of childhood, when the plasticity and impressionability of our nervous system is at its utmost, and when reactions only have to be repeated two or three times in order to last sometimes for one's entire life. If, in this period in his life, a child is forced to control and guide his behavior under the influence of false and deliberately misleading ideas and views, we can be quite certain that these views will create habits of behavior along these false directions. And when, it would appear to us, the time has come for the child to free himself of these ideas and views, it may be possible for us, by reasoning rationally, to persuade him that all those ideas we would talk to him about were false; we may even be morally justified in making excuses to him for the deception he had been subjected to for so many years, but never can he efface all those habits, instincts, and stimuli which have already evolved and which have become deeply embedded in him, and which, even in the best of cases, are capable of creating conflicts with newly implanted traits.

The basic claim is that, in the absence of behavior, the psyche does not exist, and that if we introduce into the psyche false ideas that do not correspond to truth and reality, by this very act we are also fostering false behavior. Hence we are forced to conclude that truth must become the foundation of education as early as possible, simply because incorrect ideas are also incorrect forms of behavior. If, from early childhood, a child learns to trust in "bogeymen," in little old ladies who are going to take you away, in magicians, in storks who bring babies, all this will not only clutter up his mind, but, what is even worse, it will cause his behavior to develop in false directions. It is entirely clear that children are either frightened of this world of magic or are drawn into it, but that they never remain passive towards it. In dreams or in desires, under the child's blanket or in a dark room, when asleep or when frightened, the child always responds to these ideas, responds with an extraordinarily heightened sensibility, and since the system formed by these reactions rests on an entirely fantastic and false foundation, for that very reason an incorrect and false way of behaving is methodically fostered in the child.

To this we should add that all of this fantastic world depresses the child no end, and there can be little doubt that its oppressive force exceeds the child's capacity for resistance. By surrounding the child with the fantastic, we force him to live as if in a perpetual psychosis. Imagine for just a minute that an adult were, all of a sudden, to believe in the very same things he teaches a child—how extraordinarily confused and depressed would his mind become. All of this must increase manyfold once we show the child how to think, since the child's weak and unsteady mind proves to be even more helpless when confronted by this sombre element. Psychological analyses of children's fears produce an utterly tragic impression, inasmuch as they always testify to and speak of those inexpressible germs of terror that were implanted in the child's soul by the fables adults themselves have told him.

The educational benefits produced by introducing into family lore those tales of the old man who is going to carry you away are always limited to the immediate advantage given by intimidation, in which we get the child to stop playing practical jokes or induce him to perform some task. The harm which thereby ensues may manifest itself in humiliating forms of behavior that may last for many decades.

Finally, the last argument that may be brought against the traditional view of fables is the utterly profound disrespect for reality, the excessive importance ascribed to the invisible, which such fables methodically instill. The child remains dull and foolish when he relates to the real world, he remains closed up within a stagnant and unhealthy atmosphere, for the most part in a kingdom of fabulous creatures. He has no interest in trees or in birds, and the manifold variety of experience seems to lack all substance. The result of such an education is to make someone blind, deaf, and dumb in relation to the world.

For all these reasons, we have to agree with that view which demands that all those fantastic and silly ideas children are usually inculcated with must be banished *thoroughly and completely*. It is, moreover, rather important that it is not only fairy tales which can produce the greatest harm here, but also all those silly and timeworn fictions which are used not only by nurses to frighten children with, but which not even the most highly educated teacher is entirely free of. There is almost no teacher who would be innocent of the charge of having reasoned with a child on the basis of some incongruous nonsense, simply because he knew that the child would take this nonsense for the truth, and saw that the easiest way out of problem at hand was to adapt the admonitory line of least resistance by telling the child, "Don't go there, else the house will fall down," or to say, "Don't cry, else the policeman will take you away." It is psuedo-natural-science" nonsense of this sort that has taken up the role performed by the nonsense of fantasies.

Finally, from the most general standpoint we have to say that every attempt by the teacher to "humor" the child is, from the psychological point of view, educationally harmful, since here one can never be certain of hitting the nail right on the head, and, in order to meet his teacher's expectations, the child is forced to likewise affect and distort his own reactions, and try to come as close as he can to what his teacher demands. This is simplest to understand if we think of children's speech, of those instances when adults who are engaged in conversation with a child try to imitate his way of speaking, under the impression that this will make them more then easily understood, whether lisping, or aspirating, pronouncing the sounds "s" and "z" as "sh" and "zh", or pronouncing the sound "r" as "l." For a child, however, such speech is not in the least more understandable. If a child's pronunciation is incorrect, this is not because he hears this way, but because he cannot pronounce correctly. When he then hears distorted speech coming from adults, he is totally lost and tries to approximate his own speech to this distorted speech. Most of our children speak in an unnatural way, their speech having been distorted by adults, and it is impossible to imagine anything more artificial than such affected speech.

There is also that customary false way of speaking with children in overly familiar and endearing terms, in which a "horse" is spoken of as a "horsy," a dog as a "little doggy," and a "house" as "the little house". To an adult, it might seem that the child thinks everything has to be little, though quite the contrary, he who does not belittle objects in children's imagination, but instead overemphasizes their natural dimensions, is proceeding in a far more psychological fashion. When we speak to a child of horses, which must seem a huge and massive thing to him, and talk of a "horsy," the true sense of speech is distorted, as is the concept of horse, not to mention that false and sugarcoated attitude towards everything which such a manner of speaking establishes. Language is the subtlest tool of thought; in distorting language, we distort thought, and even if a single teacher were of think of the emotional nonsense she is uttering when she tells a child, "Let's hit the little doggy," or "the little doggy is biting you," she would certainly be horrified by the mental confusion she is creating in the child's mind. And though there are things in children's literature and in children's art which are, in fact, intolerable and repulsive, this is just because adults have been falsely humoring the minds of children.

As for the need for children to gradually overcome the primitive beliefs and primitive ideas in fables, this, too, has not undergone serious criticism and slips away with the biogenetic law on which it is based. No one has yet to show that, in the course of his development, the child repeats the history of mankind, and not even science has ever had any grounds to speak of anything more than isolated correlations and more or less remote analogies between the behavior of a child and that of a savage. On the contrary, all those essential changes in the pattern of education that are a function of social circumstances and environment, more properly, as a function of the common fundament of life the child enters the moment he is born, are quite at variance with the biogenetic law, in every instance contrary to any direct translation of the law from biology into psychology. The child turns out to be entirely able to interpret phenomena realistically and truthfully, though, of course, he cannot immediately find an explanation for absolutely everything. Left to himself, the child is never an animist, never an anthropomorphist, and if these propensities develop in a child, the fault is nearly always that of the adults around him.

Finally, what is most important here is that, even if certain psychological conditions did generate atavistic tendencies in a child, i.e., where his mind reverted to stages in his history he had already passed through, even if the child did contain within his mind something of the savage, in no way would the goal of education reduce to the maintenance, sustenance, and reinforcement of these elements of the savage in the child's psyche, but quite the contrary, his propensities would subordinate these elements to the more powerful and the more vital elements of reality in every way possible.

Does this mean we have to think of fables as being ultimately compromised and that they are condemned to be banished entirely from the child's room with all those false and fabulous ideas of the world that turn out to be mentally harmful? No, not really. There can be little doubt that most of our fables, which are based precisely on such unhealthy fantasy and lack all other values, must be abandoned and forgotten as soon as possible. But this does not mean that the esthetic content of works of fantasy have to be forbidden to children.

On the contrary, the fundamental law of art demands the freedom to combine the elements of reality in any way whatsoever, an essential independence from everyday truth, which in esthetics effaces all the boundaries that separate fantasy from truth. In art *everything is fantastic or everything is real*, simply because everything is hypothetical, and the realness of art refers only to the realness of the emotions any work of art is associated with. As a matter of fact, the question is not in the least whether what is related in a fable could exist in real life. What is more important is that the child know that it never existed in real life, that it is only a story, and that he get into the habit of responding to it as a fable, and that, consequently, the question of whether such an event could be possible in real life ceases to exist for him. In order to enjoy a fable, it is not at all necessary to believe in what it speaks of. On the contrary, belief in the "realness" of the world of fables establishes such purely commonplace attitudes towards everything as to preclude the very possibility of esthetic activity.

Here we should explain the law of emotional realness of fantasy, a law of the greatest importance for our field. According to this law, regardless of whether the world we are affected by is real [*real'no*], the emotions associated with this influence and which we feel are always real. If I am hallucinating and, upon entering an empty room, see a thief standing over in the corner, this figure will, of course, be one of delirium, and the collection of all those impressions associated with this figure in my mind will not be real, inasmuch as there is no reality [*deistvitel'nost'*] corresponding to it; but the fear which I experience from this encounter and the emotion associated with the hallucination are entirely real, even if they are repressed by the comforting consciousness of having been mistaken. That we do have feelings, this is always a real fact.

Thus, fantasy justifies itself in this law of the realness of our feelings. We are not drawing children away from reality in the least when we tell them fantastic stories, if the feelings that arise thereby are brought to life. Therefore, the real emotional basis of a work of fantasy is its only justification, and it is not surprising that, though we may banish the harmful forms of fantasy, of fantastic stories tales will nevertheless remain one of the many forms of children's art. Only now it will perform an entirely different function, however; it will cease to be the child's philosophy and science, and become only an exceptionally uninhibited type of fable.

The principal value of fables is formed in the extraordinarily conceptual features of childhood. The point is that the interaction between the individual and the world, which is what all of our behavior and all of our psyche ultimately reduces to, is, in children, at its most delicate and most underdeveloped stage, and, therefore, the demand for every imaginable form that might give emotion a degree of discipline is felt in especially marked fashion. Otherwise, the vast bulk of impressions reaching the child in quantities far beyond his ability to respond would overwhelm him and make him confused. In this sense, a wise fable possesses an invigorating and restorative value within the overall structure of the child's emotional life.

The most interesting of all the recent studies on the nature of the emotions reaches exactly the same conclusions as the law we have just discussed. It has long been noted that an emotion always possesses a certain outward material expression, though only very recently has it been noted that an emotion also always possesses a certain "spiritual" or mental expression, in other words, that feelings are connected not only with a certain degree of mimicry and external manifestation, but also with imagery, with representations, and with "emotional thinking." While there are some feelings which thrive in bright colors and warm tones, there are others, on the contrary, which go better with cold tones and dim colors, and it is right here that the mental expression of the emotions manifests itself. The feeling of melancholy compels me not only to carry my body in a certain way, but to also select impressions in a certain way, and it finds its expression in sad memories, in sad fantasies, and in sad dreams. Essentially, dreams constitute a spiritual expression of emotion in pure form. Investigations have shown that a feeling which arises spontaneously, for example, the feeling of fear, is a kind of a unifying thread that weaves together the most diverse episodes and the most incongruous parts of dreams.

Hence the emotional value of imagination becomes understandable. Emotions that are not realized in one's life find their outlet and their expression in arbitrary combinations of the elements of reality, above all, in art. It should be recalled in this connection that art does not just provide an outlet and expression for a particular emotion, it always resolves this emotion and liberates the psyche from its sombre influence.

Thus does the psychological effect of the fable converge with the psychological effect of games. The esthetic value of a game manifests itself not only in the rhythm it imparts to children's movements, or in the mastery of primitive melodies in such games as square dancing and the like. It is far more important that games, which, from the biological point of view, constitute preparation for real life, from the aspect of psychology manifest themselves as yet another form of the child's creative urges. Some psychologists have referred to the law discussed earlier as the "law of dual expression of the feelings," and it is precisely this "dual expression" which games subserve. In games, the child is always creatively transforming reality. In the mind of a child, people and things readily assume new meanings. For a child, a chair does not just represent a train, a horse, or a house, but actually participates in his games as such. And this transformation of reality in games is always oriented towards the child's emotional needs. "It is not because we play that we are children, rather we are given childhood in order to play"—this formula of Karl Groos' expresses better than anything else the biological nature of games. Its psychological nature is wholly defined by the dual expression of the emotions, which is manifested in movements and in the discipline of games. Just like games, an artistically well-thought-out fable is the child's natural esthetic teacher.

Esthetic Education and Natural Talent

There is the belief that there are two entirely different systems of esthetic education, one for the gifted and talented, and the other for ordinary, average students. There is no way for such thinking to become reconciled with the fact that the esthetic education of especially gifted children shouldn't be any different than the esthetic education of ordinary children. The conclusions of science increasingly lead us away from such a view and give us ever newer proofs in favor of quite the opposite belief, that there is no *fundamental* difference between the two, and that our concern should rather lie in the development of a common pedagogical system.

As regards voice training, the view that every person is supplied with an ideal voice from birth, a voice that comprises potentialities that exceed many times over the highest achievements of vocal art, is increasingly taking root. In its normal organization, the human throat is the greatest musical instrument in the world, and if in spite of this, we always speak with terrible voices, the only reason for this is the fact that, because of shouting, improper breathing, and developmental conditions and dress, we appear to have spoiled the voice we are initially endowed with. Those who are the most gifted in terms of vocal qualities are not those who were supplied with the best voice to begin with, but those who have, by chance, succeeded in preserving it. On this point, Professor Buldin declares that "Shalyapin's voice does not constitutes a rare gift, but a rare instance of the preservation of a common gift. Once a human voice attains such musical perfection, all our conceptions of the language of angels are left far behind."

This view of the natural talents of the human organism is beginning to find more and more proponents in the most diverse fields of pedagogics. The ordinary conception of natural talent seems to have been turned upside down, and the problem cannot be posed as it used to be; one has to ask, not why is it that some people are more gifted than others, but, rather, why others are less gifted, since the high level of talent a human being is initially endowed with is, to all appearances, the fundamental datum in absolutely all domains of the psyche, and, consequently, those cases where these gifts have been lost or are in less abundance have to be explained. One can still speak of this only as a scientific premise supported quite strongly, to be sure, by a whole series of facts. However, if this is to be established as something unshakeable, the broadest imaginable potentialities open up before pedagogics, and the problem becomes one of determining how to preserve the child's creative talent.

Though this question cannot be considered solved in its final, general form, in its special application to questions of general education it may be considered already solved now in the sense that, like every form of education of creative talent, the goal of esthetic education must, in all ordinary circumstances, proceed on the assumption of the high level of talent of human nature, and the premise that the greatest creative potentiality of the human being is present, and that one's own educational influence must, thus, be accessible and guided in such a way as to develop these potentialities and preserve them. Thus, talent also becomes a *goal* of education, whereas in the old psychology it was present only as a *premise* and as a *datum* of education. In no other realm of psychology does this thought encounter such striking confirmation as in the field of art. For each of us our creative potentiality becomes the accomplice of Shakespeare when we read his tragedies, and the accomplice of Beethoven when we listen to his symphonies, and it is this which is the most striking indicator that in each of us there is concealed a potential Shakespeare and a potential Beethoven.

The psychological difference between the composer and audience of a musical composition, between Beethoven and each of us, was brilliantly defined by Tolstoy, when he pointed out the need for us to react to every impression, and emphasized the realness of art, an idea that is of the greatest importance for esthetic education.

"Of course, he who wrote at least the Kreutzer Sonata—Beethoven, that is— of course, he knew why he found himself in such a state; this state led him to undertake certain actions, so that for him, this state possessed a meaning, whereas for us it has no meaning at all. This is why music only stimulates, but does not terminate. Thus, if there is a military march being played, the soldiers will march to the music, and the music will affect them; if there is dance music being played, I'll go dancing, and the music will affect me; and if mass is being sung, I'll receive communion, and the music will also affect me; but this is only stimulation, and there is nothing I have to do in response to this stimulation. This is why music is so frightful, why it sometimes has so frightful an effect.

"For example, even though it is the Kreutzer Sonata, could the first move-ment be played, let's say, in a drawing room filled with young ladies in decollete? Suppose this movement is played, can I then tap someone on the shoulder, and then have some ice cream and talk the latest gossip? These pieces of music may be played only at certain important and significant social events and only when there are certain actions which have to be carried out and which are appropriate to this music. To play the music and to do what this music calls for, that is the point."

---

[1] So fashionable and, now, so popular a work as Chukovskii's *Crocodile*, like all of Chukovskii's stories for children, is one of the better examples of this perversion of children's poetry with nonsense and gibberish. Chukovskii seems to proceed from the assumption that the sillier something is, the more understandable and the more entertaining it is for the child, and the more likely that it will be within the child's grasp. It is not hard to instill the taste for such dull literature in children, though there can be little doubt that it has a negative impact on the educational process, particularly in those immoderately large doses to which children are now subjected. All thought of style is thrown out, and in his babbling verse Chukovskii piles up nonsense on top of gibberish. Such literature only fosters silliness and foolishness in children.

[2] "Look here, said Peredonov to the students, "we have to understand this thoroughly. There is an allegory concealed here. Wolves go in pairs, and, yes, here we have a wolf and a hungry she-wolf. The wolf is full, but his mate is hungry. The wife must always eat after the husband. The wife must obey the husband in everything." It goes without saying that, from such a view, a work of art ends up without any independent value of its own, it becomes a kind of illustration of some general moral assertion, which is where all attention becomes focused, and the work of art itself seems to fall outside the student's field of vision. And, in fact, with such an understanding not only are no esthetic habits or skills created or fostered, not only is there no flexibility, subtlety, or diversity of forms imparted to esthetic experience, but, on the contrary, the pedagogical rule becomes a matter of turning the students attention away from the actual work of art and towards its ethical meaning. Esthetic feelings are methodically extirpated as a result of such education, to be replaced by a moral element alien to esthetics, and hence that natural distaste for 99% of all of classical literature of the past which one can sense in our secondary schools. Many of those who have spoken in favor of eliminating literature from the high school curriculum take just this point of view, and claim that the best way of inculcating a dislike for some author and of dissuading someone from reading him is to introduce his works in a course in school.

[3] "Why is it that morality and truth," says the hero of the story, "have to be presented not in undigested form, but rather with extraneous elements, forever in sugarcoated and embellished form, like a pill? This is not normal ... It is a falsification, it is a deception, it is a trick ..." of art to become manifest. Once a work of art has been experienced, it may actually enlarge our view of some realm of experience, force us to look upon it as if with new eyes, to generalize and to combine together bits of information that may often be entirely disparate. The fact is that, like every powerful experience, esthetic experience creates a very tangible environment for subsequent actions and, of course, never transpires without leaving some trace that manifests itself in our behavior later on. Many writers have been quite right to compare works of poetry with batteries or devices for the storage of energy that is to be consumed subsequently. In precisely the same way, every experience of poetry seems to accumulate energy for future action, points one in a new direction, and compels us to look upon the world with new eyes. More radical psychologists have even come to speak of the purely motor environments evoked by this or that work of art. Come to think of it, we need only recall the existence of such forms of art as dance music to see that there is a certain motor impulse in absolutely every esthetic sensation. Sometimes it is realized right then and there, in rudimentary form, whether in the movements of a dance or in the beating of time, and this belongs to the lower forms of art. But there are also times when the complexity of this sensation reaches the highest levels, when, because of their motor complexity, these impulses

cannot become manifest in full and instantaneously, and then this motor complexity is expressed instead through extraordinarily subtle preliminary labor for the evolution of subsequent behavior. Esthetic experience disciplines our behavior. "From the way a person walks as he leaves a concert, we can always tell whether he had been listening to Beethoven or to Chopin"—thus writes one researcher.

(The above notes are those of Vygotsky.)

Chapter 14

EXERCISE AND FATIGUE

On Habit

Wilham James writes, "Ninety-nine hundredths or, possibly, nine hundred and ninety-nine thousandths of our activity is purely automatic and habitual, from our rising in the morning to our lying down each night. Our dressing and undressing, our eating and drinking, our greetings and partings, our hat raising and giving way for ladies to precede, nay, even most of the forms of our common speech, are things of a type so fixed by repetition as almost to be classed as reflex actions. To each sort of impression we have an automatic, ready-made response" [1]

From this alone, it is clear how important it is in education to establish habits. The process by which a certain action is turned into a habit and acquires the characteristic properties of automatic movement is called *exercise*. Behavior itself we have defined as a special mode of organization of reactions, and now it turns out that only 0.001 of these reactions are determined by something other than habit. In James' expression, man is simply a living complex of reactions, and for this reason the goal of the teacher is to accustom the student to those habits which will be of benefit to him later on in life.

Hence follows an important pedagogical rule, that we have to pay particular attention to processes of exercise. We have to look upon the process of exercise not as simple memory. Rather, we should think of exercise as creating a predisposition for optimal performance of this or that action. To investigate the capacity of exercise, one usually proceeds by Kraepelin's method, which involves the addition of one-digit numbers. "If we turn our attention," writes Gaupp, "to the number of additions produced per unit time, we see that, for the most part, efficiency increases. This becomes even clearer whenever we compare the initial efficiency from one day to the next, and do this for several days in succession. A similar increase in efficiency occurs under the influence of exercise, which is known to facilitate and accelerate every form of labor, both physical and mental. Exercise is a kind of memory. By exercise, we do not mean the retention of individual impressions, but the facilitation of the overall direction of activity, expressed figuratively, in the creation of well-worn paths."

Experimental investigations have shown that exercise at first develops slowly, and then is performed more and more rapidly, in spurts. That is, exercise induces a certain variation in the relative position of molecules in the brain. In this sense, writes James, "the great thing in all education is to make of our nervous system our ally instead of our enemy ... *For this we must make automatic and habitual as early as possible, as many useful actions as we can*, and as carefully guard against the growing into ways that are likely to be disadvantageous. The more of the details of our daily life we can hand over to the effortless custody of automatism, the more our higher powers of mind will be set free for their own proper work".[2] In this sense, that saying which calls habit our second nature expresses a profound truth:

> Could the young but realize how soon they will become mere walking bundles of habits, they would give more heed to their conduct while in the plastic state. We are spinning our own fates, good or evil, and never to be undone. Every smallest stroke of virtue or of vice leaves its never-so-little scar. The drunken Rip Van Winkle, in Joseph Jefferson's play, excuses himself for every fresh dereliction by saying, "I won't count this time!" Well, he may not count it, and a kind Heaven may not count it; but it is being counted none the less. Down amongst his nerve-cells and fibres the molecules are counting it, registering and storing it up to be used against him when the next temptation comes. Nothing we ever do is, in strict scientific literalness, wiped out. [3]

In one of Chekhov's stories, the hero, after having experienced and been deceived in love, writes in his diary that King David possessed a ring with the inscription, "everything passes." In response to this, he writes in his own diary the following words: "If I could order a ring for myself, I would select as inscription, 'nothing passes'"; and, in fact, each of our slightest steps has its own meaning for the future.

From the psychological point of view, both these contradictory assertions are equally and definitely true. Psychologically speaking, everything passes, and every repeated movement, simply because it was preceded by a first movement, has already lost something and has already acquired something new. But it is just as true that, psychologically speaking, nothing passes, that everything leaves a trace and has its own influence in the present and in the future.

With this law in mind, any teacher can see how great and significant is the meaning of even the slightest deed once it has become habitual. A careless gesture, a spontaneous movement, or an innocent prank, even if performed just once, already leaves a trace in the nervous system, and this trace may very well prove to be imperceptible to us, but will be perceptible to our organism.

William James discusses five rules for the education of habit given by the psychologist Alexander Bain in his discussion of moral habits:

1. Accumulate all the possible circumstances which shall reinforce the right motives; put yourself assiduously in conditions that encourage the new way.

2. Never suffer an exception to occur till the new habit is securely rooted in your life. Each lapse is like the letting fall of a ball of string which one is carefully winding up; a single slip undoes more than a great many turns will wind again. Continuity of training is the great means of making the nervous system act infallibly right.

3. Seize the very first possible opportunity to act on every resolution you make, and on every emotional prompting you may experience in the direction of the habits you aspire to gain. It is not in the moment of their forming, but in the moment of their producing motor effects, that resolves and aspirations communicate the new 'set' to the brain ... A tendency to act only becomes effectively ingrained in us in proportion to the uninterrupted frequency with which the actions actually occur, and the brain 'grows' to their use. When a resolve or a fine glow of feeling is allowed to evaporate without bearing practical fruit, it is worse than a chance lost; it works so as positively to hinder future resolutions and emotions from taking the normal path of discharge. There is no more contemptible type of human character than that of the nerveless sentimentalist and dreamer, who spends his life in a weltering sea of sensibility, but never does a concrete manly deed.

4. Don't preach too much to your pupils or abound in good talk in the abstract.

5. Offer something like this: Keep the faculty of effort alive in you by a little gratuitous exercise every day. That is, be systematically heroic in little unnecessary points, do every day or two something for no other reason than its difficulty, so that, when the hour of dire need draws nigh, it may find you not unnerved and untrained to stand the test.[4]

Even purely physiological investigations demonstrate how enormous is the value of repetition of actions and of the fatigue associated with repetition for the ordinary course of our behavior. Repetition turns out to be associated with the effect of virtually the most important of all our nerve mechanisms—the struggle for the total motor field. Sherrington enumerates four factors that determine the outcome of this struggle. In addition to the relative force of competing stimuli and the affective coloring of the reflexes, he refers to fatigue, which he views as possessing a dual effect.

First, fatigue leads to an attenuation of the reflex that dominates our ultimate total field; "over the course of time, the reflex, all on its own, loses the ability to preserve its relation with this field." What is most remarkable in this case is that, in and of itself, the ultimate total field almost never suffers from fatigue. Obviously, fatigue is not localized in a working organ, but constitutes an "appropriate adaptation," an exceptional prolonged dominance of one particular reflex that has been developed by the nervous system. "The organism, to be successful in a million-sided environment, must in its reactions be many-sided. Were it not for such so-called 'fatigue', an organism might, in regard to its receptivity, develop an eye, or an ear, or a mouth, or a hand or leg, but it would hardly develop the marvellous congeries of all those various sense-organs which it is actually found to possess".[5]

Second, the effect of fatigue is to facilitate the appearance of some reflex, one that is the antagonist of one that has been operating for a prolonged period of time, and even to amplify it. This phenomenon Sherrington refers to as "spinal induction," by analogy with similar phenomena in the organ of vision, which Hering had termed "visual induction."

Thus, we see that together with the biological utility of habitual actions, which we may understand as appropriate, stereotypical reactions to uniform, stable, and more or less constant stimulations that reach us from the direction of the environment, the nervous system has available one more mechanism which is no less important, biologically speaking, but one which is its diametric opposite in terms of both meaning and sense, that of the mechanism of fatigue, whose function it is to break down habits, to shut down the nerve pathways of habit, and to facilitate the appearance of new reactions.

The necessity of both mechanisms is entirely self-evident. If there were no habits, this would entail an enormously uneconomical mode of behavior. Recall that every act of thinking, i.e., every nonhabitual act of behavior, every adaptation to new conditions, every invention of new reactions, arises inevitably out of *difficulty* and is anticipated by a more or less lengthy *delay*, i.e., a cessation of all movement. An animal that possessed no habits and that made no use of this form of behavior would meet with *difficulties* in absolutely everything and would react to absolutely everything only after some *delay*.

Were there no fatigue, on the other hand, there would be no struggle for the total motor field and no transitions in this field from one receptor to the next. All the functional diversity of the animal's adaptations to the environment would vanish and be replaced by a uniform, automatic reaction.

The dialectical contradiction and the relationship between the two mechanisms is fully in accord with the general law of development of living matter.

Pedagogical Value of Exercise

Conscious behavior is distinguished by a special feature, that before carrying out any deed whatsoever, we always exhibit a disinhibiting, latent reaction which anticipates beforehand the result of our deed and serves as a stimulus with respect to a subsequent reflex. In other words, every deliberate deed is preceded by some definite thought.

Münsterberg says in this regard that, "I think of taking of the book before I move my arm toward it; and again it is fundamental that the foregoing idea of the end corresponds to the final effect. Yet it seems as if the most essential part is left out after all. Is there not a middle process, a feeling of impulse, an act of decision, between my thinking of the book and my getting up and fetching it? Is not the whole mystery of the will enclosed and hidden just here? But an exact psychology has nothing to do with mysteries. A careful analysis can disentangle this last impulse experience, too. Yes, it is easy to demonstrate that in reality this is nothing but the foregoing idea of the first movement to be performed in order to reach that final end. "If I think of taking down the book, the final stage depends upon the first step, the getting up from my chair ... The entering into the first movement decides whether the whole action is to be carried out. Accordingly, I must have in consciousness the idea of the first motion as the real cue for the whole process. This idea of the first movement preceding the movement itself is the whole content of that which we usually call the feeling of impulse...

"The impulse feeling is such a foregoing idea of the effect with reference to the first bodily movement to be performed ... In other words, the whole conscious experience of volition, including the feeling of decision and impulse, is made up of the balancing of rival ideas of ends. One of these ideas secures predominance, associates itself with the idea of the first movement to be carried out, and this mental state discharges itself into the movement. We have the feeling that it was our own will which brought it about, because that final end reached corresponds to the preceding idea of the end".[6]

Thus, all the achievements of our behavior depend on a clear idea of the goal, i.e., on how firmly and decisively the latent reaction which precedes some goal dominates our consciousness. "There is no special will faculty to be trained, no special mental power which arranges the transition between the idea of the end and its realization ... What the child must slowly learn through his development is the power to hold the end of the action steadily before his mind ... Here is practically the center of the educational influence: to do what we really will means to do our duty, and no aim of education stands higher than that of securing this power to hold before the mind that which we will with our deepest volition." [7]

The pedagogical value of exercise becomes perfectly understandable from this analysis, Münsterberg is right when he says that all the child's other functions evolve simply over the course of time, whereas the child's attention develops only as a result of methodical and careful exercise. Let us see why exercise plays such a role in the act of attention. Recall that attention involves adaptive, orienting reactions on the part of our organism. What is referred to as spontaneous attention arises thanks to an internal mental reaction. Consequently, it will appear the more frequently, the greater the number of internal stimuli with which it is associated. In other words, in order to appear, it has need for a great store of internal stimuli. To exercise attention is to induce it to function each time by means of such an internal reaction. It goes without saying that the more often we do something, and the more often we induce these instances, the more reinforced the relationship between the internal stimulus and the reactions of attention. This is why Münsterberg says that there is absolutely no way of influencing this behavior other than by strict regulation of external action, through the suppression of meaningless movements and the reinforcement of appropriate movement.

Thus, conscious behavior presupposes attention, and attention is established through exercise, i.e., through the repetition of certain movements that are reinforced by means of the method of conditional reflexes accompanied by a representation of these movements.

But this is only one side of the question. There is also the problem of habit to consider. In fact, what new item is it which habit introduces into our conscious behavior? It lengthens the foresight of our behavior, so to speak, it permits our thoughts to work with ever greater groups of interdependent movements without any effort on our part.

We only have to compare some habitual action with an unhabitual action in order to see how enormous is the economy of effort that is achieved through automatism. Just think how easy it is to count from 1 to 100, and how difficult is the process of counting if we do it in reverse order, from 100 to 1. Or think of how easy it is to read in the ordinary order, from left to right, compared to how hard is the same process when we begin to read from the end of words to their beginning, even though we are putting together the very letters. Then there is the economy we achieve when we read a sentence in the ordinary order by comparison with what happens when we read it in reverse order, which we must ascribe wholly to the economy of exercise.

Experimental investigations have shown that when we read, our eyes undergo intermittent movements, that we perceive in spurts, rather than reading with our eyes moving uniformly. By filming the movement of the eyelids, or through the use of micro-levers attached to them, we are able to clearly observe this jerky path of our eyes. Hence, we read by means of a stationary eye, rather than by means of a moving eye. In other words, we are always perceiving whole groups of letters. Once we have noticed the first letters, we guess the whole word. In contrast, when we read a word in reverse order, we have to deliberately count letter by letter. This is all the work of habit, which manifests itself in the fact that it automatically connects together a series of reactions and thereby relieves our consciousness of the need to look after these reactions. The greater the number of reactions that our habits extend over, the more distant the goal that our consciousness may set itself and focus upon. For example, if I habitually associate all those actions by means of which I get up from bed and get dressed, my conscious decision may involve just the thought, "I have to get up." If this thought is associated with the first movement, the entire process is performed without any trouble, and while getting dressed I can think about anything I feel like. But if the habit also includes having breakfast, and taking a morning walk, and going to work, then my initial conscious orientation may be expressed all at once in the thought: "I have to go to work." And, thus, the basic orientation may encompass a lengthier series of actions.

The economy of habit manifests itself in the fact that we do not possess an awareness of precisely how our movements are to be performed. "I do not know which muscles I need to take down my book from the shelf; I think of taking down the book and I perceive the movement of taking it. How one has brought about the other is no concern of my conscious volition. My will relies upon the correct play of this mechanism. But the same is true for the movements of our ideas. I may will to translate a word into another language or to solve a mathematical problem or to think about a plan; and in every case the whole array ... goes on in accordance with the end. We are not aware how an idea of the end is securing this smooth performance".[8]

The education of habit provides our will with increasingly more powerful mechanisms and permits it to pose for itself ever more distant goals. Habits relieve the will and, thus, allow it to turn to higher goals. "If the process of reading and writing never become habitual with us, it would absorb all of our volitional energy,"[9] leaving nothing left over for concentrating on meaning, which we have to bring to bear every time in these processes. The broader the range of activity embraced by habit, the lower the level of volitional energy we have to bring to bear to achieve our desired goals.

The only danger is that habit always denotes a mechanical mode of behavior, and therefore may be useful only where there are uniform conditions. Habitual behavior may prove to be harmful whenever a new and anticipatory adaptation is needed. "Hence habits enrich us and make us free to give our efforts to higher aims, but habits also enslave us and resist our efforts. Education must be most careful to consider both aspects of habit formation"[10]

The dual nature of habit becomes quite clear if we recall the indisputable relation that exists between processes of exercise and processes of memory. Memory functions purely reflexively, and automatically. "Nothing is recalled without cue," says James. A cue, this entity that serves to initiate a memory reflex, may possess a dual nature. If it is one of the more or less constant and stereotypically functioning stimuli and requires just as patterned and template-like a response, the habitual action will be a commendable and routine response to the cue which corresponds to the conditions of the reaction. But if the cue relates to novel, unanticipated, and unforeseen circumstances, if, moreover, it includes a kind of obstacle against the routine course of stereotypical reactions, the habitual action will be the worst response to it and will only serve as an obstacle against thinking.

There is one more psychological rule that is extraordinarily important for a proper understanding of exercise. Exercise turns out to be successful only when it is accompanied by internal satisfaction. Otherwise, it turns into tiresome repetition the organism will rail against. A successful effort is the most essential condition for progress. Every complete satisfaction with the result evidently brings about a new setting and settling in the nerve adjustment. This is full of pedagogical significance. It suggests that the mere repetition alone does not secure progress, inasmuch as only the successful practice helps toward the desired setting of the central nervous system. If the same movement is simply repeated and repeated, fatigue will bring unsuccessful results, which directly interfere with the forming of the new paths of least resistance".[11]

The Study of Fatigue

Fatigue, says Gaupp, is the antagonist of exercise. The point is that the process of exercise may require the concerted activity of several of our organs simultaneously. For example, when we write or walk, the movements of our hands or of our feet are regulated and determined by the work of our eyes, and everyone knows how difficult it is to write or walk with one's eyes closed. Thus, all of our activity induces work not only in just this or that organ, but in several organs together, and, in every act of attention, is accompanied by an intentional delay and inhibition of all other reactions. This is also because of the fact that, in addition to purely muscular fatigue, which develops in a working organ, for example, in the writing hand, there is also the phenomenon of general nervous fatigue, which may spill over and make our body incapable of further activity.

There are three basic concepts that have to be distinguished at this point: exhaustion [*ustalost'*], fatigue [*utomlenie*], and overwork [*pereutomlenie*]. We will understand exhaustion to refer to the nervous state that may arise in us whenever there is no other physiological basis for the onset of fatigue. Exhaustion may also occur after a good night's sleep, or following hypnosis, or as a consequence of a loss of interest or boredom in those processes we happen to be involved in. Under ordinary conditions, exhaustion signals to us the onset of fatigue. Fatigue is a purely physiological factor, and certain researchers believe it is associated with the introduction of special intoxicants into the nervous system.

For some time, it was even believed that there exists a special "fatigue drug" that intoxicates our tissues when we are engaged in intense and prolonged work. The existence of such a drug could in no way be proved, however, and the physiological nature of fatigue has yet to be fully disclosed. In any case, the rather simple and generally well-known fact that every nervous action is performed through the effect of certain physical substances that are found in us in our nervous system, and that, consequently, the depletion of these substances will, sooner or later, have to put an end to the work occurring in our body, cannot be denied.

Then the nervous system, in its need to replenish spent nourishment, falls into a kind of torpor, which, in its diffuse forms, may assume the nature of sleep. In his investigation of these phenomena, Pavlov came to the conclusion that sleep constitutes of broadly diffuse processes of internal inhibition in the large cerebral hemispheres. Thus, fatigue is an entirely healthy and essential condition that regulates our behavior in the sense of inducing us to cease effort whenever it has become harmful to the organism. In this sense, too, the ordinary onset of fatigue amounts to a mandatory law of absolutely all types of work. The educator not only must not be apprehensive of fatigue, rather he need be concerned only with those instances when an extraordinary degree of fatigue sets in without any exhaustion. This may happen whenever we exert our will by suppressing our exhaustion and overcoming it, for example, when we have to do some complex and difficult task, or, when, because of great straining, we experience such excitement that we can't get to sleep.

Thus, it is self-evident that exhaustion is a subjective reaction, whereas fatigue is an objective state of our organism. Fatigue does not manifest itself all at once, but gradually and may become paralyzed by the slightest interruption in a task or by a change in the form of work. Hence, it is extraordinarily important for the educator to determine how long a child may work without stopping or becoming fatigued.

In very small children, the sense of fatigue is much greater than in older children, and for this reason we cannot but recognize how great a pedagogical error we are committing when we allow lessons for younger children to last the same length of time as those for older children, despite the fact that the onset of fatigue occurs at far from the same point in eight-year old children as in 16-year olds.

Hence the need for intermission, i.e., frequent interruptions in work, and the need to change from one type of work to another, in order that the uniformity of work not lead to fatigue too early.

In and of itself, fatigue is the worst condition in work. It is like a protest of the organism against work, it disturbs the organism, slows it down, reduces its accuracy, and diminishes the performance and results of exercise.

A special pedagogical restorative mode of work represents, therefore, a most important need, where the child's tasks would be distributed in such a way as to lead him to become fatigued in a healthy way, but would not so overload him with work when he is already fatigued. In this sense, fatigue, in and of itself, is a desirable factor, since it creates powerful stimuli for tranquility, rest, and sleep, and, thus, promotes the restoration of consumed forces in the most energetic way possible. In this sense, work that brings the child to the very threshold of fatigue, rather than leaving him several steps short of it, is far more useful.

On the other hand, overwork denotes an abnormal consumption of forces in which it is no longer possible to completely restore these forces. Then there always arises a certain deficit, an irreplaceable consumption of energy that threatens to bring with it unhealthy consequences for the organism. Labor which induces overwork creates the most profound contradictions for the entire organism.

---

[1] William James: *Talks to Teachers*, page 48.

[2] *Ibid.*, page 48, quoted from *Principles of Psychology*.

[3] *Ibid.*, pages 53-54.

[4] *Ibid.*, pages 49-50, 52-53.

[5] Hering: *Integrative Action of the Nervous System*, pages 223-4.

[6] Münsterberg: *Psychology and the Teacher*, pages 184-5.

[7] *Ibid.*, pages 187-8, 188-9.

[8] *Ibid.*, page 187.

[9] *Ibid.*, page 194.

[10] *Ibid.*, page 194.

[11] *Ibid.*, page 193.

Chapter 15

ABNORMAL BEHAVIOR

The Concept of Abnormal Behavior

The concept of the average is among the most difficult and indefinite of all scientific ideas. In the real world, there is no average at all, since an infinite set of different variations and deviations from the average are encountered, and it is often very difficult to tell where one deviation has crossed the boundaries beyond which the domain of the abnormal begins. There are no such boundaries anywhere, and in this sense the average constitutes a purely abstract concept having to do with a certain mean value, the concept of the most frequent instances of a phenomenon and, in fact, is not encountered in pure form, but always with a certain admixture of abnormal forms. Therefore, there are no exact boundaries between normal and abnormal behavior.

However, these deviations sometimes attain such quantitatively impressive dimensions as to fully justify our speaking of abnormal behavior. Such forms of abnormal behavior may also be encountered in ordinary people, constituting temporary and transitional forms of behavior; but they also may be encountered in the form of more prolonged and even permanent patterns of behavior. From this point of view, the different patterns of abnormal behavior may be divided into the following groups: (1) short-term and random patterns (slips of the tongue or of the pen, forgetfulness, delirious ravings, intoxication, etc.); (2) lengthy and persistent states (neuroses, psychoses, certain forms of mental illness); and, finally, (3) permanent and lifelong defects of behavior. We will first speak of these latter forms, though the reader should be forewarned that the older view, according to which abnormal forms of behavior constituted a total aberration from the healthy forms, is false. We will oppose this view everywhere below, and always try to show how narrow are the boundaries that demarcate the healthy from the abnormal, and how frequently ordinary behavior is studded with psychopathological features.

Physically Disabled Children

Physical disability may be either congenital or acquired, and may assume the most diverse forms, depending on how the disability is expressed. It may be expressed either in the absence of certain organs or limbs, for example, arms or legs, and then it manifests itself in that particular defect in behavior which distinguishes a crippled person. The whole group of reactions associated with the particular organ or limb slip out of the child's behavior. That the child's behavior is, in fact, abnormal then becomes clear from the fact that the organism confers new functions on its other organs and limbs, and organizes its behavior in a way that differs from how other people behave, in an attempt to compensate for its deficiency and to make up for absent forms of behavior. For example, if one has lost one's legs, one's hands are given the responsibility of helping out when it is a matter of moving one's body about in space.

A second consequence of this disability will always involve the consciousness of one's own deficiency, which isolates the child from the entire social unit and places him in a less advantageous position than all the other children. Hence the teacher must be concerned with ensuring as healthy a resolution of the different consequences of the particular disability as is possible. If the child's life is properly organized, there is no way a physical disability can make the child feel utterly inadequate, nor does a physical disability have to turn someone into a public charge as an invalid, in view of the modern differentiation of social functions.

The whole point is simply that educational techniques have to be individualized in these cases, depending upon each special case, and as for methods of compensation, on the one hand, and methods of adaptation, on the other, the question can be solved without any trouble. As for the crippled person himself, with the proper education it is possible to preserve the sum total of his value to society, to the extent, that is, that the influence of his disability can be reduced almost to nil.

It is not so long ago that crippled people were banished from society because of their deformity, and their social functions confined exclusively to a parasitic existence which depended on the pity of others.

The miracle of public education is that it teaches the crippled person how to work, the mute person how to speak, and the blind person how to read. But this miracle should be understood as simply a perfectly natural process of educational compensation of these disabilities, as will be shown below.

Abnormal behavior assumes far more intractable forms when it is associated with impairments in the organs of sense, the analyzers. Children who are congenitally blind or who are congenital deaf mutes represent more complex pedagogical problems than all the other forms of disability. In this case, it is not any one of the child's functioning organs which is impaired, but rather the perceiving organs through which the enormously important relations with the environment are established.

Here everything depends on how important is the corresponding analyzer within the context of the overall system of behavior. Where such functions as the sense of smell or the sense of taste degenerate, the consequences for the overall structure of our behavior may not be very great, and, under the contemporary conditions of our existence, the result may represent a barely perceptible and, perhaps, even an entirely insignificant disability. In the modern world, there are extraordinarily rare instances when the sense of smell has to be employed, and its biological function is becoming increasingly negligible.

It would appear, however, that the isolated functions of the sense of smell and of taste virtually never degenerate, and instances where the sense of touch or of motor sensibility degenerate are just as rarely encountered. On the other hand, congenital forms of blindness and of deaf muteness are encountered extremely often. It is easiest to show what constitutes the principle of the education of disabled children using these forms of disability as illustration.

Let us first consider the blind child. A disability of blindness, in which all the other forms of behavior remain unimpaired, denotes the disabling of the most important of all the analyzers, that which enables us to establish the subtlest and most complex of all relations with our surroundings. Accordingly, the blind child proves incapable of undertaking all those forms of movement in which the sighted person excels. Hence, the pitiful social role of the blind, which has been their lot in all epochs and in all societies, on the one hand, and the inner sense of oppression and their depressed state, both of which have been the constant companion of the blind for many long years, on the other.

The belief that one has to "feel sorry for beggars and cripples,"[1] that it is necessary to provide them with public subsistence and assist them in barely eking out a miserable existence, served as the principle of education, according to which virtually everything was put in the hands of charity. For the blind themselves, the thought suggested itself at every turn to look upon one's misfortune as divine punishment or as God's way of testing them, and to accept it with the greatest of humility. There was never any attempt made to go beyond being simply reconciled with one's disability, and the adaptation of education to the particular disability, rather than to its conquest, became the fundamental pedagogical rule. And instead of the conquest of disability, there were created psychological myths of the seemingly extraordinary and secret sixth sense of the blind, a sense that allows them to see in the dark, by some wise providence, and of the extraordinary development of the sense of touch among them, which seems to exceed in force and subtlety the sense of touch in ordinary people.

All of this was profoundly false. The point is that the behavior of the blind obeys precisely the same sort of rules as does the behavior of perfectly ordinary people, except for the fact that the analyzer organs they lack (i.e. those associated with the eye) are replaced by other analyzer pathways in their accumulation of experience, for the most part by tactile and motor pathways.

It is in this sense that the process of reading employed by the blind is extremely curious. Books for the blind are printed with ordinary letters, which, however, bulge out, as embossed type, as if extruded out of the paper, so that from early childhood a blind person is taught to associate the reaction of pronouncing a particular sound with the tactile sensation that originates in his touching a particular extruded letter. The whole difference from the way sighted people read is simply that, here, visual sensation is replaced by tactile sensation. But we have to always remember that, in educating a conditional reflex, it makes absolutely no difference which new stimulus we will be dealing with. The dog's salivary reflex turns into a conditional reflex and settles into a new relation whether it is stimulated by a blue light, by being stroked with a brush, or by the beating of a metronome.

Blind people are far more likely to make use of the special type created by Braille, a type that involves a special alphabet. In this alphabet, each letter is formed from different combinations of six dots, which are inscribed in paper in embossed format. If a sighted person who is not accustomed to this type tries to touch the page with his hand, he will feel a set of raised dots arranged haphazardly, and will receive a series of meaningless sensations and not even be able to say how many dots there are or what is their relative position. For the blind person, these dots are associated with the idea of sounds, sounds for the blind person are put together into words, words are connected into sentences, and thereby is a definite meaning produced.

It is not too hard to understand with this in mind that every act of reading bears a purely conditional, reflexive character, and that any system of sensations may serve as an alphabet for recording human speech. For this purpose it is only necessary to associate the new stimulation with the old sound as a conditional reflex. Hence, it is understandable that the sense of touch in the blind is in no way any better or any subtler than in sighted people, except for being associated with a far greater number of relations and except for having far greater accumulated experience than in the sighted. To see this is so, just think of how a literate person might look at a printed page of our text as compared to how an illiterate person might. A literate person has no trouble at all in orienting himself quickly and precisely to the thousands of letters there. To someone who is sighted but illiterate and who is looking at a book for the very first time, each page will seem like a haphazard agglomeration of thousands of signs in which his eyes become helplessly lost. Thus, order and meaning are introduced not by the acuteness of vision and touch, but above all by accumulated experience, above all by the already established relations of our conditional reactions, which bring together and link up the aggregate of external stimuli. In teaching the blind, the whole problem is to replace relations between one set of stimuli by relations between another set, though all the other psychological and pedagogical laws that constitute the foundation of education remain in force.

Bear in mind that the ultimate goal of every effort at settling these types of conditional relations is the acculturation of the blind person to the social environment of other people, and that this acculturation will have been achieved once we have succeeded in causing the aggregate of the blind person's conditional sensations to converge as closely as possible to generally accepted social systems of intercourse. Thus, although the Braille script is highly efficient and convenient, from the psychological point of view it is not the right approach, since its use isolates the blind person from the general mass of people. A letter written in Braille will be understandable only to someone who is blind and, thus, will not serve as a basis for broad intercourse between the blind person and the sighted population, but only for the narrow and closed world of the blind. Moreover, in absolutely all of our requirements we have to strive towards bringing the blind person's realm of experience out of the narrow constraints of his disability and to relate his experience to the social experience of mankind in as broad and intimate way as possible.

It is for this reason that we have to suggest a possible reduction in programs of special education for the blind, and insist on bringing the blind child into ordinary schools, both secondary and post-secondary, as early as possible. The isolation of blind children in private and specialized schools cannot lead to good results, in this form of education everything focuses the students' attention on their blindness, instead of guiding them in other directions. Such schools intensify the psychology of separatism that is natural to the blind and locks them up in a tight and narrow little world. There is the widespread belief that the blind are different from other people also by possessing a spiritual constitution all of their own. There is that special sensitivity of the blind, their passion for philosophizing, their gluttony, and forth. To the extent that all of this springs from reliable observation, it is not too hard to turn it into a truism. However, it would be a short-sighted view for us to conclude that blindness, understood as a congenital disability, is the real cause of all these features. There can be no doubt that they are defects not of the student, but of education itself, i.e., secondary developments in the behavior of the blind. They originate far more out of the particular social environment in which the blind person grows up and is educated, than out of the inherent structure of his personality.

It is in this sense that Korolenko's story, *The Blind Musician*, is odd. The hero of the story is always suffering from (and is always tormented by) an instinctive striving towards light and from the consciousness of his disability. Shcherbina, himself blind, is entirely correct when he points out how incorrect is such a judgement on the part of a sighted person regarding the blind, adding that blind people lack any sort of sense of living in some kind of darkness. To imagine that blindness is a state where one lives permanently in a state of darkness is to reason about the blind from the standpoint of a sighted person. There is, however, some truth in Korolenko's story, which coincides entirely with the psychological theory. The blind musician languishes in endless torment so long as he is closed up in the narrow circle of his personal and self-centered suffering. But after wandering about with blind beggars, he submerges his own personal grief in the ocean of pain of everyone's suffering and only then does he become enlightened, i.e., find himself as a man, spiritually and inwardly. What is extraordinarily curious is that the very same music now saves him, that previously could not teach him anything, other than new forms of suffering; when his mother had tried to convey in the language of sound the world of colors, this had only served to underscore and sharpen his feeling of being disabled. But once music had become for the blind man a source of broad social experience, it actually helped him overcome his disability.

Social compensation for the defect of blindness is the fundamental principle for the education of the blind. Here as nowhere else do we see the utter impotence of individualized forms of education in comparison with the healthy resolution of the problem of blindness within the context of public education.

Children who are deaf mutes represent an even more complex problem. In most cases here we are dealing basically with deafness, which is a congenital defect, while muteness represents a secondary phenomenon, as a consequence of the fact that the speech of the child who has not been nourished by any sort of verbal models from without, and is not under the child's own control, becomes fixed at the stage of the reflexive shout. From the moment he is born, the deaf child hears neither other people's speech nor his own speech, and consequently *becomes* mute, though his speech centers and his speech apparatus are not in the least impaired. Thus, in the case of deafness we are dealing with an entirely different type of defect than blindness. Though the entire external world manifests itself for us more through our eyes than through the ears, and though sounds play a comparatively negligible role in the total picture of the world, nevertheless deaf muteness represents an incomparably greater and more terrible defect than blindness.

To the blind person the world of nature is closed, though, in return, the social world is open to him, whereas for the deaf person, in contrast, the perception of the world of nature is preserved nearly entirely, though all possibility of social intercourse is excluded. Here we see quite graphically how much more essential and important are social relationships than are natural relations in the modern world. Essentially, only the need to hear human speech is associated with sounds, though this turns out to be entirely necessary for the inner development of personality. Nowhere as in the case of deaf mutes is it so clear that our consciousness has a purely social origin and evolves in the mold established by our intercourse with other people.

Mimicry develops very early in deaf mutes, so that audible stimuli are very often replaced by visual stimuli. Mute people converse by means of a manual alphabet. They converse by means of this alphabet in just the same way as we converse by means of sounds, and in both instances we find systems of conditional stimuli used to denote our reactions. Their language of mimicry, however, represents the lowest stage and narrowest form of the development of speech and of consciousness. It only allows the deaf mute to communicate with other deaf mutes and locks deaf mutes up within the narrow and restricted circle established by their disability. Moreover, this form of speech bears the traces of primitive thinking, and is therefore incapable of serving as a means of expression or of cognition of any sort of complex and subtle phenomenon. Finally, what is most important is that speech, in addition to fulfilling the functions of social intercourse, possesses yet another function, that of the construction of consciousness. We have seen that all of our mental reactions, all of our orienting acts, constitute, for all intents and purposes, inner speech. Thus, muteness also points to the absence of fully developed thinking as well.

The principle of education of deaf mutes may be stated in the form of the very same rule as for the blind, that of compensation for the disability through an expansion of social experience, and by leading the deaf mute to engage in healthy [*normal'nyi*] forms of behavior.

This may be achieved through more complex pedagogical techniques. It's not enough to simply replace the system of auditory stimuli by visual stimuli. What is needed here is to also restore the impaired mechanism of the feedback reaction. The point is that to develop a purposiveness to speech and the capacity to control speech, it is necessary that one's own reaction revert back to the individual himself, in the form of a new stimulation. What usually happens is that when we speak, we hear ourselves, and an awareness of our speech develops thereby. In the deaf mute, this mechanism of the feedback reaction is realized by means of the kinesthetic sensations that arise in speech and which supplant the act of hearing. Only when the speech mechanisms arise in the mind of the student does he learn to control his own speech and to construct it deliberately. He learns to relate it to the visual inscription of the word and to the visual impression of someone else's pronunciation. As a result, the deaf mute may be taught to speak, and to understand the speech of other people, by correlating speech with the movements of the lips in the same way we might correlate someone else's speech with a text written down on a sheet of paper.

It is only such a development of speech that can guarantee the social rebirth of the deaf mute and that can ensure his mental development. Left to himself, without the means of speech, the deaf mute is condemned to remain at a stage of extraordinary mental retardation and underdevelopment. The history of the development of deaf mutes is extraordinarily instructive both psychologically and educationally. There is the well-known case of Helen Keller, who has achieved such a stage of consciousness as to have succeeded in writing several interesting books on a number of different topics.

The machine used in communication between the blind and deaf mutes is a good indication of the state of the entire educational process. Communication is based on the use of the six dots of the Braille code, which are embossed by depressing the six corresponding buttons of the machine; by depressing the buttons, the blind person produces the desired combination of dots and forms words out of them, which the deaf person then reads. For his part, the deaf person performing the same task leads the blind person to feel the raised dots and thereby to grasp his meaning. Here we see how easy it is for education to triumph over physical disability and create an opportunity for social intercourse, and, consequently, for individual development, through the formation of new conditional relations.

Mental Disability and Psychopathology

The education of children with mental disability represents a more complicated problem. There are three groups of children involved.

In the first group are children with different forms of congenital imbecility differing in terms of severity, beginning with idiocy and ending with mildly severe retardation. These manifestations tend to be associated for the most part with certain organic defects in the nervous system or with congenital endocrine illnesses and the associated disabilities are expressed in attenuated forms of accumulation of individual experience. Children in this group usually turn out to be slow in acquiring new conditional reflexes and, consequently, are limited from the very start in their capacity to develop a sufficiently rich, diverse, and complex pattern of behavior.

The natural goal for education in the case of children in this group, therefore, is the formation of the most essential of all those vital reactions that could assist these children in attaining a minimal adaptation to the environment, make them useful members of society, and make their lives meaningful and focused on work. The teaching methods to follow with these children are generally the same as those used with normal children with only the pace of instruction slowed down somewhat and instruction itself somewhat less intense. From the psychological standpoint, it is extraordinarily important not to isolate them in special closed groups, but to give them as much opportunity as possible to practice interaction with other children. For pedagogics, practical considerations regarding the feasibility of education in this area sometimes are in contradiction with the psychological requirements, for example, when the principle of the auxiliary school was put forward. Some educators believe that it is not always useful to isolate retarded children in special schools, though, from the standpoint of carrying out the educational program, it is desirable to relieve the public schools from the burden of having to teach retarded children.

In severe instances of retardation, however, there can no longer be any doubt of the need to entrust the educational process to schools that are specially adapted for this purpose. The full range of pedagogical features of such schools may be encompassed by a single general psychological rule. That is, such schools must constitute a *facilitative* social environment, i.e., one that will not overwhelm the child's weak mind with a multitude and heterogeneity of relationships, but will instead give him the opportunity to acquire essential conditional relations slowly and patiently.

Children who are nervous, who are epileptic, who suffer from hysteria, and so on represent pathological deviations in their patterns of behavior and are more in need of therapy than education. Nevertheless, it is here that Zalkind's idea assumes special force, that, essentially, there can be no sharp boundary between education and therapy, between pedagogy and psychotherapy. The two are simply different forms of "social hygiene" [*sotsiagogika*], i.e., methodical and planned social construction. And in fact, by observing children who are mentally ill, we see, ultimately, that the way to properly educate them lies through an organization of the environment that would make it possible for them to acquire desired relations by means of education. The pedagogical requirements that may be imposed on this type of education once again reduce to adapting the environment to the particular nervous disease the students are suffering from. If these children cannot stand harsh and noisy stimuli, their lives should be so arranged as to ensure the child's organism peace and quiet. No one could be such an optimist as to think that every kind of abnormal behavior might be ultimately redirected and made to flow in healthy channels through the techniques of this form of education. We are only saying that we still don't know one-hundredth of all the possibilities which public education can provide, and if one cannot speak of completely overcoming every disability, there is nevertheless every reason for declaring that, without such education, no other form of education is capable of imparting socially useful patterns to this type of abnormal behavior.

There remains for us to discuss the last group of the various patterns of abnormal behavior, that of psychoneurosis in children. By infantile psychoneu- rotic forms of behavior, we usually understand a transient and temporary illness. It has been suggested that psychosis should be distinguished from neurosis by the following sign. Psychosis arises out of a conflict between the environment and personality, out of the fact that an inner drive of the personality comes into collision with the conditions of the environment. Neurosis, on the other hand, springs from a conflict within the ego itself, when certain inner drives are in contradiction with the fundamental moral level of personality. In any case, in both there is mental illness arising out of an inner conflict and attesting to the fact that there is a certain unhappiness in the interaction of the individual with the environment. It goes without saying that displacement of the conflict entails the elimination of the causes that have generated it and, in this case, therapy of a child suffering from psychoneurosis reduces to re-education.

Such re-education may be achieved through new inter-relations which are established between the environment and the child which make it possible to gradually overcome conflict painlessly. This becomes especially self-evident if we consider as an example the nature and character of infantile psychopathology during wartime. War, always an enormous social upheaval, induced in our society vast shifts and vast breakdowns and, naturally, created a whole series of nervous conflicts. Out of this soil there grew what came to be called the "flight into neurosis," i.e., the attempt on the part of personality to overcome its own conflict, its own deviation from the environment, expressed in different kinds of delirium, imagination, and abnormal behavior. Social hygiene and therapy, i.e., imposition of a compulsion to overcome conflict in socially acceptable and useful forms of behavior, is the only correct way out of these forms of psychopathology.

Re-education of psychoneurosis is, in general, fully in accord with all the other laws of public education of the conditional reflexes. It is not only a matter of supplying a certain outlet for inhibited and bottled up energy. Present-day psychology is, therefore, inclined to look upon infantile psychopathology as a social phenomenon, and to see it as a matter of antisocial manifestations in children. This is how Zalkind puts it: "Just as 'circulars [patients with manic depression, as in Ernst Kretschmer's typology—trans.] lost their cycles under the influence of external conditions, so did the schizophrenics not only not continue to experience a breakdown, but even made up for their own past losses, so that one must reject the idea that one is fated to be psychopathological on the basis of a diagnosis of psychopathology except, possibly in really severe cases. And even in severe cases, explicit and particularly clear-cut forms of psychopathology would be subject to an entirely different rate, an entirely different depth of development under other social and pedagogical conditions, as we may more often than not verify." Thus are the different forms of infantile psychopathology dissolved in public education without leaving anything over.

Psychopathology of Everyday Life

But abnormal behavior manifests itself not only as congenital disability or transient illness. It also takes root and seeps into our everyday lives and is encountered at every turn, and in every person. For a long time, these phenomena escaped the notice of science, inasmuch as science and popular wisdom took them to be accidents and did not attach any value to them, since it did not seem they played any sort of major role in a person's life.

Sigmund Freud has referred to these phenomena as the "psychopathology of everyday life," and has subsumed under this term different forms of our behavior, such as accidental forgetfulness, when we forget the last name of someone we know well or the name of some location on a map with which we are well acquainted with; next are instances of accidents, or when we cause damage to certain objects; there are cases when we forget our own intentions and symptomatic actions where we, while engaged in conversation, play with some object, tear a piece of paper into small pieces; there are slips of the tongue, slips of the pen, misreadings [ochitki], and so on. If a careful approach is undertaken, these instances are all revealed upon investigation to be strictly deterministic processes. The very concept of chance has to be banished from scientific investigation, since we have to suppose from the very start that there are no random actions that are without cause, that the most accidental and slightest forms of our behavior are essentially determined by and conditioned upon profound causal relations.

For example, if we were to ask someone to give the first number that comes to mind, and he says, for example, 3448, it can be shown by means of psychoanalysis almost always why just this number was given, and not some other number, and what are the reasons for this choice. It may be shown just as precisely what are the causes responsible for all of our little mistakes, our forgetfulness, slips of the tongue, and so forth. It turns out that these forms of behavior are always based on certain subconscious desires or drives that burst forth in these instances. Such, for example, is the meaning of slips of the tongue, which give away a speaker's concealed thought or unconscious intention, very often without the speaker himself expecting it.

What is clear is that, in such cases, we are dealing with rudimentary forms of psychoneurosis, since every slip of the tongue and every forgotten name constitutes just as much a consequence of conflict as does every major neurosis, except for the fact that here conflict is induced by an insignificant collision of two insignificant thoughts. The study of these forms of behavior is of profound importance, however, not just to explain the general foundations of mental causality, but also to gain an understanding of the actual mechanism which directs neurosis in its simplest form. In his everyday activity, the educator should not have to be overly concerned with these phenomena, though he must know what he is dealing with, and has to always understand that in every slip of the tongue, he may discern the subconscious showing through as if through a crack.

Hypnosis

Hypnosis is one of those forms of behavior which are not of much practical interest to the educator, but which are extremely important in the study of the fundamental forms of behavior. By the term, "hypnosis," we understand a state close to sleep which is induced artificially in some person, differing from sleep only by the extraordinarily vivid manifestation of suggestibility which nearly always accompanies it. A special relation is established between the hypnotist and his subject, called *rapport*, which places the subject in a kind of subordinate position relative to the hypnotist. By his own devices, the hypnotist can usually induce hallucinations, and negative hallucinations, in his subject, and to suggest he carry out this or that action or deed.

The nature of hypnosis has yet to receive sufficient study, despite a wealth of observations that have been made in this area. In most general outline, however, it may now be assumed that hypnosis denotes nothing other than a broadly diffuse inner inhibition in the cerebral hemispheres which the hypnotist disinhibits through his words, first in one direction, and then in another, and first in one area, and then in another. It is therefore not remarkable that hypnosis is induced either by any sort of sharp and powerful overwhelming sensation, or by a peaceful and quiet, prolonged and monotonous sensation applied to some perceiving organ.

Post-hypnotic suggestion represents the most curious form of hypnotic behavior. While he is asleep, the subject is given the suggestion that when he awakens, he will perform some deed, but only after some appreciable length of time has elapsed. The hypnotist might suggest to him, for example, that in three months he is to write a letter dealing with this or that topic or go somewhere, or, on the other hand, when he leaves home, he will perform some harmless, though odd deed, or, in response to some sign, or upon hearing someone utter the word, "water," or call out some number, will move in a certain way. The subject is then told he has to forget what it is that was "suggested" to him. And in fact, upon awakening, and during the intervening time period, the subject will have no memory of what he has been told to do. Once the time period has elapsed, or once the stipulated sign has been made, however, the suggested action is quickly carried out to the letter.

What is most curious is that the subject usually feels it's as if he's being drawn into performing the particular deed, and will think up pretexts which he uses to try and justify the strangeness of his deed. Thus we see that the conditional reflexive relation which we may cause to settle in in a hypnotized subject may be entirely unconscious and that it may not be correct to ascribe it to him. A person may not even suspect the existence of the relation, which nevertheless may have an effect on him with unerring precision.

Quite often, hypnosis resembles education, and some educators, for example, Guyau, are inclined to declare that education, in general, constitutes only a series of coordinated hypnotic suggestions. Hence, all forms of suggestion are made out to be hypnotic, and then it is proposed that genuine hypnosis be used in certain instances with children who are hard to teach.

It has to be admitted that, in fact, hypnotic suggestion plays an extraordinarily significant role in education, though it differs from ordinary educational techniques by the fact that it often creates artificial and alien relations in the student's nervous system instead of allowing these relations to arise in a natural way in the course of experience.

The theoretical value of hypnotic experiments is that they disclosed for the very first time and with perfect clarity the *realness of the unconscious*; they demonstrated that we can carry out certain deeds without knowing anything at all of the true cause of these deeds—i.e., suggestions concealed in the unconscious—and instead possess an awareness of a false, surrogate motive.

And in general, abnormal behavior harbors a host of possibilities for the investigator. "The nursery," writes Karl Buhler, "lunatic asylums, and schools for the mentally deficient, are places where one can learn most about the structure of the human mind and the general lines of its development".[2]

---

[1] The Russian word for "beggars" or "cripples" which Vygotsky uses here, *ubogii*, literally means "those who are of (or belong to) God" (trans.).

[2] Bühler: *The Mental Development of the Child*, p. 33.

Chapter 16

TEMPERAMENT AND CHARACTER

The Importance of Terms

From the earliest development of psychology, aside from special topics in human behavior, the subjects of temperament and character have been proposed as disciplines whose study encompasses all of human behavior as a whole. Throughout this entire period of time, the content of these terms has changed repeatedly, and even now when we use them we can never be certain of being understood properly, simply because certain investigators have invested in these terms the most diverse content and have used them with different meanings. In all these instances, different understandings are being combined together, nothing more, and the use of the same words to denote different concepts is being justified; this general rule expresses the idea that every individual human organism has a special character and mode of behavior as a whole inherent to him alone, and, despite their particular differences, these distinctive features of behavior may nevertheless be reduced to certain special types.

In other words, it is believed that the full diversity of these distinctive features may be reduced to certain fundamental classes of typical cases. If this were in fact so, it would mean that all individual manifestations are subordinated to a special law and could be encompassed by certain general laws.

This question is of extraordinary importance for the educator, inasmuch as he actually has to always deal, not with the child's individual reactions, but with the child's behavior as a whole. And to what should we ascribe the evolution of the overall composition of the child's personality—whether his inherited features or aspects of his personality that have evolved or were acquired in the course of education, in other words, whether temperament and character are the givens of education or are its results—is a question which has given rise to the most discordant ideas imaginable and it is these ideas which have come to dominate the field of pedagogics.

In our subsequent presentation, both these terms will be used with the meaning which is most commonly employed in modern psychology. Thus, by "temperament," we will understand the distinctive features of the aggregate of innate and inherited reactions, the inherited constitution of the organism. Thus, temperament is a concept which is, for the most part, physiological and biological in nature, encompassing that sphere of personality which manifests itself in instinctive, emotional, reflexive reactions. Throughout that realm of our behavior which is usually acknowledged to be involuntary and inherited, it is temperament which is the dominant concept.

By "character," on the other hand, we will understand that special aggregation of personality which develops under the influence of acquired reactions, in other words, character will denote the very same thing as regards the individual superstructure that is built up on top of innate behavior which temperament denotes as regards the unconditional forms.

Thus is the discussion divided up so that temperament becomes a given precondition of the educational process, and character the ultimate result of the educational process. Of course, this usage is somewhat arbitrary, though it is entirely legitimate, since, on the one hand, it does not involve a sharp break with psychological tradition, which has always ascribed character to the sphere of the will, and temperament to the sphere of the feelings, and on the other, since it distinguishes two radical layers in human behavior, that which is innate from that which is acquired. In other words, linguistic usage is legitimate, since it accords with everyday reality.

Temperament

Even ancient teachings of temperament conflated it with the structure of the body and established which tissues or fluids in the organism seemed to constitute the bearers of temperament. Thus, the dominance of one temperament was ascribed to the dominance of bile in the organism, and the dominance of another temperament to the dominance of the blood, and so on.

Subsequently, other observations of the same order have been made; for example, Lesgaft pointed to the decisive importance which the width of the passageways and thickness of the walls of the blood vessels in different people holds for temperament. Other writers have conflated the concept of temperament with various internal tissues in the organism, though despite all the differences between these views, they are unified by a common belief that the sources for distinctive features of temperament must be sought in certain features of bodily structure.

There are investigators who have abandoned these teachings and have thoroughly forgotten them, and in their place have advanced a theory which ascribes a purely mental essence to temperament. By means of this theory they have attempted to attribute differences in temperament to different relationships between mental forces in the organism, for example, between the higher and lower passions, between ideal and sensual desires, or between abstract and concrete ideas. It must not be forgotten that, whereas the former attempts at explaining temperament did not bear any fruit simply because these attempts could never confirm in graphic fashion the relationship which they suggested, nor could they defend this relationship, the latter attempts proved illusory by their very nature, since they took the unknown to be the solution, and made of the problem an answer.

The point is that explaining temperament in terms of different combinations of mental properties means an explanation *idem per idem* [i.e., on the basis of synonymity—trans.], since the whole problem of temperament is only a matter of explaining the existence and dominance of certain passions and ideas in one person's psyche, and of other passions and ideas in someone else's psyche. Thus, a vicious circle is the inevitable defect of virtually all psychological theories of temperament. It was because of this fact that the subject of temperament ended up as a back-water of scientific psychology, and became the subject of semi-fictionalized and semi-anthropological description and (or) lacked any status at all in serious psychological systems, or was interpreted incidentally and without sufficient depth.

Structure of the Body and Character

> In the mind of the man-in-the-street, the devil is usually lean and has a thin beard growing on a narrow chin, while the fat devil has a strain of good-natured stupidity. The intriguer has a hunch-back and a slight cough. The old witch shows us a withered hawk-like face. Where there is brightness and jollity we see the fat knight Falstaff—red-nosed and with shining pate. The peasant woman with a sound knowledge of human nature is undersized, tubby, and stands with her arms akimbo. Saints look abnormally lanky, long-limbed, of penetrating vision, pale, and godly.

Thus begins Kretschmer's *Physique and Character*. As is clear from these lines, as regards temperament and character, Kretschmer returns to the ancient teachings, according to which there exists the closest imaginable dependence between character and bodily structure, and in this regard, he gives a helping hand to the popular view of the human body, which sees in it the truest signification of temperament. His theory is now only in a rudimentary state, though the material which he has discovered indicates rather convincingly that there is a grain of truth to it.

His investigations began with the mentally ill, and he succeeded in showing that the structure of the face and the skull, the outer surface of the body and its constitutional structure are in a direct and clear-cut relation with the particular form of mental illness the patient is suffering from.

Kretschmer proceeded from an assumption that there exists two basic forms of mental illness, the *cyclothymic* and the *schizophrenic*, and established a correlation between an individual's constitution and his character in these cases. Since both these forms of mental illness are accompanied by extraordinarily acute and heightened forms of character formation, as well as by explicit features of bodily structure, as in the popular case of the devil and the saints, in this case as well a dependence could be established with exceptional graphic force. The conclusions that Kretschmer reaches, however, go far beyond psychiatry. His idea is to pass beyond the boundaries of psychiatry in order to encompass within his purview absolutely all human traits, by claiming that all of them are based on the same two types, the cycloidal and the schizoidal character, which are essentially distinct and which in their extreme expression yield mental illness, though they are encountered also in everyday life in more or less dilute and attenuated form.

It is in this sense that it becomes extraordinarily important to grasp Kretschmer's fundamental classification. Three concepts underlie his study. By "constitution," he understands the aggregate of all particular properties which are due to heredity, i.e., that are genotypically fixed. By "character," he understands the aggregate of all affective and volitional capacities of human reactions in the form in which they manifest themselves throughout a person's lifetime, i.e., thus from among those traits which are passed down, or given, by heredity and all the exogenic factors, the somatic influences, the education of the mind, the environment, and experience. Thus, the concept of character encompasses the mental personality as a whole together with its affective aspect, and it is impossible to set it apart from intellect, however one tries.

Finally, for Kretschmer the expression of "temperament" is no longer an isolated concept, but becomes just provisional notation. Though he does not yet know what is its scope, nevertheless it is his belief that it must be a starting point for the principal differentiation of biological psychology. For now, he distinguishes two principal, intersecting realms of action:

1. The psychic apparatus, which is more or less what one calls the system of psychic refex-arcs, that is to say the factors which, by means of a train of happenings which probably has some phylogenetic foundation, bring about the perceptual and imaginal digestion of psychic stimulation, from the moment of sense-impression to the effective motor impulse. Their bodily correlates are the brain-centres and paths in inseparable combination with the sense organs and motor events, that is to say the sense-brain-motor apparatus.

2. The temperament. It is, as we know certainly from empirical observation, co-determinated by the chemistry of the blood, and the humours of the

body. Its physical correlate is the brain-glandular apparatus. The temperament is that group of mental events which is correlated with the physical structure, probably through the secretions. The temperament works in with the activity of the psychic apparatus, providing feeling tone, inhibiting, and pushing forward. The temperament, so far as our empirical investigations go, has a clear influence on the following psychic qualities: (A) On the psychaesthesia, abnormal sensitivity or insensitivity to psychic stimulation; (B) on the mood-colouring, the pleasure or pain colouring of the psychic content, particularly on the scale which lies between gay and sorrowful; (C) on the psychic tempo, the acceleration or retardation of the psychic processes in general ... ;(D) on the psychomotility; on the general movement-tempo (mobile or comfortable) as well as on the special character of [psychic-] activity (lame, stiff, hasty, vigorous, smooth, rounded, etc.)[1]

Kretschmer also allows for the possibility that the humeral influence of the hormones extends to the anatomic structure of the brain, and likewise to the structure of the rest of the body as well, "...so that," he writes, "the question assumes an almost dizzy complexity. We shall therefore do well to sum up under the notion of temperament such psychic elements as experience teaches us to be particularly, readily and frequently responsive to acute chemical influences of an exogenous (alcohol, morphine) as well as of an endocrine nature, that is to say effectivity and general psychic tempo.[2]

Thus, Kretschmer proceeds by ascribing paramount importance to the internally secreting [endocrine] glands for bodily structure and the evolution of temperament.

We have already remarked that together with glands which discharge their secretions externally (tears, saliva, gastric juices, perspiration, etc.), there also exist in the organism a number of glandular bodies of precisely the same structure though lacking any external outlet duct. For a long time, the function of these organs could only be conjectured about until, that is, scientists succeeded in establishing by empirical means and through experimental excision and grafting that these bodies were apparently glands which discharged their secretions directly into the blood stream. They have therefore been termed phlebotomic glands, or endocrine, incretorial, or internally secreting glands. Here the material for observation consisted, first, of pathological cases of congenital or acquired glandular deficiency, or the overdevelopment of some gland; second, experimental excision and surgical grafting of glands from one animal to another; finally, third, surgical experiments at the rejuvenation of human beings which have been carried out quite recently. These observations are all in agreement in demonstrating that the activity of these endocrine glands, which discharge into the blood stream certain still unknown stimulants, usually called "hormones" (from the Greek meaning "I excite" or "I move"), alter the chemical composition of our blood in direct fashion, and, through the medium of the blood, exert a paramount and unimaginably powerful effect on absolutely the entire organism and on all the processes which occur in it.

It must not be forgotten that further investigation revealed a third type of gland, one which seems to "function on two fronts," in the words of one Russian scientist, i.e., possessing, on the one hand, external secretion discharged directly through a special outlet duct, and on the other, internal, hormonal secretion. Among these glands, incidentally, are the sex glands of men and women.

The activity of internal secretion regulates the growth and structure of the body, the size and shape of the bones, cartilage, muscles, and tissues, the functioning of the brain and nervous system, developmental changes in the human body, and the sexual features in the body. Where there is congenital absence of the thyroid gland, cretinism and idiocy inevitable ensue, from which a complete cure may be achieved by grafting of a new gland onto the patient. Castration leads to a change in the structure of the entire body, where in men the body assumes effeminate features and in women masculine features. There then follows degeneration of the voice and of all the features of temperament, which, according to the testimony of all observers, changes beyond recognition. By grafting the sex glands of the opposite sex onto castrated animals, experimental biology has been able to achieve a kind of experimental change in sex, i.e., a total regeneration of absolutely all the secondary sexual features. Such an experimental hen in Zavadovskii's experiments lost all the features of its sex, comb and spur grew out, a cock's crow appeared, an attraction for females sometimes manifested itself, and, in general, in terms of behavior and bodily structure, it displayed an unmistakable resemblance to a male. Experimental transformations of sex in the opposite direction are also possible. Similarly, hypertrophy of a cerebral process or of the hypothalamus brings with it gigantism and the disfiguring efflorescence of individual organs. Underdevelopment of the gland leads to diminutive growth.

Finally, rejuvenation experiments have demonstrated that all those changes in our body and character which are associated with particular developmental periods in the life of man constitute essentially a direct consequence of the internal secretions of the sex glands. By regulating the activity of the sex glands through surgical intervention, by increasing its internal secretion at the expense of external secretion, we may achieve rapid and startling rejuvenating effects in the body and character as a whole.

In cruder experiments on animals and in man, direct transplantation of this gland, placed somewhere in a neutral organ, for example, behind the ear, have produced the same effects in even more striking forms. A direct and intimate relationship between the internally secreting organs and chemical secretions and the chemical composition of the blood due to these secretions, on the one hand, and between absolutely all of man's psyche and his bodily structure, on the other, may be considered to be fully established.

Until now, investigations have succeeded in establishing only this one single dependence, though the subject has entered a different phase of development, and the question has become one of establishing a correlation between bodily structure and character, since the two possess common generating causes, i.e., the functioning of the secretory apparatus.

In this sense, we return to the ancient view of the soul, as we already pointed out, and in accordance with this view we are inclined to also localize the soul in the blood stream and to claim that man's blood stream is actually of paramount importance for the psyche; it is the blood stream which is the "organ" that unifies the functioning of the brain, the nervous system, and the endocrine glands.

Four Types of Temperament

For a long time now, the description of temperament given in traditional psychology has usually encompassed four types, and this classification was itself based on even more ancient teachings of the fundamental types of human behavior. These types are described in the most varied way imaginable, though despite all the differences in their various definitions, two fundamental elements have remained unchanged, first that each of these types possesses a certain bodily expression, that temperament may be illustrated by a picture; and, second, that movement, and the rate of movement, possesses a certain character, a thesis that constitutes the basis for making an interpretation of a person's psyche on the basis of his outward behavior. Here is a brief summary of these four types, given by Kornilov with respect to children:

A detailed description of these temperaments is as follows:

> There is the child who possesses a sanguine temperament; he is
> thin, well-built, and graceful. In his movements, he is jumpy and
> too quick, even fidgety; he takes up every new activity
> impulsively, but, not having the persistence to see it through to
> the end, quickly grows cool towards it. His mind is keen and
> lively, though it lacks sufficient depth, and he is not thoughtful

enough. His feelings quickly build up, though they grab him too superficially; he is overflowing with life, loves to have fun, and seeks it out. Overall, he is a nice, charming child, without cares for of the future, and without profound regrets for the past.

A somewhat different constitution is presented by the phlegmatic child. In physical appearance he is plump, and in his movements slow, even lazy and sluggish. His mind is logical, he is thoughtful and observant, and is so filled with knowledge as to lack originality and creativity. He is not fervent in his feelings, but constant; overall, he is a good-natured, even-tempered child who doesn't give his parents or teachers much trouble.

The other two types, the 'strong' types, are the opposites of these two types (what we may call the 'weak' types). There is the choleric type, the child who is thin and well-built, but too hasty and critical, and therefore often precipitate in his movements. He is audacious, persistent, and hasty in carrying out his intentions. His acute, penetrating, and derisive mind is too categorical in reaching conclusions. In his feelings he is too passionate and hasty in displaying his likes and dislikes. He is ambitious, vindictive, and inclined to every imaginable type of conflict. Such a child is most restless and least well-balanced of all children, giving his parents much to worry about, though, for all that, where educational conditions are favorable, promising much for the future.

The child who possesses a melancholic temperament represents a different picture. Such a child is gloomy and forever serious, he is slow and dogged in expressing his will. Possessing a strong, profound, and thoughtful mind, he is inflexible and persistent to the point of obsession in his most cherished opinions. Extremely impressionable, gloomy, and reserved, he rarely expresses his own feelings. Such a child grows old before his time, there is little in him that recalls the *joie de vivre* of the child, and he inspires his parents with involuntary deference and suppressed fears for his future.

In order to move on from such overly general and abstract descriptions of temperament to more exact investigation, it is necessary to find some sort of basic feature in which temperament would be realized with exhaustive and unmistakable completeness and certainty. Thus we return to the objective study of these external manifestations of temperament.

From the foregoing discussion alone, it is perfectly clear that, ultimately, temperament is determined on the basis of the type of movement which our organs perform, put differently, in terms of the capacity or readiness to undertake movements which we divine in the features of the body. Consequently, our observations have to be based on the epiphenomenon of reaction as the fundamental and integral element out of which all patterns of behavior are composed. By relating temperament to the various types of reaction, we at once acquire a vast store of material from experimental psychology on the transient dynamic characterization of reaction for use in the determination of an individual's temperament.

It has long been established that each of us possesses a customary rate of response that is inherent to us, and in this sense people may be distinguished as fast or slow in terms of the nature of their reactions. Further differentiation may be achieved if a new component is introduced into the description of reaction, that of dynamism or force. By taking a cross-correlation of these two components, we then obtain in a natural way the four fundamental types of human behavior, which Kornilov describes thus: (1) individuals with a natural disposition towards a strong and rapid mode of response, or active-muscular type; (2) individuals with a natural disposition towards a weak and quick mode of response, or passive-muscular type; (3) individuals with a natural disposition towards a strong and slow mode of response, or active-sensory type; and (4) individuals with a natural disposition towards a weak and slow mode of response, or passive-sensory type. It is not too hard to see that these four types, which have been determined entirely independently of the science of temperament, are, in their ultimate conclusions, entirely identical with the classical teachings of temperament.

It is also not hard to see that the passive-muscular type of person, the sort of person who reacts quickly and who is easily excited, but whose reactions do not attain their full force and expressiveness but are extinguished just as quickly as they flare up, have usually also been referred to, and usually continue to be referred to, as individuals who possess a sanguine temperament. The characterization of the choleric personality is identical to that of the active-muscular type, with both types defined by quick and strong reactions, and it is not without reason that such a temperament has been ascribed to great and vigorous historical figures, people of great persistence and will. The melancholic type reacts slowly and strongly, and is the same as the active-sensory type.

Hence, what seems like a permanent state of sluggishness and obstructiveness, or one of delay and tension, is observed in melancholic temperaments, their capacity to attach themselves to a single idea or thought for many years, and their seemingly unexcitable state, associated in an individual with a kind of stern resolution and manly tension. And, finally, the phlegmatics, those with a natural disposition towards weakened and slowed rates of reaction, correspond to the passive-sensory type.

We gain an indisputable advantage by stipulating the existence of such a system of four types, no matter how many faults we see in it and even if we regard it only as a preliminary and rough scientific scheme. That is, with such a scheme the question of temperament assumes an objective ground, and it becomes possible to study it from the aspect of its complaisance to the influence of education.

Any decision as to the actual limits of the re-education of temperament is a matter of extraordinary complexity, and only by undertaking to study temperament from the standpoint of the reactions does it become possible to study experimentally the possibility of transforming a person who possesses a natural disposition towards one of the above four types of response into someone with a different type of temperament, whether as a result of educational training, exercise, a change in surroundings, and so on. General conclusions of experimental investigations have shown that all the rules of the re-education of temperament may be comprehended by a single general law, a law which is of paramount importance for pedagogics.

It is not hard for anyone to assume an intensified mode of response starting from a weakened type, i.e., to turn from a passive mode of response to an active on, and from a slowed rate of response to one which is speeded up. A change in the reverse direction, from a quick rate to a slow one and from a strong type of response to a weakened type, proves to be extraordinarily difficult and in a whole series of cases virtually impossible. Hence, it is entirely understandable that it is easiest to re-educate people of the passive-sensory type, i.e., phlegmatics, inasmuch as individuals in this type have no trouble mastering the form of behavior which is typical of active choleric natures. Such, in fact, has been the distinguishing mark of all so-called figure-heads in history, who, as one psychologist has put it rather wittily, were phlegmatics who pretended to be choleric. The intermediate switch, from a phlegmatic temperament to melancholic or sanguine, is also possible, since each of these types is associated with a change in only a single characteristic component in one of the possible directions which is amenable to re-education. Phlegmatics readily change into sanguines when they begin to move more quickly, and then their reactions become more intense, and they begin to resemble the melancholic type.

The group of choleric temperaments are the most difficult to re-educate. What one can never make of a choleric is to train him to be cool and composed regardless of the circumstances he confronts. But forms which are transitional with respect to the phlegmatic type remain nearly inaccessible to the choleric, and such a child is nearly always among the most difficult of all children to educate. In the pedagogical literature it is just these children which one speaks of as not fitting into their environment, or as being rebellious by nature.

The two other temperaments, which, roughly speaking, may be assumed to be only partially amenable to re-education, occupy an intermediate position in terms of re-education; in other words, a melancholic temperament can be easily turned into a choleric temperament if the individual's reactions are speeded up, and the sanguine temperament, also under certain conditions, may be easily conflated with the choleric temperament if the individual's reactions become more intense. The sanguine individual who has learned to have strong feelings and to speak in a commanding tone and who had, at some point in the past, recognized what it means to have powerful desires and to manage on his own, is no longer distinguishable from a choleric in any way whatsoever.

Whereas the pedagogical conclusions may seem to possess too great a degree of generality and the conclusions may seem overly diffuse, the very same scheme may possess far greater value for making decisions and for arriving at judgements in vocational psychology as regards a person's occupational suitability.

The Problem of Career and Vocational Psychology

Every type of labor is formed out of particular combinations of reactions which are inherent to it. Though one occupation may differ from another, this happens not because of the overall character of their psychological composition, but because of the nature and order of the reactions which are typical of the occupation. It is for this reason an extraordinarily simple matter to decompose every form of occupational labor into several primitive constituent elements, i.e., to reduce all of labor activity to a series of known types of reactions and to combinations of these reactions.

It is extraordinarily important to establish whether this or that person is suitable for a particular occupation. This is a requirement which is not only a matter of concern to the business itself, but also for the sake of a proper development of personality. Thus do we arrive at a determination of someone's suitability by considering both of these points of view simultaneously. Initially, vocational psychology arose out of a concern for ensuring the proper management of a business, and business confronted the practical problems of what became known as "negative selection."

The task of negative selection is to choose from among all the applicants for a job those who are absolutely unsuitable on the basis of psychological tests, i.e., those who could not handle the job under any conditions no matter what and who would only be a drag on the enterprise. Accordingly, vocational psychology began by devoting all its attention to the development of the minimal requirements of a job which, if not met by some applicant, would be equivalent to saying he was unsuitable for the job. The range of concerns of this scientific discipline then expanded, and one began to speak not only of negative, but also of positive selection, i.e., deciding which psychological tests would make it possible to judge not only the unsuitability for an occupation, but also a positive degree of talent, and a calling, for this occupation. Accordingly, instead of the development of a minimum quantity of necessary and sufficient conditions, psychology came to be concerned with the compilation of a detailed "psychogram" for each type of professional labor, i.e., a detailed psychological analysis of all the constituent parts of the particular type of labor. It was not possible to base such a psychological analysis of the most varied types of professional labor on the overall typical gamut of labor processes involved, i.e., establishing certain basic types under which the full diversity of different occupations could be subsumed.

According to the scheme proposed by Kornilov, there are several different types of labor processes. First is the natural type of labor process, which corresponds to those occupations which require neither strenuous physical effort nor intense mental effort. Among such occupations are household work and the labor of technical attendants, hall porters, watchmen, maids, and so on. In all these occupations, the labor reactions are formed out of a series of movements which are more or less customary to every one of us in our everyday life. The working conditions are such that the entire job transpires more or less stereotypically and automatically, requiring no particularly intense level of attention, and, finally, what is most important, such occupational labor occurs nearly always in a more or less natural and untrammeled state, requiring on the part of the worker no special straining of effort and no particular celerity. Naturally, it is easiest to select suitable applicants for these natural types of labor processes through the use of vocational psychology, since, although any worker reveals a definite natural propensity towards a particular reaction, nevertheless no worker should have any difficulty handling the functions of this type of work.

The second type of labor, what are known as muscular labor processes, requires concentrated attention focused not on the object of labor, but mainly on the movements peculiar to it. This kind of work represents a more complex type. Work of this sort entails enormous muscular strain and significant peripheral consumption of energy. The jobs involved include stone quarrying, and the occupations of blacksmith, miner, blacksmith's striker, wood-cutter, and others.

Here the vocational psychological requirements dictate in entirely exact and clear-cut fashion that we decide in favor of those temperaments which would be conducive to the expression of muscular and vigorous types of reactions. In other words, phlegmatics and sanguines whose reactions are customarily weak, i.e., individuals whose actions manifest an insignificant release of energy, are out of place in such occupations. What is even more important, such individuals find themselves in real conflict with the basic proclivities of their own organism if, in the course of their life, they nevertheless take on such work.

Of the two remaining types, the most appropriate is the melancholic behavioral pattern and temperament, since the slow rate of perception typical of this temperature provides an assurance of a degree of accuracy, insatiability, a calm and orderly state of mind, and a persistent attitude on the job. Indeed, the enormous force associated with every movement assures a desired effect. In contrast, cholerics, who die down just as quickly as they flame up, are restrained and less persistent in their work in this regard.

The third type of labor process may be provisionally denoted the sensory type. It is characterized by totally opposite features from the preceding types. Attention here is focused mainly on the object of labor, with the reactions involved entailing, as their *sine qua non*, a minimal external release of energy, though an extraordinarily slow and complex perception of external sensations. These occupations include those of watch-maker, mechanic, lathe operator, tailor, and others.

It is again obvious that the most appropriate types of applicants are those with a temperament type characterized by just these features, i.e., slow and weak reactions. Phlegmatics can become excellent watch-makers and rather good tailors, with a far greater chance of success than people with any of the other types of temperament.

People who possess an inappropriate reactive composition are especially destructive in a particular type of occupation, a fact which had been established by simple observation long before the advent of vocational psychology. For example, there are people who, before they have reached the point where they are ready to engage in some powerful and vigorous reaction, prove to be entirely incapable of grasping, for example, the art of clock repairing, despite the fact that their overall intellectual development is entirely adequate, and this may go on for years and years. Thus, they inevitably bend some spring or cannot bend it back, though they are in no way capable of tempering their movements and imparting to them the subtle and delicate aptitude which would make them uniquely useful and effective on the job. In this sense ordinary observation coincides with the results of vocational psychology. There are people who can never be entrusted with washing glasses, since they are, in general, incapable of holding anything fragile and breakable in their hands without squeezing it with such force as if it were a vessel made of copper.

Those which require complex types of reactions, called discriminating reactions, constitute the fourth type of labor process. Such processes are typical of printing and typesetting; before engaging in a labor movement, a printer or typesetter must accurately discriminate between all the stimuli on a sheet of type and in his case of type and must not produce a response before this act of discrimination has been performed accurately and correctly. Obviously, it is not possible to determine someone's suitability for this type of labor process in an unambiguous fashion on the basis of just a single feature of temperamental constitution, as we did above for all the simpler types of occupations.

Obviously, here the reactions are more complicated due to fact that the demand for central processing is so great that such complex central processes as thinking, attention, and so forth turn out to play a far greater role in any assessment of the effect of labor than do all the elementary properties of a reaction which may be discovered in temperament. In view of the natural diversity of individuals and their variable suitability with regard to these occupations, these occupations have to be described by a far more complex scheme than that which is used to make the roughest selection of applicants on the basis of vocational psychology. Here we are in the realm of those complex mechanisms whose functioning is more a matter of character than of temperament, i.e., more due to learned and acquired reactions than of hereditary reactions.

Therefore, as a general rule, one which is equally applicable to all succeeding types of temperament, it may be assumed that, in general, no matter what temperament someone has, he will be equally suitable to a particular type of occupation depending upon the functioning of the most complex types of mechanisms which go to make up his character.

However, here we may also point to the most likely vocational suitability of all those people whose reactions occur slowly and in attenuated fashion, all other conditions being equal. That is, the sensory component is, without a doubt, amenable to appreciable intensification in these occupations, whereas the motor component is relatively neutral towards the ultimate effect of labor. Nevertheless, reactions which proceed weakly usually become more closely associated with intense thought and guided attention than in the opposite instance.

Incidentally, this rule expresses, in general, a tendency of all of human labor, which is increasingly being transformed so that in place of enormous and wasteful releases of mental energy, it is now characterized more by weak, though complex and intelligent reactions. The general pedagogical rule, therefore, says that if we wish to teach a child the proper reactions for the higher forms of labor, we have to teach him weak movements, because weak movements are the most "intelligent," moreover this rule holds true in any given instance.

Fifth are those labor processes which involve making choices, requiring discrimination not only in the perception of stimuli, but also in the course of producing responding actions. In these types of labor, it is necessary to discriminate between and take into account in precise fashion two components, first that of stimulation, and second, that of response. The occupations in this group include those of chauffeur, conductor, streetcar driver, typist, pilot, and others. A streetcar conductor has to perceive in accurate fashion the objects in front of him which lie in the path of the vehicle, but it is even more important for him to make an unerring and proper choice between the decision to turn the engine handle to the right or to the left, thus between a movement which involves applying the brakes versus one which involves increasing its speed. Thus, here there is a kind of double discrimination or choice reaction in its purest form.

The element of response rate is of substantial importance here, since one can hardly say it doesn't matter at what rate the brakes are applied or released when danger is spotted, or how quickly a typist will be done with a particular text, or how many instants it will take a pilot to respond by turning the rudder towards the side of the plane which is listing.

In our analysis of the elementary properties of temperament, we do not get a clear enough idea of the suitability of a particular applicant, and again have to defer the decision pending a more rigorous analysis of complex behavioral reactions. However, here we already can see the general path we have to follow if we are to reach a correct decision, a path which involves the experimental investigation of all those types of reactions that are required in a particular occupation. In other words, if we are dealing with the reactions of a streetcar conductor or of a pilot, in which the essential element of the job is that of a choice reaction, we always have to test to see how the choice reaction manifests itself in the particular subject, and at what speed and intensity, if we wish to determine this person's vocational suitability. Likewise, it should be perfectly clear to the reader that if there are two applicants who are equal in all respects, other than in terms of the rate at which they produce their choice reaction, i.e., one of them responds with the correct and necessary movements to a properly perceived stimulus in 0.120 - 0.130 seconds, and the other in 0.160 - 0.180 seconds, of the two candidates the first is the more suitable one for the given occupation.

This principle also holds true of all types of complex labor processes which vocational psychology is in the habit of investigating on the basis of tests of the integral functioning of the organism in the course of some complex reaction.

Sixth are the recognition type of labor processes, i.e., those which require the recognition of a particular stimulus as an anticipatory condition of a given reaction, where this stimulus is not previously known to the worker. This type differs from that of simple discrimination only by the fact that the act of discrimination presupposes potential stimuli which are known beforehand to the entire group, whereas it is a matter of recognizing an indefinite and vast quantity of stimuli which the candidate could not previously take into account. Such, for example, is the work of a proof-reader who is not supposed to make any movement before he notices and recognizes a particular error in a printed text. Here it is clear that this type of labor will differ from that of a typesetter only by the fact that the typesetter deals with a pre-defined quantity of alphabetic elements, whereas a proof-reader can never tell ahead of time just what kind of error he will encounter next.

Last are the most complex labor processes, those involving associations, under which it is most appropriate to subsume the intellectual occupations. In these occupations, the most diverse operations on a specific subject are required on the part of the worker, either by means of free or constrained association, or where some sort of work has to be undertaken involving a mental selection to achieve of some goal which had been decided on once upon a time. These types of processes are the most complex of all and, quite naturally, require the most complex techniques of vocational psychology in order to decide on a candidate's suitability.

The overall conclusion of all the investigations which have been carried out in vocational psychology may be reduced to a single rule which has been given by Kornilov in roughly the following form. Every transition from a peripheral consumption of energy to central processing involves greater effort than the transition in the opposite direction. Put differently, the transition from mental labor to physical work is always easier to realize than the reverse process, that of the transition from physical work to mental labor.

The pedagogical value of vocational psychology is, of course, not confined to the sort of elementary analysis we have just presented; such an analysis, however, is entirely sufficient for obtaining a general idea of the subject of vocational psychology in the field of pedagogics and of its basic methods of application.

Bear in mind that the content of vocational psychology is not confined solely to the determination of vocational suitability, and instead plays a far more substantial role in teaching and in education. It always allows us to get an idea as to how successful the reactions of our students have been trained and have developed in the particular direction we have selected as the goal of our labors. Thus, in vocational psychology we possess not just a precautionary counselor and masterful judge at the start and end of the educational process which together give us a basis for deciding whether it is worth the effort to teach this or that occupation to a given student, and, second, whether a given student has learned a particular occupation.

But in addition to this, we possess in vocational psychology a constant companion and guide in our educational process, one which can show us every day with objective precision what point we have reached as regards the reactions we are teaching that very day, what has been achieved so far, and what must be achieved, and which aspects of these reactions, and in what sequence, have to be the object of our concern and of our educational responsibility.

We have to note that in the ordinary understanding, the subject of vocational psychology assumes a quite narrow and limited meaning, since as the saying goes, there is far more to life than the particular vocation we choose to pursue. Education possesses much broader goals than the training of a professional. After all, it is often of profound indifference which occupation a particular person chooses, so long as he turn out a fully developed and completed personality.

Such a view, since it proceeds from a fairly low opinion of the choice of vocation, is the most damaging legacy of the Tsarist school, which steered the basic goals of education to a point "somewhere off in the distance," to certain ideals of a harmoniously developed and perfected personality which had never been realized anywhere in the world, and missed the point of work and, accordingly, arranged the daily routine under close watch in the feeblest and crudest way imaginable, with all those daily lessons, all that busy work which, after all is said and done, filled up all the student's time and sapped all of his strength.

The complete and basic failure of every student was, in this way, sanctioned and foreordained. Students were not prepared for the life they actually lived, and this real life was declared to be a matter of indifference to them, whereas there was no other life whatsoever possible or feasible for them to lead. Such complete and basic failure usually assumed the form of a melodrama, a dissatisfaction with one's own work, the idea that life had lost all meaning, together with all those features which characterized the mental outlook of the Russian intellectual of the not too distant past, who was the typical pupil of such schools.

The emptiness and futility of abstract and farfetched ideals, meanwhile, accorded with the disgrace and narrow-mindedness of a petit bourgeois existence, and work, which has always determined the most important aspects of individual existence, was condemned to assume the most humiliating, the most brutish, and the most servile forms. From the standpoint of occupational education, therefore, vocational suitability has to be evaluated in an entirely different fashion. From a side issue and a slight matter of pure practicality, the general theoretical problem of deciding which specific and concrete goals should be made part of the education of each individual student has to assume paramount importance.

It is when, on the basis of general pedagogical reasoning and approaches, we have reached a point where we are thinking of one student in particular and are concerned with this student's individual personality, that we have most assuredly moved from problems which are purely pedagogical in nature to those which involve vocational psychology. Thus, for us the subject of vocational psychology encompasses nearly the entire field of personal pedagogics, though we will have to speak of it separately in a chapter on the study of giftedness and the measurement of the individual features of each student.

Endogenic and Exogenic Features of Character

Accurate discrimination between *endogenic* and *exogenic* features of character is of decisive import for the educator. Here it is a matter of distinguishing between those features which are determined by the mental and nervous organization of the child and which function in fully prepared form from the time of birth, on the one hand, and those features which constitute a product of external influence and are of most recent acquisition, what we may term the *taught features*, on the other. In other words, the question is to decide what it is in character which belongs to the innate constitution of the organism, and what it is which is due to education.

This topic still represents a subject of the most passionate and bitter dispute, and, depending on the fields in which they carry out their observations, investigators are inclined to point to one aspect as being the dominant one rather than some other aspect. In particular, biologists and physiologists are inclined to discern the decisive importance of the physical and innate component, and to associate in a direct relationship the most complex forms of character with various physiological processes. For example, Kretschmer whose theory was set forth in brief above is all for reducing those groups of characters he refers to as the "silent good-tempered man," "the formal aristocrat," "romantics fleeing from the world," "the cold, masterful natures," "the egoists," and so on, and so on, exclusively to biological components of constitution.

Hence the view whose essential core reduces to the claim that heredity determines absolutely the entire composition of our personality in the most important and subtlest way imaginable. The role of education and, in particular, that of the social environment to which personality assumes its orientation and in which it evolves, becomes virtually nil.

The opposite view is taken by psychologists of a sociological bent whose investigations have penetrated to the realm of concrete historical and sociological reality and who are led to conclusions that possess a diametrically opposite meaning by drawing on the thousands of bits of information they come upon day in and day out. These observations show with indisputable persuasiveness that not only the final strokes in the overall picture of our personality, but even the most fundamental outlines of this picture, those which define its very look, develop in no other way than under the sovereign influence of the environment

Between these two extreme points of view there would appear to be no compromise attainable, and science confronts the option of acknowledging either heredity or the environment, and so the dispute always goes on in just this plane. Only with the development of the science of conditional reflexes has it been possible to shed light on this question, and made it possible to test an entirely novel formulation of the question. This science has reconciled these two extreme points of view and determined the true role of each of these two components with the precision of experimental natural science.

There is nothing more misguided than the idea of the child which dominated the old Tsarist pedagogics, according to which the child was imagined to be a clean sheet of paper, i.e., an absolutely pure complex of potentialities which had not been realized in any way. To think in this way is to expunge not only all the processes involved in embryonic development and the birth of the human infant, but the entire limitless path of organic evolution, which has led to the creation and development of human nature. It is clear in advance that neither may be excluded from attention, though it is quite unlikely that just a single unadorned potentiality, in which there would be nothing that would be foreordained by the nature of these processes, would be obtained as a result of these processes.

On the contrary, we are now inclined to take account of all these influences in the most absolute fashion imaginable, and come closest to scientific truth when we say that there is absolutely no fact from the life of man or his animal ancestors or from the influences which a mother and fetus are subjected to that occurs without leaving a trace for the organism of the newborn infant, and that the latter comprises within itself the lengthy aggregate of accumulated genetic experience whose final links are the infant's mother and father.

In this sense, we would have to speak not so much of heredity in the narrow sense as it settles in within the family circle, as of the broadest forms of inheritance of the experience of mankind. In this sense, too, we are inclined to ascribe to the component of heredity absolute importance in the behavior of the child and to declare that not even the slightest movement in the child's future life arises from any source other than that of the capacities and reactions which have been passed down to the child by heredity. Without the slightest exaggeration, we may assert that absolutely every movement and every mode of behavior which this future adult and citizen of the world will have available to him throughout his entire life had already been given to him when he was in the crib and helplessly flailing without being able to focus his eyes or to hold still.

In fact, where do all those movements, with all their new potentialities, come from that appear later on in life? There is nowhere they could come from, just as there is nowhere that new organs in the body could come from. However, there cannot be the slightest doubt that this inherited experience, once it has been reduced to certain entirely conventional and stereotypical forms of behavior in all the individuals of a given species, does not constitute something permanent and congealed, but rather something which is prone to constant change.

And just as our preceding remarks hold true, so does our second assertion, that absolutely none of those movements which the child has at its disposal while still in the crib remain in precisely the same form throughout the individual's subsequent lifetime and continue to function in precisely the same way in which they were passed down by heredity. The mechanism of education of the conditional reflexes also reveals those laws under whose influence inherited experience is adapted to the particular conditions of the environment, and if the behavior of the adult differs from that of the child, this is only because into that chaotic melange of the newborn infant's uncoordinated and disorganized movements, discipline, meaning, order, and succession are introduced through the methodical educational influence of the environment. The infant's helpless flailing is transformed into the adult's struggle with the world and with himself in an utterly tragic and profound sense.

The point of public education may be defined with scientific exactitude as that of a kind of social selection which education produces from out of the wealth of potentialities contained within the child, allowing only one potentiality to be realized. The child, say Frank, plays at being a soldier, a pirate, and a horse because there is really concealed within him the propensities of a pirate, soldier, and horse. The point of education is that from out of this multitude of personalities there is realized through methodical influence and selection one and only one personality.

Thus, the educational process loses that tranquil and joyous character of a concern for the child and an interest in "lending a hand to nature," which is what had been prescribed for it in previous times. It manifests itself from a new angle as a dialectical and tragic process of unceasing atrophy of certain social potentialities for the sake of the realization of others through the unceasing struggle of different parts of the world for the individual, and through an unceasing struggle within the individual, without the clash between the most diverse forces within the individual himself ever abating.

This struggle, just like its outcome, is, as we showed in the early chapters, determined in its most essential respects by the very order of the world in which the child finds himself from its very first moments. Thus, a well-balanced point of view proceeds from a recognition of both components, though not through a settlement of all questions that bears the impress of a compromise and of irresolution, whereby this or that half or this or that sphere of influence is allotted to one or the other of the two conflicting sides, but in the sense of a dialectical confluence through the full recognition of their contradictoriness.

In other words, we are also not denying the existence of the contradiction between heredity and the environment, it is just that it seems to us that this contradiction exists not just in the mind, but in life itself. And it is just this fundamental point, this contradiction, which education takes as its foundation. If the child were to be born with all those forms of behavior which correspond to its life in the future, as if it were a plant, there would be no need whatsoever for education. The very demand for education arises, in Thorndike's expression, from the fact that "what exists is not what should exist." Therefore, education always denotes change and, consequently, the negation of certain forms of behavior in favor of the evolution and triumph of others.

Only in this light does education disclose itself as a process which possesses a meaning that gives it absolutely the same status as all the other processes of life. And in this sense, too, that assertion is profoundly true which points to the tragic character of this process, a feature which it holds in common with all the other processes of life. "Without pain no mother could give birth to a child, nor could a star come into being."

It is in this sense, too, that character has to be understood not statically, as a kind of foreordained aggregate of features, regardless of whether these features happen to be innate or acquired reactions, but instead as a dynamically flowing stream in which the two types struggle against each other. In other words, character arises not from the inherited features of the individual taken as such, as they actually exist, and not from the social influences of the environment considered independently, but from a discordant clash between the two and out of a dialectical transformation of inherited behavior into personal behavior.

Hence that assertion which requires from us a recognition of the presence of both types of elements in character, becomes understandable. Hence, too, does the solution to the problem of re-education of character become plain to see. Whether character is wholly amenable to education, or whether education has to be considered together with it as an invariable and foreordained condition—this is not the way to ask the question in scientific psychology. That which we provisionally denote by character constitutes an unceasing disruption and clash of individual life and inherited experience, and in this process of disruption and struggle the teacher may intervene at any time, and one can actually see that both assertions are simultaneously true.

Struggle is created not by education, it began before education and proceeds independently of it. Hence, it is understandable that any intervention in this struggle presupposes the most highly perfected and the most exacting measurement of absolutely all the elements that define the status of the struggle at any given moment. But by this very circumstance educational passivity may be overcome and, by organizing in a novel way all the elements of the environment in whatever way we wish, we throw into the struggle ever new forces or, on the other hand, take out of this struggle and disable all those forces which we feel are undesirable.

Thus do we attain the greatest results imaginable often by means of the most negligible doses of intervention. In order to start up a body at rest, an immeasurably powerful thrust is required. In order to exert an influence on a complex system of moving forces, slight intensification or relaxation of a single one of these forces is often sufficient in order to impart a new direction to the entire resultant force and give it a new meaning. Thus, in war a little force is sometimes enough to decide the outcome and to give the victory to one of the combatants. It is in this sense that William James likened the art of education to the art of war and declared that, in some sense, to educate means to engage in a battle. In some sense, pedagogics also denotes a science of strategy.

Thus, the general educational rule remains true in this case as well. There can be no direct intervention of any sort in the formation of character, all talk of moral influences on the development of the student's character, all talk of the good teacher fashioning, as if from wax, the soul of his students and imparting to it desirable forms—this is all either foolish talk which should not be trusted, or it overlooks what is most important and ascribes to moral influence that which is, in reality, realized by quite different forces.

For the educator to exert a direct influence on the formation of character is just as incongruous and ridiculous as a gardener would be who takes it into his head to promote the growth of a tree by pulling on it mechanically from the ground up. But the gardener influences the growth of plants, not directly by pulling on it from the top of a plant, and thus dragging it up from out of the ground, but indirectly by changing the environment appropriately. He moistens the soil, applies fertilizer to it, creates a perimeter about the tree, alters the temperature, light, air, and so on, and through all these effects actually attains the results he desires. In the same way, too, by influencing the surroundings and organizing it appropriately, the teacher determines the character which is assumed by the clash between inherited forms of behavior in the child and the environment, and, consequently, gains the ability to influence the evolution of the child's character.

Bear in mind in this connection that here as everywhere else nothing happens and nothing passes without leaving a trace, and that the teacher has to forever deal not only with the influence of heredity, but also the influences of all of previous experience, i.e., the accumulated capital of all the child's reactions which had been acquired previously.

In this sense, for the sake of clarity we will introduce for the term, "temperament," as if a parenthetical definition, first, all those purely hereditary elements of character which are given from the very start in the form of the elementary properties of character. Next is what we may term "static character," i.e., the customary form of behavior which develops as a result of individual experience and represents a kind of summary of this experience. Finally, we have to make a special distinction of "dynamic character," that fluid something which in science has yet to acquire any exact name, but which constitutes the most genuine, the most authentic and essential reality in the child.

---

[1] Kretschmer: *Physique and Character*, pages 259-260.

[2] *Ibid.*, page 260.

Chapter 17

THE PROBLEM OF GIFTEDNESS

Individual Goals of Education Personality and Education

Constant reminders of the social character of the educational process should by no means be taken as denoting the abolition of personality in the school or as mandating a spirit of indifference toward it. Ultimately, education always has to do with the individual personalities of students, and the social environment is composed, or more properly, is realized in the ranks of separate individuals.

It goes without saying that the role and guiding importance of the student's personality in the educational process in no way recalls that "pedagogical sing-song" in which individualistic education sometimes reduces the process that exists wholly between teacher and student. Where the student's personality formerly amounted to the focus of the educational world, now it has acquired a new sense and a new meaning.

The subject of personality may refer to several separate topics in public education simultaneously. First are all those individual differences which are inherent to each student. In view of the natural generality of the structure of the human body and of human behavior, every human constitution is distinguished by special, unique, and isolated properties and qualities which belong to this one individual alone, and, essentially, constitute a variation of the average type of "man in general." The latter has to be looked upon as only a convenient methodological technique, as an abstraction, and nothing else.

Man in general, like his separate parts and aspects, say, the human skeleton, human psychology, and so on, exists only in an abstract sense; in fact, in genuine reality there exists only this or that person, the skeleton and the psychology of this or that person. And it goes without saying that concern for these concrete features of each individual person has to become obligatory for the educator and the psychologist.

The construction of education is never undertaken in a void, education never undertakes to forge entirely novel reactions, it never makes the first thrust. On the contrary, it always issues out of already prepared and given patterns of behavior, and only intends to alter these patterns, always seeks to replace them, and not to create something entirely novel. In this sense, every form of education constitutes a re-education of what has already been realized. Every form of education, therefore, has as its first requirement the demand for entirely exact knowledge of hereditary forms of behavior. It is upon this foundation that the personal realm of experience must be constructed. And it is precisely here that knowledge of individual differences manifests itself with especial force.

This is particularly striking whenever we are dealing with very clear-cut and very explicit deviations of personality from the general average type. Just think of a child who is blind, or one who is deaf mute, or one who has some congenital organic defect of the central nervous system, say, suffers from mental retardation. It should be clear to the reader that every form of teaching and upbringing, though it must also not run counter to the fundamental laws of pedagogics, must nevertheless be guided in one particular direction or another, and possess some one particular meaning with regard to these children. In blind children, for example, conditional reflexes evolve that are just as accurate as in sighted children, it's just that they involve the sense of touch, and not vision, and accordingly, the blind person reads with his fingers from embossed type, i.e., he touches and feels letters, rather than perceiving them with his eyes. Thus, the whole process of reading and the events associated with it assume an entirely special character and slant.

For the deaf-mute child and children who are mentally retarded, all processes of training and adaptation to the workaday world likewise involve explicit differences which the educator cannot but take into account. Deaf children, for example, usually do not learn to speak from birth, since they do not hear the words spoken by other people, nor do they hear the very sounds they themselves make. To help them interact with each other and with normal children and also to accustom them to human speech, it is necessary to focus their attention on those movements of the lips which we make every time by pronouncing a particular word, and to teach them to connect each of these movements with a particular mode of inscription of the word and with a particular referent. Then we have to teach them to read off human speech with their eyes, from the lips of other people, just as we might read off a passage of text from a sheet of paper. To train a deaf child how to speak, it is necessary to give him the opportunity to perceive his own motor speech reactions and to control these reactions. Since this usually cannot be done by means of the ear, in this case hearing has to be replaced by kinesthetic and tactile stimulation. By placing the student's hand on his throat, we thereby teach him to sense those movements he performs in the course of speaking and which, once they have been reflected back to the speaker himself, help him develop the capacity for deliberate speech. In those of us who are not mute, speech develops by means of the ears, by virtue of the fact that we not only utter words, but also hear them and, consequently, evaluate what we have uttered.

In the education of children who are mentally retarded, we must likewise resort to psychological techniques in order to reinforce and settle in the child the same conditional reactions as when we are educating other children, and it is often necessary to employ the most primitive instincts and needs in such a child in order to teach him normal forms of behavior. For example, in order to teach certain mentally retarded children how to wash up or get dressed, we have to relate these acts with that of food, since it is only under the pressure of the very powerful stimulation of hunger that such a child is capable of overcoming a state of immobility and forcing himself to engage in some activity.

Thus all those techniques that might merit the severest censure were they to be employed with children who do not suffer from any disabilities turn out to be the only reasonable ones, and necessary, when it is a matter of educating children who are mentally retarded and who suffer from other disabilities.

Similarly, if we think of some other extreme example, say children who are specially gifted, here we come up against the need to alter certain general techniques and principles of education just for their sake. Once again, this becomes is easiest to see and is most pronounced in certain special forms of giftedness, for example, in children who have a special gift for music or art, or dance, where only early special education beginning at a very tender age can ensure the normal development of the capacities with which the child is endowed.

It is for this reason that the education of abnormal children, whether those who are impaired in some way or those are gifted, has long been thought of as seemingly outside the field of pedagogics, as constituting a realm which the general laws of education do not reach. We have to say that that such a view is profoundly mistaken, and that there is no justification for thinking of the field as falling outside pedagogics, and indeed such a view was arrived at only by error, out of a natural misunderstanding of phenomena which had not been subjected to investigated. The general laws of pedagogics can become scientific laws only when they remain applicable to every sphere of education equally. The laws of pressure and of gravity are entirely the same whether we are laying rails in a mountain tunnel or in marshaled. The physics is absolutely the same in both places, though the practical labor connected with the laying of track will always assume an entirely different form at one site as opposed to another. The fact that the labor involved at one site as opposed to the other assumes, of necessity, distinctive forms scarcely means that there exist separate laws at each site, but only points to the fact that the same laws may be expressed differently and may possess different quantitive meanings.

Thus, when they are children both the genius and person who is mentally retarded constitute just as much a subject of education as does every other child, and the general laws of pedagogics hold just as well for them as for all children of the same age. Only by proceeding on the basis of these general pedagogical laws are we able to discover correct ways of realizing the process of individualization which has to be imparted to the process of educating every child.

Likewise is it false to think that the problem of individualization arises only in relation to that which goes beyond the average. On the contrary, in every individual child we confront certain forms of individualization, of course not so sharply pronounced and not so sharply expressed as in blindness, genius, deaf-muteness, or mental retardation. But a phenomenon does not cease being itself if its quantitative expression is diminished. The demand for individualization of educational methodology, therefore, also amounts to a general demand imosedon pedagogics and extends to absolutely every child.

Hence, the educator confronts two problems, first, the individualized study of all the particular traits of each individual student, and, second, the individualized accommodation of all of educational methodology and all the effects of the social environment to every student. To force everybody into the same mold represents the greatest of all the delusions of pedagogics. The fundamental prerequisite of pedagogics inevitably demands an element of individualization, that is, conscious and rigorous determination of the individualized goals of education for each particular student.

Modern psychology is increasingly beginning to be imbued with this idea of the specificity of the individualized goals of education, and is thus inclined to review the traditional concept of giftedness, as abstract and general capacity, or in any case to introduce major correctives into this concept. Cyril Burt, for example, replaces the concept of mental giftedness by that of academic readiness, and in just this way imparts to the entire subject a vocational bias. The child is then viewed in terms of the extent to which he is in compliance with all those practical goals which the school places before him, in absolutely the same way that vocational psychology studies the worker in terms of the extent to which he is in compliance with the demands of a particular occupation. In place of abstract capacities, this point of view suggests concrete and practical investigations and testing of genuine skills, whether in writing, in arithmetic, or in reading.

Yet another major corrective is to replace the concept of *general* and *abstract* giftedness with that of *special* and *concrete* giftedness. This corrective justifies itself with equal clarity in the case of the disabled child and in the case of the gifted writer. Every form of giftedness is unfailingly a special form of giftedness toward some one thing. Tolstoy, for example, would be first in any list if it was giftedness in writing which was under study, though he would occupy a very modest position, perhaps one of the last spots, if it was musical abilities, suitability for engineering activity, or mathematical talent which was being investigated. Chekhov was a very average physician and a great writer. Instances in which semi-retarded people may be blessed with such phenomenal memory as to make them seem like geniuses are not at all that uncommon. All these examples only go to show that there does not exist any kind of "giftedness in general," rather that there exist special predispositions to certain types of activity.

Chapter 18

BASIC FORMS OF INVESTIGATIONS
OF THE PERSONALITY OF THE CHILD

C ontemporary psychology makes use of three basic techniques in its study of the personality of the child. [1] First is what may be termed *scientifically ordered observation*, which involves the observation of the particular characteristics of any one of our students, but only in a scientifically ordered way. To comprehend the meaning and goals of this method, we have to recall the difference between scientific observation and ordinary observation.

All of us observe an extraordinary breadth of facts every day, and scientific observation differs from such observation in only several essential features. First, unlike ordinary observation scientific observation presupposes a pre-defined selection of facts which are subject to observation. Let's suppose a solar eclipse has been observed by an average person, by an astronomer, by a zoologist interested in animal behavior, by a psychologist, and so on. The observations which are scientific will always identify a special series of facts out of the set of phenomena associated with a solar eclipse. And whereas the average person will be guided by his own interests and the random sequence of facts, and will shift his gaze from the frightened cow to the person making the sign of the cross, and from the darkened solar disk to its ash-gray reflection in the water, the scientific observer will always limit his observation to just a single group of facts, striving to avoid going beyond these facts even for one minute. The astronomer will follow only the gradual darkening of the sun, the zoologist only the behavior of the animals, and so on.

Thus, the first skill which is the mark of the scientific observer is in knowing which group of facts is to be isolated from all the others.

The classification of observed facts would have to be acknowledged as the second condition of scientific observation. By this we mean the ability to place similar facts together into groups, as if transcending the individuality of each, and to discover some characteristic sense and reference which it shares with other facts. The tallest stack of entirely reliable observed facts will still never amount to the even the most primitive elementary datum of science. It is necessary to know what purpose is served by the collection of these facts. In other words, we have to make a new, second selection of essential properties within these facts and pick out those facts in which these properties stand out and manifest themselves with unmistakable clarity.

Finally, the third rule of scientific observation is the demand to establish a certain relationship between individual groups of facts, i.e., the ability to construct a connected and integral picture of some one aspect of a process under investigation that would draw into itself a whole fragmentary group of facts.

And the very last feature, the fourth one: the capacity of scientific observation to not only describe facts, but to also explain them, i.e., discover the principles and relationships which constitute the foundation of these facts.

The same kind of general conditions must be imposed on the form of scientific observation peculiar to psychology as well. We have to insist that our concern here should not be with the general question of technique in psychological observation, but the special question of deciding which of the techniques of psychological observation are proper to pedagogics, i.e., the sense and reference which psychological observation represent for the teacher. Moreover, the assumption is that we are always working not with a psychologist, but with a person who has turned to psychology only for auxiliary assistance.

And it is in this sense only that all those schemes, programs for the observation of personality, and plans for the study of the child's mind come to the teacher's assistance. Though they go under different names, they all have the same goal, that of placing in the teacher's hands a means whereby he could subordinate the mass of observations which he makes on a daily basis to the above four rules and to thereby transform his own observations of the student's personality into scientific psychological observations.

Without concerning ourselves with the particulars of each of these plans, let us note the general principles and fundamentals of each. In fact, every such plan seems to be in the form of a series of questions directed towards the teacher and applies to this or that individual chapter, subchapter, section, or subsection. Say Chapter 5 is composed of material that responds to questions having to do with memory, touching on different aspects of this function, for example, the duration, accuracy, and volume of memory, and so on. In turn, each of these subchapters may be subdivided into a series of passages that respond to various specific questions which direct the teacher's attention to those symptoms which may be ascribed to the given instance and be indicative of it. Here is how a question might be posed: "How long does a student retain material he has mastered and has absorbed?, or "How much repetition does a student require in order to memorize a particular poem? The plan usually is produced in the form a notebook or workbook printed on one-half of the page so that the teacher may enter the appropriate observations opposite each question in the space left blank.

A printed version of this type could also be used for an entire school if entries were to be made in separate notebooks next to numbers printed in each notebook that would correspond to each of the questions, sections, and chapters. The teacher would have to be familiar with the plan in all its particulars beforehand in order to know how to work with it.

Then the process of gathering psychological observations goes on in an entirely unremarkable fashion in daily life at home or in the school. In such a process, the teacher, tutor, or parent enters each fact (datum) relating to the child's behavior which he or she has observed in the notebook, after first determining where it belongs and which question it corresponds to, in terms of number. If there is no appropriate question for the particular datum, this means that this datum is not supposed to be observed and noted down. Such a mode of record-keeping and such a process of gathering observations goes on for a long period of time, say six months or even a year, and much material is gathered as a result. It also turns out that we have thereby realized in fully mechanical fashion the first two conditions of scientific observation. First, a selection of all the essential observations has been achieved as if all by itself, and, second, because of the very existence of a plan, any datum which is of little or no significance has been absolutely banished from the focus of our attention. Finally, thanks to the system of record-keeping adopted, facts are not simply gathered, but are classified in mechanical fashion, inasmuch as they are placed in an appropriate place and, consequently, the meaning of each datum is thereby determined in prototypical and generic sense.

With this in mind, a daily log serves as a kind of collection box into which observed data are placed as if into compartment set aside for them beforehand. Thus, the teacher is left with the responsibility for the final two components of scientific observation, that of systematizing all the observations which have been gathered, and then explaining them. In view of the unusual difficulty of the fourth component, even in the case of a rigorously formulated scientific investigation, and the particular obstacles in the way of any complete explanation of observed facts, we have to admit that this condition may be satisfied only partially in those areas which are most amenable to interpretation, while only the goal of systematization of observations is fully achieved.

There exist several techniques of such a process of systematization, though once again the feature which is common to all of them consists in a transition from a series of specific observed data to certain general conclusions and formulations regarding a particular aspect of behavior. Let's assume that after a year we have gathered several dozen observations which support the hypothesis that this or that student always recalls exceptionally large and significant masses of material. But there will be virtually no one datum we might have happened to have taken note of in the course of the year which reinforces the length of recall in our case. It goes without saying that by systematizing our observations, it is natural for us to conclude that the reinforcement of reactions in our student has to be acknowledged as having achieved an incredibly high level of development and vigor in the sense of the volume of reactions mastered and embraced, though it represents an extraordinarily modest quantity if we bear in mind how long this reinforcement will last.

This example makes it entirely and clearly obvious that, essentially speaking, systematization does not involve anything new. In any process of systematization it is extremely important to avoid any kind of strained interpretation, or contrived explanation whatsoever, or to construct from it any sort of fantasy or wild conjecture, and so on. There must be nothing present in the systematization other than what is present in the facts themselves, though it must proceed only from a description of individual facts to general formulations.

Then a causal explanation becomes desirable and even conceivable here, only when the actual compilation of the individual groups of observed data which crop up in the course of systematizing these observations suggests the existence of a causal dependence between two groups of observed data. If in the section characteristic of the receptive component of some reaction, we are led to the conclusion, on the basis of the observed facts, that the visual receptors in our student function in weakened and slackened fashion, and if at the same time in our characterization of memory we are also able to actually establish that, of all the different types of memory, it is visual memory which is the most poorly developed in our student, then it is natural for us to conclude that in this instance we are dealing with causally connected phenomena, and it just for this reason that the student's visual memory is underdeveloped, that his visual perception is weak.

Among the advantages of this mode of scientifically ordered observation, we may note, first, the natural quality of the observations that are obtained, second, the scientific classification of the observed data, and, third, the simultaneity of observation and work in school.

Come to think of it, we are always observing the student in a natural setting, i.e., while he is working, and the observed facts we gather always refer to those direct methods of work that are customary methods for the particular student. Second, facts such as those we are classifying again fit within the natural setting of schoolwork, simply because this is how they appear. And, finally, the last point is that never and in no way does the student suspect he is a subject of observation. For our part, we never cease our instructional labors to make any special observations, but incorporate these observations as a constituent part of the overall process of educational methodology.

This system also possesses a whole series of very major drawbacks, however. The first, and most important, point is what may be thought of as the indeterminacy and the spontaneity of such a system of observation. We are not the master of the situation in such instances; on the contrary, we are left to wait calmly until the datum we need to observe appears all by itself. We might, therefore, have to wait a long time, sometimes for years, for the desired observation, and it may sometimes happen that it does not disclose itself in the student's schoolwork at all. That various facts relating to one area or another are missing in the case of some one student, therefore, is hardly an indication that that student lacks these forms of behavior, but instead says only that they cannot be observed in a school or family setting.

The second drawback lies in that duplication of attention which is required on the part of the teacher or tutor when, functioning simultaneously as psychologist and educator, he not only has to be involved in what he is doing, but he must also observe. It should be clear to the reader that with such a duplication of attention both areas readily suffer, the accuracy of observation as much as the intensity of pedagogical creativity.

Third and finally, such a system also suffers from the drawback that it distracts the teacher with the need to attend to several students, indeed a mass of students all at once. Now when observations are carried out over a lengthy period of time, the teacher doesn't have a chance to recall which aspects, belonging to which students, have already been reinforced sufficiently in the observations and which are still not represented in his daily log at all. Because the process of observation is haphazard and unsystematic from one moment to the next, and from one day to the next, observation is deprived of all effective, deliberate character.

In an effort to avoid these drawbacks, another form of psychological observation, one which is also extraordinarily popular and which is closely connected with the study of giftedness, has appeared. It may be termed the experimental investigation of the personality of the student.

Experimental Psychological Investigation of the Personality of the Student

In the experimental psychological method of investigation, the student is placed under special conditions which involve presenting him with various problems so as to evaluate individual aspects of his personality. Of all the different techniques which may be used for this purpose, there are two which, in our experience, are the most popular, and these we shall now discuss. Bear in mind, though, that all the different methods of psychological experimentation may be easily broken down into three basic groups, the first consisting of methods of stimulation, in which the force, composition, and interdependence of the elements of a stimulus are varied to determine particular relations and connections between an external cause and the reactions induced by it; the second, methods of expression, which are intended for the study of those physical manifestations, such as changes in pulse rate, respiration, facial expression, and speech through which various mental states are manifested; and the third, or methods of reaction, in which previously conditioned reactions are induced upon some signal.

In pure form, none of these methods is applicable to children. What is needed from such an investigation is not a detailed analytic description of observed facts, but a more or less integrated determination of complex articulated groups and patterns of behavior. Accordingly, any one reaction is always associated with a whole series of other reactions, and behavior is studied in its integral and connected form.

Binet and Simon constructed a measurement scale for the investigation of giftedness in children as a function of age. The scale consists of a series of tests or problems that are geared to each age group. It is assumed that the correct solution of all the required tests is indicative of a level of development in the particular child which is normal for that age. One has to admit, however, that the accuracy of Binet's tests in terms of age represents only a gross approximation. It assumes that 50% of all the children at a given age will solve all the tests correctly, 25% will be ahead of their age group, and 25% will lag behind it. And in general, a child's age is not a quantity which expresses itself in his development with such precision as to allow us to make judgements about children's development in an entirely objective and precise fashion. This is not, however, a serious drawback of the system, since here, as in any measurement, the unit may be selected in an entirely arbitrary fashion. For us, what is important is to have some sort of exact standard in order to make comparisons between children, and moreover, such a standard can only partially correspond to the real stages of a child's development.

The examination process itself consists in asking the child to complete all the tests that belong so some one age level. It is necessary to find the boundaries between which his solution ranges, i.e., on the one hand, to find out at which age level he is no longer able to solve any problem, and on the other, to determine the age level at which he is able to solve all the problems. For this purpose, we have to move forward and backward by age levels, beginning with the level corresponding to the child's physical age. Those levels at which some of the problems can be solved, and some cannot be solved, will be located between the two boundaries.

The calculation is then performed in the following way. Say a boy has solved all the problems appropriate to an age of eight, and then three problems appropriate to an age of nine, one problem appropriate to an age of 10, two problems appropriate to an age of 11, but none of the problems appropriate to an age of 12. For each problem solved at any one level, one-fifth of a year is counted up for the child. Thus, the whole calculation takes the form: $8 + 3/5 + 1/5 + 2/5 = 9\ 1/5$.

These figures also determine the child's "mental age." Now we only have to find the difference between the mental age and the physical age, and to say whether the child is lagging behind or is ahead. It is this which is given by the difference between mental and physical age. Thus, in our example $9\ 1/5 - 8 = 1\ 1/5$, which means the child is $1\ 1/5$ years ahead of his age. The ratio of mental age to physical age is then computed, a ratio that is also an index of the child's giftedness or his backwardness.

Finally, it is also important to keep in mind the number of age levels between the boundaries. A child's mental age may correspond to his real age or even be ahead of it, yet it may nevertheless not be possible to think of the child's development as being normal. It might be that the figure for mental age has been derived from individual problems that are scattered among so many age levels that the child would have to be acknowledged as possessing a clearly uneven development.

Thus our brief presentation of the Binet-Simon method. The method's distinguishing feature is that it attempts to apply its own tests to the investigation of complex mental processes, taking individual patterns of behavior in the form in which they are encountered in the real world, and not broken down, where we study memory, attention, and other functions separately. Binet selects those actions in which a combination of reactions that is typical of a given age level is expressed. Binet's tests, therefore, may be easily adapted to different countries, and may represent a concise rough guide until new tests to replace them have been constructed. Such a guide allows us to analyze three new areas. First, it allows us to select from out of the mass of normal children a group whose members have to be acknowledged as being abnormal simply because they are lagging behind, and thus have to be placed in special educational institutions. Next, it serves to convince us that the development of the rest of the kids is more or less genuine. And, third, it allows us to keep track of the overall course of each child's development by supplying us, from one year to the next, with measurements that tell us how far this one child has progressed.

Rossolimo's method, which the author refers to as reducing to the creation of a "psychological profile," pursues the same goals. The choice of name emphasizes the fact that it is not integral patterns of behavior which are investigated, but rather isolated psychological functions, such as memory, attention, will, receptivity, acuity, and so on. Each function is subjected to a total of 10 tests. A test that has been solved is denoted by a plus, and an unsolved test by a minus, and the overall total of pluses for any one function then characterizes its height. Next, this result is plotted in the form of a graph on a sheet of paper which has been subdivided into 10 squares; the number of tests that have been solved is indicated by means of dots entered at the corresponding height.

The arithmetic mean is then computed, and taken as characterizing the child's overall giftedness. The mean of each of the three basic groups, that of volitional processes, of memory, and of associative processes, is also computed separately.

Versions of tests that are just as much an approximation exist for the investigation of elementary representations in very young children. The general drawback of these types of experimental investigations is the fact that they rest on the entirely false idea that there exists some sort of general mental giftedness. Undoubtedly, this doctrine is based on ideas, already out-of-date scientifically, which are echoes of the psychology of capacities. The very concept of mental giftedness has to be replaced by that of special adaptability.

Moreover, we cannot but emphasize the relationship between these systems and the old Tsarist school, where all the educational techniques were based on mental training. These systems, therefore, involve nothing more than an investigation of intelligence, but not an investigation of the emotional nor the volitional sphere of the student.

These systems intellectualize the personality of the child in one-sided fashion and, therefore, represent it in a false light. Finally, all these systems suffer from the drawback inherent to any experimental investigation, that of artificiality, since the subject is forever being placed in an extraordinary situation. There is no guarantee, moreover, that the student's memory or attention will function in school in precisely the same way it functions in the laboratory. Despite the fact that any experimental investigation presents extraordinary opportunities from the standpoint of the opportunity it affords for the production of any change in the student's behavior which one might wish for, nevertheless, it suffers from all those drawbacks that are inherent to any experiment. It places the student under new conditions, moreover, there can never be any certainty that the conclusions which are obtained are valid. Thus, an experimental method, while avoiding the drawbacks of observation, bears within itself new defects.

A way out of these and other defects is supplied by the third system of psychological investigation, called *natural experiment*.

For purposes of illustration, we now present Binet's method in the form set forth by K.P. Veselovskaya.

Binet-Simon Method

To determine the levels of giftedness and backwardness of children of different ages, Binet and Simon outlined the following sequence of questions:

For three-year old children: Show me your or her mouth, nose, and eyes. Repeat a sentence consisting of six syllables. Repeat one of three pairs of numbers. Call out the names of several objects in a picture.

For four-year old children: Tell me whether you are a boy or a girl. Name three objects in common use in the home, e.g., knife, key, coin. Repeat a series of three digits. Compare two lines (5 and 6 centimeters in length) and tell me which one is longer.

For five-year old children: Compare two pairs of boxes, one pair of 3 and 12 grams, and the other of 6 and 15 grams, and tell me which one is heavier. Draw a square. Repeat a sentence consisting of 10 syllables. Add up four single sou pieces. Construct a parallelogram from two line segments.

For six-year old children: Tell me what time it is. Give me a definition or simple description of five objects. Draw a rhombus. Add up 13 identical coins. Compare two faces from an esthetic point of view (pictures taken from special albums provided in the Binet-Simon test).

For seven-year old children: Show me your right hand and left ear. Copy a picture. Perform three small assignments. Add up three simple sums and three double sums. Tell me the names of three colors.

For eight-year old children: Compare from memory three pairs of objects. Count from 20 down to 0. Tell me what are the missing parts in the faces in the pictures in front of you. Tell me what is today's date. Repeat a series of five digits.

For nine-year old children: Tell me how much change is left over if 16 coins are subtracted from 20. Tell me the definitions of five objects. Express all the coins of our country's monetary system in terms of a single unit. List the months of the year in order. Respond to three simple abstract questions.

For 10-year old children: Arrange five boxes of different weights in order. Draw from memory a simple picture. Find something out of place in four sentences. Respond to more difficult abstract questions. Construct two sentences using three given words.

For 12-year old children: Teach the child to resist a suggestion, for example, show him six pairs of lines, the first pair 4 and 5 cm in length, the second 5 and 6 cm in length, and the third 6 and 7 cm in length, with all the lines in the remaining pairs being 7 cm in length. If a subject who is attempting to compare the fifth and sixth pairs keeps on saying that the longer lines are the ones which lie to the right, this is counted as a suggested response. Construct a single simple or compound sentence using three given words. Say at least 60 words in three minutes. Define three abstract concepts. Place words that have been deliberately mixed up in the right order.

For 15-year olds: Repeat a series of 7 digits. Select two rhyme schemes for a given word. Ask him to construct a sentence consisting of 26 syllables. Explain the meaning of three pictures. Derive a conclusion from a series of facts.

---

[1] In reading the present chapter, it will be useful to bear in mind that at the time the book was written Soviet schools were the scene of very large-scale programs of psychological testing; cf. Bowen, *Soviet Education*, page 58 (trans.).

Chapter 19

PSYCHOLOGY AND THE TEACHER

The Psychological Nature of the Work of the Teacher

Until now we have been concerned with the psychology of the pedagogical process from the point of view of pupil and student. We have tried to explain those laws and influences to which education is subordinated in terms of how this process depends on the child. The psychological well-springs of the educational process, insofar as they are embedded within the child's psyche, have constituted the subject of all of our preceding discussions. This, in fact, is how things go in the majority of modern courses in educational psychology.

Such an approach is, however, extremely incomplete and one-sided. To get a complete idea of the entire integral process of education and to represent all the most important aspects of the overall process in the light of psychology, it is not only necessary to take into account the psychology of the work of the teacher; we also have to show what sorts of laws it is bound by. But we cannot make this the subject of the present concluding and brief chapter; only in a complete and fully developed course in educational psychology, which is a project for the future, could it find its proper place.

Science has yet to achieve the sorts of results and discoveries which would help it discover the key to the psychology of the teacher. Instead, we have only scattered data, only fragmentary remarks which have yet to be reduced to a system, and on top of that, certain attempts of a purely practical nature to assist in the vocational psychological selection of teachers. Do not forget that the development of a psychological profile for teachers within the realm of vocational psychology presents far greater difficulties than in other occupations.

Accordingly, we have to acknowledge the fact that it is hardly possible to write a scientifically rigorous chapter on the work of the teacher within the framework of educational psychology. Thought has been given to the most general considerations in this area more than once, however, so that the present volume would be incomplete without some discussion. Therefore, some space must be given over to a discussion of these basic considerations for the purpose of completeness and conclusiveness of the presentation.

There is no denying the fact that every theory of education imposes its own conditions on the teacher. In the pedagogics proposed by Jean-Jacques Rousseau, the teacher is only the child's guardian and keeper, protecting him against bad influences and from becoming spoiled. For Tolstoy, such a person has to be an unfailingly virtuous person who arouses the child by own personal example. For ascetic pedagogics, an educator is someone who knows how to fulfill the precept, "Break the child's will so that he does not perish." In *Domostroi*, [1] once again new capacities are required of the parent or teacher when it is prescribed, "Punish your son severely from the time he is a little boy, and you will be at peace in your old age and have some pleasure. And do not ease up when you are striking a small child, for he will not perish if he is beaten with a rod, but become wiser. Because by striking his physical body you will save his soul from death." For Guyau, the teacher is a hypnotist, and, according to Guyau, only he will be a good teacher who is able to convey ideas to someone else by means of hypnotic suggestion and to subordinate someone else's will to his own. For Pestalozzi and Froebel, the educator is a kind of gardener who works with children. For Blonskii, the educator is an engineer who makes use of "anthropolotical methodology" [*antropotekhnika*], of a science of "child engineering," that is, an engineer whose science of the cultivation of human beings operates just like plant-growing and animal husbandry, as if of the same type.

There have been many who have compared the work of a teacher with that of an artist, assigning paramount importance to all questions of individual creativity. On the other hand, there have been those, Kamenskii, for example, who have declared that "we have to hope that the method followed in the education of human beings would become mechanical, i.e., that it should be prescribed in such definite form that everyone, whatever he is learning and whatever he is involved in, cannot but succeed." Kamenskii has referred to this kind of teaching as reducing to a "teaching machine" [*didakticheskaya mashina*]. A similar view was maintained by Pestalozzi.

Thus, we see that every individual conception of the educational process is associated with a particular view of the nature of the work of the teacher. We can therefore well understand that new point of view which has now been put forward in pedagogics that attempts to construct a new system of education, thereby creating all at once a new system of educational psychology as well, i.e., a new scientific discipline that serves to justify it. And it stands to reason that a new system of educational psychology, i.e., a new view of the nature of the educational process which attempts to explain absolutely every single one of its aspects and all its elements from a unified conception, leads to a new understanding of the work of the teacher.

We have already pointed out in one of the early chapters that, from the standpoint of his own work, the teacher represents a person engaged in what is essentially a dual phenomenon, just like any type of human labor. A teacher can seem like a mere fount of knowledge, a reference volume or dictionary, a manual or illustration, in a word, an auxiliary aid and tool of education. It is not very hard to see, meanwhile, that it is just this aspect of the work of the teacher that made up nine-tenths of the content of the labor of the teacher in the Tsarist school, as we have shown earlier. Now this role is increasingly disappearing, and is being replaced in every way imaginable by the active energy of the student himself, who, at all times, has to himself seek and obtain knowledge on his own, even when he gets it from the teacher, and not gulp down all that stuff [*pishcha*] the teacher is filling him up with.

We have already taken leave of that prejudice which seemed to demand that the teacher educate. Consequently, we are also far from that view which supposes that a person has to carry heavy loads all by himself. It is in this sense that we are quite right in saying that the real secret of education lies in <u>not</u> teaching. The process of development is subordinated to the very same iron laws of necessity as is everything else in nature. Consequently, parents and teachers "have just as much power or right to prescribe to this new being as to tell the stars what path to follow."

The student educates himself. A lecture that has been presented by the teacher in finished form may teach many things, but it inculcates only ability and drive, and everything it makes use of comes from the hands of others, without accomplishing anything or checking anything. For present-day education, it is not so important to teach a certain quantity of knowledge as it is to inculcate the ability to acquire such knowledge and to make use of it. And, like everything else in life, this may be achieved only in the very process of labor and in the very process of attaining this knowledge.

Just as you cannot learn how to swim by standing on the sea shore, that to learn how to swim you have to, out of necessity, plunge right into the water even though you still don't know how to swim, so the only way to learn something, say, how to acquire knowledge, is by doing so, in other words, by acquiring knowledge.

Thus, the teacher must shoulder a new burden. He has to become the director of the social environment which, moreover, is the only educational factor. Where he acts like a simple pump, filling up the students with knowledge, there he can be replaced with no trouble at all by a textbook, by a dictionary, by a map, by a nature walk. When the teacher presents a lecture or explains a lesson, in these instances he is only partially acting in the role of teacher, say, in that area of his labor which establishes the child's relationship to all the elements of the environment which affect him. Where he is simply setting forth ready-prepared bits and pieces of knowledge, there he has ceased being a teacher.

The greatest danger associated with the psychology of the teacher is that it is just this latter side of the teacher's personality which might begin to assume the dominant role there. Thus, the teacher begins to think of himself as a tool of the educational process, as a record player, without a voice of his own, singing what some record suggests to him. Quite frankly, there is no denying the fact that every kind of occupation which contains an element of teaching superimposes characteristic indelible features on its practitioners, and creates pitiable figures that assume the role of propounders of commonplace truths. It is no accident that the teacher, this walking storehouse of sayings, has always seemed like a comic figure, the object of laughter and mockery, and has always been a funny character beginning with the comedies of ancient Greece right down to modern stories. Chekhov's "straitlaced man," or that hero of his who would be forever saying, "The Volga flows into the Caspian Sea," and "Horses eat oats and hay," was for this reason alone a terrible sight, constituting a vivid example of the utter absence of personality, of someone who had finally lost all feeling and thought.

That the Volga flows into the Caspian Sea is an extremely important scientific fact of vast educational import, and there is nothing funny about it. What is funny is that this fact is made into a roll of wool the individual wraps himself in, that it consumes his entire life, and that for this fact the person has entirely ceased to exist. Truth is not a very wise thing if those who are its heralds are, for the most part, stupid, thus says a character in one old comedy about such a straitlaced person.

What is seen here in caricature basically constitutes a permanent feature of the teacher so long as he is treated as a tool of education. It is extraordinarily curious that the very same picture Chekhov drew of teachers may be seen in all those professors who, 30 years ago, would give lectures on esthetics without understanding anything about esthetics and who were being profoundly convinced that it is not Shakespeare who is important, but the commentaries on Shakespeare. The point, that is, lies not at all in some little bit of knowledge, in a circumspection of outlook, and in how insignificant are the facts themselves. The point is not that man always swims in shallow waters and knows very little, rather that the very transformation of a person into a "teaching machine" represents an extraordinarily willful misrepresentation of man, in terms of a human being's own psychological nature.

Thus, the fundamental requirement imposed on the teacher under our new conditions is the utter rejection of all woolly thinking and the development of all those aspects which breathe of movement and life. In all those forms of work which teachers would engage before the revolution, there was a certain musty and stale odor, as in stagnant and undisturbed water, And this did not help along the ordinary doctrine of the teacher's sacred mission, of the teacher's consciousness of his very own ideal goals.

Psychologists have demanded of the teacher educational inspiration, and it is this which defined in their eyes the personality of the teacher. The concern has been with the teacher's inner warmth. "A teacher who does not feel the beauty and the sacredness of his mission and who has entered the school, not because his heart was full of the desire to teach the youth, but just to have a job and to earn a living, is doing harm to the pupils and greater harm to himself," says Hugo Münsterberg, [2] the writer who has given the clearest expression of this view. What is required of the teacher is enthusiasm, and it is with such inspiration that the teacher may nourish the students.

Continues Münsterberg, "For the teacher at his desk it holds as true as for the minister in the pulpit, that without belief in his heart, he is doomed ... And if the enthusiasm has touched the soul, everything will become living and inspiring ... There is no need for a distorted perspective. It is not necessary to teach the irregular verbs as if they were the center of the intellectual universe. Everything may remain in its right place ... On the other hand, the pupil's interest is absorbed because his interest in the enthusiastic teacher is projected into the indifferent material taught". [3]

These are the words of Hugo Münsterberg, one of the founders of the field of vocational psychology, and he has discovered nothing better than an inspired faith in the value of human ideals upon which the work of the teacher may be based. Truth in this view is mixed up with error. Münsterberg is quite correct when, speaking in the language of psychology, he demands of the teacher a certain innate emotional temperament. Whoever is neither ardent nor cold, but only lukewarm, can never be a good teacher. He is also right when he points to the danger of placing the work of teaching increasingly in the hands of women. "To put the education of boys in the years in which their manhood is developing, essentially into the hands of women cannot be without danger to the best interests of the community". [4]

It is also true that, because of the economic balance of forces, the occupation of teaching has become a place where all those who are maladjusted or unlucky, all those who have suffered defeats in every area of life huddle together. We can think of school as a refuge which life allots to vessels that have suffered shipwreck. It is for this reason that a natural selection of delicate, unfit, and crippled human material has been created for the vocation of teacher. It says something that there was a time when retired soldiers would take up teaching. Those who have retired from life's battleground now, in fact, make up three-fourths of the ranks of teachers. "It is terrible," writes one educator, "that there are so many spinsters and bachelors and, in general, every imaginable type of failure, among our teachers. How can someone teach a child to have faith in life if his own life has been a failure?" So perhaps we should come right out with it and admit that far from everyone should be a teacher, but only those who are most suited to the profession.

With this the present-day point of view is fully in accord. Moreover, it is also in agreement with the demand that the teacher has to know a lot. He must possess a complete grasp of the subject which he teaches. "The teacher must draw from a full spring," writes Münsterberg. "It is not enough that he know what he wants the pupils to know and that he hastily supply himself in the morning with a reserve fund to answer the questions of the next morning. He alone can give information in an interesting way who might give a hundred times more than he has a chance to give. If a teacher interprets a single poem, it makes all the difference whether he is versed in the whole literature or not; and his nature study may be confined to the elements in the class room and yet those elements demand that the wide perspectives of real modern science be open before his eyes". [5]

This may be compared with the process of walking, when we can take a step with confidence only when we can see 1000 steps ahead of us, and it is only the path which our very next step is to follow which remains to be discovered. This example also elucidates for us quite well the role which has to be assigned to specialized knowledge in present-day pedagogics. The point is that to take a real step forward, to place our foot down somewhere, an extraordinarily narrow space is needed. Why, then, do we need a wide and open road? It is needed not so much for the foot, as for the eyes, so as to steer and regulate the movement of the foot. In just the same way, the teacher who has been relieved of the obligations of having to instruct must know far more than before. Ultimately, in order to instruct, one need know very little, but one must know it clearly and distinctly. In order to guide the student's own knowledge, one must know far more than he knows.

Until now the student has always stood on the teacher's shoulders. He has looked upon everything through his teacher's eyes and judged everything by the way his teacher thought. The time has come to place the student on his own two feet and to recognize that there is not very much knowledge the teacher can impart to the student, just as one cannot teach a child to walk by means of lectures and the most painstaking demonstration of skillful perambulation on the part of the teacher. The child must himself be made to walk and to fall, to suffer pain from injuries, and to decide what direction to follow. What is true as regards walking, that it can be learned only on one's own two feet, and only by one's own tumbles, is equally applicable to all aspects of education.

But there is a profound divergence between the reasoning taken by the old Tsarist pedagogics and today's pedagogics as regards the teacher's idealistic inspiration. Münsterberg is profoundly correct when he speaks of the relationship between every particular fact and the overall value of an entire subject, and points out that the experience of value has to be imparted to the student even in the study of the irregular verbs is profoundly true. The error lies only in the determination of the means through which psychologists have hoped to achieve the success they are aiming for.

Psychologists have seen as the guarantee of this success the enthusiasm that the teacher is imbued with, in the background which forms in the teacher's own mind, and in the interest which arises in the student towards an inspiring teacher. All of this constitutes the greatest of psychological delusions. Inspiration, first of all, is psychologically so rare an event and so difficult a process to guide as to make it impossible to construct on its foundation any one thing of vital importance whatsoever. Either we end up with false inspiration, that image of false pathos where the teacher speaks of irregular verbs as if they were actually the center of the universe. Or, there is the inspiration which is not contagious, just like the actor who experiences sincerely and who cries real tears, but who makes the audience laugh. There is no counting how many times an inspiring teacher finds himself in such a situation.

Nor can we forget yet another noble type of teacher, the Don Quixote idealist who is infinitely enraptured with Livy's style, or the contours of the island of Madagascar, to the greatest amusement of his students.

Whether someone is an inspiring teacher is not the point in the least. Nor is the problem the fact that this inspiration does not always reach the student. The real point is that the student must be made to become enraptured by the very same thing. It is even worse when inspiration does not succeed, and, like the case of the cold actor, there appears in the teacher that contrived, rhetorical pathos which found a rather splendid expression in the style of some of the textbooks from before the revolution, where history or geography was set forth in an exceedingly bombastic tone as a way of reaching the student's feelings and inspiring him. But even when inspiration reached the student's consciousness, it was always misguided, turning into veneration of the teacher after having assumed profoundly anti-pedagogical forms.

Nowhere did the sickness of the Tsarist pedagogics exhibit itself with such special clarity as in those instances when, in place of open warfare between teacher and student, there sprang up friendly relationships. The deification of the "favorite teacher," which assumed the form of adoration, represents, in fact a genuine psychological problem that recalls that which in psychoanalysis is referred to as "transference." By the term, transference, the psychoanalyst is referring to that special false relationship which springs up between the patient suffering from a neurosis and the doctor who is treating him when unhealthy, neurotic interest is focused on the doctor's personality, when the interests nourishing the neurosis are associated with him, and the doctor's personality turns into a wall that separates the patient's inner world from the world outside.

Thus, the problem is, instead, to induce in the student inspiration of his own, and not to tell the teacher how to go into raptures when presenting the country's history, as was done in the regulations distributed by the Prussian Ministry of Education.

Enthusiasm is akin to fraud, and inspiration to risk-taking. There is an age of enthusiasm even in poetry, this eternal refuge of this dark force. There is hardly a single American manufacturer who would entrust the management of his own factory to the enthusiasm of a manager, or an admiral who would entrust a ship to the enthusiasm of a captain. The preference is always for the experienced engineer and the skilled seaman. It is time that pedagogics, too, followed this road and sought out people who possessed an exact knowledge of laws and the methodology through which the child's own sense of inspiration could be aroused within the confines of his own soul, making use of whatever means were available, by whatever means possible, the child's own inspiration.

Thus, *exact knowledge of the laws of education—this, above all, is required of the teacher.* It is in this sense that we can avail ourselves of Munsterberg's expression, that there must exist many different types of teacher, though the true teacher is always the same, is applicable. And the true teacher is that teacher who constructs his own educational work not by inspiration, but on the basis of scientific knowledge. Science is the truest path to the mastery of life.

In the future, every teacher will have to construct all his own work by psychology, and scientific pedagogics will become an exact science based on psychology. Scientific pedagogics must be based, says Blonskii, on scientific psychology, i.e., on sociobiological educational psychology. Thus, in place of quacks we will get scientists.

Thus, the first condition which we impose on the teacher is that he or she be a scientifically trained professional, that he or she be a true teacher before he is a mathematician, or a teacher of literature, or whatever. Only exact knowledge, exact calculation, and sober thought can become the true tools of the educator. In this sense, the primitive ideal of the educator *qua* nursemaid, which demanded of the teacher warmth, tenderness, and concern, is not quite to our tastes. On the contrary, for the psychologist the Tsarist school must be condemned just from the fact that it made the very profession of educator into one that demanded little talent. It reduced the educational process to such monotonous and negligible functions as to have methodically corrupted the educator in the most profound way possible.

And it was no psychological paradox that grades and detention rooms, examinations and inspections, corrupted the educator even more than the student. The *gymnasium* exerted a greater educational influence on the teacher than on the students. No psychologist can write a single page that would hold any interest if his subject is the psychology of the teacher of the Tsarist school. Now, in the light of psychoanalysis we can say without flinching that the pedagogical system as organized before the revolution was a place for the education of every possible type of mental illness in the teacher, and in the full sense of the word, created a kind of neurosis peculiar to the teacher. In this sense, Sologub's hero, Peredonov, does not constitute any kind of absurd or monstrous fiction.

Now with all the problems the teacher has to deal with, which become more complex from one day to the next, the number of instructional techniques required have become so infinitely varied and their complexity so great that any teacher who would like to be a scientifically trained educator must master an extraordinarily large volume of knowledge.

It used to be that one only had to know one's own subject, the curriculum, and, of course, how to raise one's voice at the class in a difficult situation. Now pedagogics has become a real and complex art that grows out of a scientific foundation. Thus, what is required from the teacher is enhanced knowledge of the subject, and enhanced knowledge of the methodology of his craft.

Moreover, the very method of instruction demands of the teacher that same sense of activity, that same sense of group spirit, with which the soul of the school must be infused with. The teacher must live within the school collective, as if an integral part of it. It is in this sense that the relationship between teacher and student can attain a force, a transparency, and a depth without equal in the entire social scale of human relationships.

But this is only half the problem. There is also the fact that the teacher has to satisfy a requirement that is of an absolutely opposite order. He must be a teacher through and through, but he must also be not only a teacher, or to put it somewhat more properly, he must be more than just a teacher. Strange as it may sound, if we think of it as a profession teaching constitutes, from the psychological point of view, a false reality, and there can be little doubt that it will vanish in the near future. This, of course, does not mean that rejecting what was said above regarding the extraordinary complexity of the specialized areas of knowledge the teacher has to possess. And though there can be little doubt that the teacher of the future will be not an instructor, but an engineer, a seaman, a political worker, an actor, a worker, a journalist, a scholar, a judge, a doctor, and so forth, this, however, does not mean that the teacher of the future will be a dilettante when it comes to pedagogics. Our only concern is that there exist within the very nature of the educational process, within its psychological essence, the demand that there be as intimate a contact, and as close an interaction, with life itself as might be wished for.

Ultimately, only life educates, and the deeper that life, the real world, burrows into the school, the more dynamic and the more robust will be the educational process. That the school has been locked away and walled in as if by a tall fence from life itself has been its greatest failing. Education is just as meaningless outside the real world as is a fire without oxygen, or as is breathing in a vacuum. The teacher's educational work, therefore, must inevitably be connected with his creative, social, and life work.

Only he who exerts a creative role in real life can aspire to a creative role in pedagogics. It is just for this reason that, in the future, the educator will also be an active participant in society. Whether in theoretical science, in the sphere of work, or in practical social activity, he will always relate the school and the real world through the subject which he teaches. Thus, pedagogical work will inevitably be linked to the broad social work that the scholar or political leader, the economist or the artist, pursues.

In the city of the future, there will not be any one single building from which one might hang the sign, "school," because the very word, "school," which denotes in the rigorous sense of the word, "leisure," and which has meant setting aside a special building and the assignment of particular individuals for "leisure" [6] activities, will be absorbed altogether in work and in life, and schools will be held in factories, and in the public square, in museums and in the hospital and the churchyard.

As Münsterberg says, "There are windows in every class room; the right teacher will look out from his desk into the wide world, into the turmoil of men, into the joys and duties of life ..." [7]   And in the school of the future, these windows will be opened as wide as can be, and the teacher will not only look out, but also actively participate in the "duties of life." That which was responsible for the mustiness and spiritual stagnation in our schools, was due to and sprang from the fact that all the windows to the outside world in our schools had been tightly shut and shut, first and foremost, in the teacher's own soul.

To many it seems that in our new system of pedagogics the teacher will have a negligible role to play, that it is a pedagogics without an educator, and a school without a teacher. To think that in the school of the future the teacher will have nothing to do is just like thinking that the role of man in mass production has diminished or been reduced down to nothing. One might even think that in the school of today the teacher has been turned into a mechanical mannequin. But on the contrary, the role of the teacher increases beyond all bounds, the school of today requires of the teacher a *higher test for life* in order that he possess the capacity to turn education into the creation of life.

Life as Creation

There has existed until now, unfortunately, the conviction that since the educational process is expressed in a relationship between teacher and student, it is confined for the most part to imitation alone. Even in the latest systems of Marxist pedagogics, there are writers (e.g., Zalkind) who sometimes speak of a reflex of imitation as if it were a kind of foundation stone of education. "And the teacher has to seduce, he has to attract the individual who is to be educated," Zalkind goes on, "with the tempting content of the example of his own example, else all attempts to set the student's reflexive machinery in motion will come to naught."

This is all basically false. To the extent that the pedagogical process is itself transformed in the light of scientific knowledge, all idea of the foundation and nature of education has been altered. Above all, the very concept of education has expanded. The concern is not simply with education, but with the "reforging of men," in Trotsky's expression. And this reforging requires, above all, as we have indicated repeatedly, the greatest possible use of the innate substance of behavior.

Therefore, none of the child's reactions must go to waste. William James has said that

> Respect then, I beg you, always the original reactions, even when you are seeking to overcome their connection with certain objects, and to supplant them with others that you wish to make the rule. Bad behavior, from the point of view of the teacher's art, is as good a starting-point as good behavior; in fact, paradoxical as it may sound to say so, it is often a better starting-point than good behavior would be.[8]

Thus does the creative character of the educational process manifest itself with full clarity. Thus does the creative nature of the educational process, directed not towards the simple cultivation of natural data, but towards the creation of "supra-natural" human life, becomes understandable.

In this sense, present-day pedagogics radically diverges from the theory of natural education, which sees the ideal of education in the past. For Tolstoy and for Rousseau, the child constitutes the ideal of harmony, and all subsequent education only spoils the child. For scientific psychology, the child is disclosed as a tragic problem, what with the terrible imbalance and disharmony of his development. Without saying a word of biogenetic parallelism, we may nevertheless declare that the newborn infant is a clot of previous experience, he is unclothed biology, and in the several years of his development he actually has to go through the entire path which mankind has gone through from the apes to the airplane.

The whole difference is that the child has to travel this road on his own two feet and not at all in parallel with the paths of history. Once we bear in mind the incredible vastness of this path, however, it becomes entirely understandable that the child will have to enter into a brutal struggle with the world, and that in this struggle the teacher has to have the final word. That is when we get the idea that teaching is like warfare:

> The science of psychology, and whatever science of general pedagogics may be based on it," says James, "are in fact much like the science of war. Nothing is simpler or more definite than the principles of either ... there would be nothing but victories for the masters of the science, either on the battlefield or in the school-room, if they did not both have to make their application to an incalculable quantity in the shape of the mind of their opponent. The mind of your own enemy, the pupil, is working away from you as keenly and eagerly as is the mind of the commander on the other side from the scientific general.[9]

Thus does pedagogics disclose itself from the standpoint of the battlefield. Zalkind says that since the goods of three-fourths of modern social reflexive installations constitute, because of the chaotic structure of mankind under capitalism, a collection of sociophobias. For this reason the inculcation of a concrete social force in any one individual is *a bitter struggle, now concealed, now explicit, between teacher and student*. Therefore, "sociogogy" (pedagogics, psychotherapy) must not and cannot be politically indifferent. The true sociologist, i.e., teacher is always politically involved. The education of social reflexes constitutes the education of all the individual's social patterns of behavior, i.e., political education. Pedagogics (sociogogy) is never and was never politically indifferent, since, willingly or unwillingly, through its own work on the psyche (social reflexes), it has always adopted a particular social pattern, i.e., political line, in accordance with the dominant social class that has guided its interests.

Therefore, the borders of education have never before spread so far apart as today, when the revolution has undertaken the task of re-educating all of mankind and has created in the midst of its very being a clear-cut direction for education. Bear in mind that the sociogogics of the individual reduces the production of consistent and profound changes in all its socially reflexive settings, i.e., in all its reflexes without exception, since all of them are diminished by the social elements. The education of opinions, of sensations, of knowledge, of drives—all of this is only a partial and improper expression of a single common conception of the education of the individual as a whole, in all his functions, and especially in the social portion of these functions, since the inculcation of definite knowledge, sensations, and so on is, at the same time, the education of a definite *social type of breathing, of digestion, and so on*. Opinions and feelings cannot be isolated from the "organs", neither in a theoretical sense nor in a practical sense, and it is necessary to be done with this fictionalizing as soon as possible.

Let us add to this the fact that such functions of the organism as growth, the formation of bone, and so on also depend to a large degree on public education. Thus, education reveals itself as the greatest problem in the world, the problem of life as creation. It is in this sense that Zalkind is correct when he merges artistic creativity together with every other mental act.

Zalkind also said that other than in quantitative strength, the basic elements of the process of artistic creation do not differ whatsoever from any of the other mental acts, even the simplest. Every impulse in man's mental machinery, the slightest shift in the chain of so-called thoughts, sensations, and so on constitutes an act of social adaptation of the individual, the manifestation of the individual's social struggle for self-preservation. Only a state of social discomfort will induce a change in the mental machinery. Utter happiness would submerge it in deep slumber. The source of every movement of the soul, from the slightest thought to the discovery of a genius, is one and the same.

Every thought that has ever been expressed, every picture that has ever been drawn, every sonata that has ever been composed, has been born out of a state of unease in their originator, who has sought through re-education to change this state of unease into that of the greatest contentment. The greater the intensity in this sense of unease and, at the same time, the more complex the individual's mental mechanism, the more natural and the more insurmountable the peda-gogical eruptions of this unease, the more powerfully do they force their way outside.

The creative person is always from the race of the discontented. This is why education can never be limited to a single faculty. For such dislocations and snags, an inner affinity is needed between teacher and student, they must be close in terms of feelings, and in terms of thinking. Education is a process of mutual and continuous adaptation of both camps, where sometimes it is guide or leader which represents the most active and the most original effective side, and sometimes those who are being led.

A pedagogical process of this sort comes to be a real social world, like the shifting of victory from one side to another in a field of battle, like a tense battle in which the teacher is, in the best of cases, the embodiment of a small part of the class (often he is in a class all by himself). All his personal traits, his entire experience of feelings and thoughts, other than the will, he makes continuous use of in this atmosphere of tense social struggle, this inner pedagogical effort. The chain of his personal dissatisfactions, his discontent, his strivings is adapted and the pedagogical revelations which ensue consequently constitute all told that very chain of artistic creativity which we have sketched just above. The teacher as educator cannot but be an artist. Pure objectivity in the educator is utter nonsense. A teacher who is sober-minded teaches no one.

It should be clear to the reader that the more intense this discontent, which provides the initial push for all movement of the soul, the more intense is the movement itself, and therefore education and creativity are always tragic processes, inasmuch as they always arise out of "discontent," out of troubles, from discord. The world evolves without any particular purpose in mind. It is just for this reason that childhood is the natural time of education, that it is the time of the greatest tragedy, discord, and incompatibility between the individual and the environment. The harmony of education arises out of dissonance, which it thereupon strives to resolve. The older we become and the greater is our sense of fitting in and the greater is our feeling of contentment in the world, the less that remains in us of the creative spirit and the less amenable are we to education.

None of that pedagogics which sugar-coated the "golden time of placid childhood" and sweetened the educational process with rose-colored water lies along our road. On the contrary, we know that the tragedy of childhood is the greatest motive force for education, just as hunger and thirst are the inspirers of the struggle for existence. Education, therefore, must be guided in such a way as not to conceal and not to mask the stern features of the true "discontent" of childhood, but to push the child into a confrontation with this discontent in the sharpest way possible and as often as possible, and to force him to conquer it.

Life then discloses itself as a system of creation, of constant straining and transcendence, of constant invention and the creation of new forms of behavior. Thus, every one of our thoughts, every one of our movements, and all of our experience constitutes a striving toward the creation of a new reality, a breakthrough to something new.

Life becomes creation only when it is finally freed of all the social forms that distort and disfigure it. Questions of education will have been resolved when questions of life will have been solved.

Then man's life will become one of continuous creation, a single esthetic ceremony that will arise not out of a striving toward the satisfaction of isolated little needs, but out of conscious and brilliant creative eruption. Eating and sleeping, love and play, work and politics, every feeling and every thought, all will become the subject of creation. What is now realized within the narrow confines of art will thence infuse all of life, and life will become creative labor.

The infinite potential for the creation of life in its infinite diversity discloses itself to the teacher. Not in the narrow confines of his own personal life and his own personal affairs will one become a true creator in the future. It is then that pedagogics, as the creation of life, will assume the foreground: "Alongside technology," writes Trotsky, "pedagogics, in the broad sense of psychophysical formation of new generations, becomes the domain of social thought. Pedagogical systems will gather about themselves powerful camps. Socially inculcated experience and the competition of diverse methodologies will assume a scope that now cannot even be dreamed of."

Man, finally, has taken it upon himself to make a serious effort to discover a sense of inner harmony. He has given himself the task of instilling in the movement of his own limbs, whether in labor, in walking, or in play, a degree of intelligibility, appropriateness, and economy of the highest order, and, thereby, elegance. He wishes to become master of all the semi-conscious processes in his organism, and then all the unconscious ones as well, such as breathing, the coursing of his bloodstream, digestion, and reproduction, and, within necessary limits, to subordinate them to the dominance of reason and the will.

The human species, which crystallized in the form of *homo sapiens*, once again enters into a process of radical redevelopment and becomes the subject of the most complex methods of artificial selection and psychological conditioning at man's very own hands. This is fully within the realm of development. Man first banished the dark elements from industry and from ideology, supplanting brutish routine with scientific technology and religion with science. Next he drove the unconscious out of politics, having toppled the monarchy and class-conscious democracy and replaced them with apologetic [*ratsionalisticheskii*] parliamentarianism, and then at one fell swoop, by the transparent Soviet dictatorship. The blind element had firmly lodged in economic relationships, but man chucked it out through the socialist organization of labor.

Finally, in the deepest and darkest corner of the unconscious, in the spontaneous well-springs, in the underground of our soul, we find the nature of man himself concealed. Isn't it clear that the greatest efforts of analytic thought and of creative initiative will be led in just this direction? The human species did not cease crawling about on all fours in front of god, tsar, and capital just so that it could then bend down submissively before the dark laws of heredity and blind sexual selection! The free man wishes to attain the greatest sense of balance in the workings of his organs, the most uniform development and use of his own tissues, in order to, at one fell swoop, bring the fear of death within the realm of the organism's appropriate reactions to danger. For otherwise there can be little doubt that man's extreme disharmony, the extraordinary anatomical and physiological unevenness in the development and use of man's organs and tissues impart to living instinct an unhealthy, pinched, hysterical fear of death which obscures reason and feeds foolish and humiliating fantasies of life after death.

Man has set himself the goal of becoming master of his own feelings, of lifting the instincts to the heights of consciousness and making them transparent, of stretching the thread of will into what is concealed and into the underground, and to thereby lift himself up to a new stage, to create a "higher" sociobiological type, a, so to speak, super-man.

---

[1] Collection of rules of behavior composed in the mid-16th century for people living in towns to guide them in their dealings with the church and secular authorities, with family members, and with their servants; cf bibliography (trans.).

[2] Hugo Münsterberg, *Psychology and the Teacher*, page 316.

[3] *Ibid.*, page 317.

[4] *Ibid.*, page 320.

[5] *Ibid.*, page 321.

[6] The Russian word for school, *shkola*, like its English cognate is derived from the ancient Greek *scholé*, which originally meant a "halt, hence a rest or leisure, hence employment for leisure" (Eric Partridge, *Origins* New York, Macmillan, 1959, page 594) (trans.)

[7] *Op. cit*, page 317.

[8] William James, *Talks to Teachers*, page 45-46.

[9] *Ibid.*, page 16-17.

HISTORICAL NOTES

The following biographical notes on writers referred to in the text have been drawn from a variety of secondary sources, in English as well as in Russian, French, and German. They are intended to give the reader an idea of the intellectual climate which served as the background for the present book, as well as the source of many of the thoughts the author wove together in this study of educational psychology from minds in the then-new field of educational psychology as well as from researchers in psychology, physiology, philosophy, and literary criticism. Poets and short story writers also provided inspiration to Vygotsky's thought.

Aall, Anathon (1867-1943), Norwegian anti-Hegelian philosopher specializing in the history of philosophy and psychology. Aall viewed psychology as an empirical science.

Aikhen'vald, Yuli, Russian literary critic, author of studies on Tolstoy and Pushkin, a monograph on Russia writers, and another monograph on Western writers. Vygotsky's professor at the pre-revolutionary Shanyavsky People's University, a non-degree granting community established by scholars who had resigned from Moscow Imperial University in protest against widespread expulsion of student protestors. Aikhen'vald was sent into exile in 1922 together with other non-Marxist writers (see *Literary Gazette International*, 1:11, August 1990, page 8).

Andreev, Leonid Nikolaevich (1871-1919), Russian short story writer, playwright, and novelist, friend of Gorki and member of Znanie group. His early work was in the trend of critical realism and expressed a sympathy with democratic hopes, though his later stories and other works evinced a loss of faith in reason and in the chance of a restructuring of life. His heroes' dissatisfaction with life gradually turned into passivity or anarchist and nihilist revolt, and in his last dramas irrational forces triumph, and reason is helpless.

Bekhterev, Vladimir Mikhaelovich (1867-1927), Russian and Soviet physiologist, neurologist, and psychologist. Constructed a science of behavior that viewed behavior as a system of reflexes underlying both mental and social activity. Bekhterev referred to this science first as objective psychology, then as psycho-reflexology, and finally, as reflexology. The latter he also opposed to empirical, subjective psychology. See, in English translation, *General Principles of Human Reflexology*, London, 1933.

Binet, Alfred (1857-1911), French psychologist, concerned with thinking processes in children and with the notion of intelligence and individual differences. With Theodore Simon, devised a scale for the measurement of intelligence for the French Ministry of Public Instruction in 1904. See, in English translation, *The Psychology of Reasoning*, Chicago, 1899.

Blonskii, Pavel Petrovich (1884-1941), Soviet psychologist, educational reformer and historian of ancient and modern philosophy. Author of studies on child psychology and the development of memory and thinking, and pedagogy. In educational psychology, he was a follower of William James. He wrote of the need to replace scholastic methods of instruction with methods that answered the needs of industrial society, and suggested industrial work as the basis of Soviet education. In *Trudovaya Shkola (The Labor School)* (1919) he set forth the concept of a trade school. He viewed learning as involving the development of new qualities on the foundation of the child's innate capacities.

Bühler, Karl (1879-1963), Austrian psychologist, adherent of the Wurzburg trend in psychology, specializing in the psychology of thinking and perception, and developmental psychology. Bühler viewed behavior as consisting in triads, believing that Freud's conception of pleasure as consisting in satisfaction presented only one-third of the phenomenon, the two pleasures of functioning and of creating being the other two thirds, and defined speech and behavior in general as likewise triadic. He maintained the teleological orientation of the Würzburg school, seeing a biological orientation in the development of the child's psyche.

Buridan, Jean (1295-1356), French philosopher and scientist, attempted an "axiomatic derivation of the laws of valid deduction". The quandary of Buridan's ass referred to in the text (Chapter 9) is not found in his writings, but is based on an analogy from Aristotle that Buridan commented upon. See the article on Buridan in *The Encyclopedia of Philosophy*, Paul Edwards, ed., I, 428.

Burt, Sir Cyril Ludowic (1883-1971), British psychologist in the area of intelligence. Much of the data on which his results relied have since been shown to have been deliberately falsified. (*"Burt Affair"*, *Encounter* 12/89)

Ebbinghaus, Hermann (1850-1909), German experimental psychologist in the area of learning and memory, developed methods for the study of memory based on an associative approach. His results involving the use of nonsense syllables played an important role in the study of association and learning. He discovered a law that describes the rate at which learned material is forgotten.

Frank, Semyon Lyudvigovich (1877-1950), Soviet philosopher, author of The *Soul of Man* (1917).

Froebel, Friedrich (1782-1852), German educator who saw the goal of education in the development of the individual's innate potentiality, with the teacher responsible for assisting the child as guide in reaching his or her potential without coercion or reliance on pre-conceived molds. He viewed play as a spontaneous expression of thoughts and feelings, and as critical for learning, and was thus led to develop kindergartens. See, in English translation, *Friedrich Froebel: A Selection From His Writings*, Irene M. Lilley (ed.), Cambridge, Cambridge University Press, 1967.

Gershenzon, Mikhail Osipovich (1869-1925), Russian historian in the area of literature and social thought, author of works on Russian revolutionaries and the conflict between Western and native influences in the development of Russian culture. In studies on Pushkin and Turgenev, he presented a theory of creativity which viewed it as originating in the irrational, and also discussed a method of "slow reading."

Goethe, Johann Wolfgang (1749-1832), German poet, visionary, and natural scientist. Author of a study of visual perception.

Griboedov, Aleksandr Sergeevich (1795-1829), Russian Playwright, diplomat, and author or the comedy, *Gore ot uma* (translated as *Wit Works Woe* (1933), which is considered among the greatest of Russian works of literature, both in terms of style and content. It is one of the major sources of the modern Russian literary language and many of its lines have even become popular idioms. A sympathizer of the Decembrists' aborted revolution of 1825 against the Tsarist regime, he was jailed for several months on suspicion of active involvement, though upon release was permitted to rejoin the diplomatic service, and two years later was sent on a sensitive mission to Teheran, where he was killed when a mob instigated by local mullahs and British agents sacked the Russian legation. His play, *Wit Works Woe* was censored and could not be published in full until 1862, circulating instead in thousands of manuscript copies. It satirizes the upper classes of Tsarist Russia, where the barbary, pomposity, and careerism of the serf owners comes up against the progressive movement in the person recently returned from several years stay abroad who, consequently is able to see through the pretense of the aristocracy, as an "outsider," or "superfluous man." Griboedov was also the author of a number of other plays that espoused the ideas of the Decembrists.

Groos, Karl (1861-1946), German psychologist in the area of genetic psychology, developed a theory of play, according to which games constitute a school that prepares the individual for critical experiences. See, in English translation, *Play of Man*, New York, Appleton, 1901.

Guyau, Marie Jean (1854-1888), French philosopher, proponent of positivism and utilitarianism, author of studies on aesthetics, morality, and religion. He viewed art as a biological phenomenon, the result of an excess of vital forces which nevertheless requires intense labor. He believed the measure of a mental phenomenon could be found in its usefulness for biological functioning, similarly that morality ensured the balance of vital forces.

Haeckel, Ernst Heinrich (1834-1919), German zoologist and philosopher, among the first to propagate the theory of organic evolution in Germany. He formulated the "biogenetic law" in his book, *The Riddle of the Universe*, which in English translation (New York, 1900) became a best-seller. He was opposed to "pure metaphysics," as well as "pure empiricism," holding that empiricism and rationalism are both necessary for knowledge.

Herbart, Johann Friedrich (1776-1841) German philosopher, psychologist, and educator. In opposition to the psychology of capacities and Kantian doctrines, he conceived of the mind as consisting of an apperception mass of mental states, and the unconscious as consisting of ideas existing in a static state but with a force associated with each; an unconscious idea could reach consciousness if the force associated with it was strong enough to counter forces in the apperception mass; he believed that this interaction could be measured mathematically. See, in English translation, *Application of Psychology to Science of Teaching*, New York, 1898.

Hering, Ewald (1834-1918), German physiologist and psychologist who studied the nature of visual space perception and the theory of color vision. He also discovered that the judgement of warm vs. cold in an object was based on the relative, rather than absolute, temperature of the skin. He was the author of a study that conceived memory to be a special function of organized matter. See, in English translation, *On Memory and the Specific Energies of the Nervous System*, Chicago, 1905.

Ivanov-Razumnik pseud, (Ivanov, Vasil'evich) (1878-1946), Russian literary critic and historian, leader of Scythians, a literary group, and editor of the literary journal *Skify*. Author of studies on Blok, Belyi, Russian social thought, the relationship between literature and society, and the intelligentsia. For comments on his works, see *A Soviet Heritic: Essays by Yevgeny Zamyatin*. Edited and translated by Mirra Ginsburg. Univ. Chicago Press, 1970.

James, William (1842-1910), American physiologist, philosopher, and psychologist. He viewed the mind as consisting in functional, adaptive mental processes that aid the person in adapting to his or her surroundings, and suggested studying mental and emotional activities as processes, rather than static elements. James (and, independently, Carl Georg Lange) developed a physiological explanation of the emotions and feelings whereby the latter were viewed as the consequence of organic changes in the form of reflexes in response to stimulation.

Kerschensteiner, Georg (1854-1932), German educator, author of works on vocational education that presented vocational education as a tool for the government to reconcile the conflict between the different social strata. He believed that schools for the children of the poor should foster a spirit of diligence, and obedience and subordination, and that trade schools are needed for workers' children who leave regular school early to take up work, in order to counter the influence of the "unhealthy" ideas they meet up with on the job with patriotic sentiments. Selected works of his were translated into Russian early in the First World War.

Köhler, Wolfgang (1887-1967), German and American zoologist and psychologist, and founder of gestalt psychology. In his book, *The Mentality of Apes* (1917), which Vygotsky (with A.L. Luria) reviewed extensively in the book, *Studies in the History of Behavior - Ape, Primitive Man, Child* (1930). Köhler showed that gestalt theory could help in understanding the behavior of apes, particularly as seen in their problem-solving behavior. He also carried out experimental studies of perception.

Kornilov, Konstantin Nikolaevich (1879-1957), Soviet psychologist. He led the struggle against idealist psychology, reflexology, and American behaviorism in Soviet psychology. The theory of reactology or reaction psychology which he developed consisted of an eclectic mixture of Marxist principles together with mechanistic and energy-based concepts, in which reaction, a biosocial phenomenon, was understood to refer to all response movements rather than just a reflex, including, in particularly, complex forms of human behavior, and in this way he was able to distinguish between psychology and physiology.

Kraepelin, Emil (1855-1926), German psychiatrist who broke down the range of mental disorders into dementia praecox and manic-depressive psychosis, further subdividing them into subtypes. He believed mental disorders to be predetermined, basically biological in nature, with physiological malfunctioning, rather than psychological factors, constituting the principle cause.

Kretschmer, Ernst (1888-1968), German psychiatrist, constructed a typology according to which four basic types of body structure and physiology were correlated with different forms of mental illness, and, thereby, personality in general. He also wrote on child and adolescent psychopathology. See, in English translation, *Physique and Character*, New York, 1926.

Krylov, Ivan Andreevich (1769(8)-1844), Russian author of fables and plays. His early works ridiculed the corruption of the upper classes and despotism, and he was consequently forced to flee Moscow and live incognito for several years. Upon his returning, he started to write satires of the nobility's francophilism, but shortly afterwards turned to fables. In his fables, which employed a highly picturesque style, satire was usually uppermost rather than there being any definite moral present. They tended to express popular views of social injustice and attacked the autocratic rule and predatory nature of the Czarist bureaucracy, and the evils of egotism. An English translation of a collection of his fables may be found in xxx.

Lange, Carl Georg (1834-1900), Danish physician and psychologist, author of a theory of the emotions that resembled that put forward by William James in his *Principle of Psychology*, though unlike James for division between "emotion" which Lange saw as consisting in joy, sorrow, fear, anger, and the like, as opposed to passion, for example love, hate, admiration, and so on. For Lange, emotional experience followed the perception of the activity of the circulatory system. See, in English translation, *The Emotions*, Baltimore, 1922, originally published in 1884.

Lange, Nikolai Nikolaevich (1858-1921), Russian psychologist, proponent of a natural science approach in the investigation of mental functions such as perception and attention. He propounded a genetic and biological approach to the study of these functions, formulating a law of perception relating phase character of perception and the direction of phase shifts from generalized sensory images to increasingly differentiated images and developing a motor theory of attention according to which attention was a motor reaction intended to improve the conditions of perception.

Lazarev, Petr Petrovich (1878-1942), Soviet physicist, biophysicist, and geophysicist, worked out a physico-chemical theory of sensation, called the "ionic theory of the sensations," and the thesis that the central nervous system adapts to external stimuli, and investigated the process of physiological adaptation in vision, hearing, and taste.

Lesgaft, Peter Frantsevich (1837-1909), Russian educator and physician, leader in the development of public education and night schools for workers, and in opening up public education to women and in the development of centers of physical education. His conception of physical education assumed a unity of man's mental and physical development and a unity of form and function which he viewed as fundamental in his theory of functional anatomy. The relation between neuromuscular activity and mental signs led Lesgaft to view directed exercise as a means of mental, moral, and aesthetic education. He attempted to base pedagogy on the foundations of anatomy, physiology, and psychology, and thereby to turn it into a science.

Meumann, Ernst (1862-1915), German educator and psychologist. He carried out experimental studies of memory in children, and also constructed a synthesis of different psychological concepts of the development of the child for use in a theory of education. Meumann was also the author of studies in aesthetics.

Münsterburg, Hugo (1863-1916), German and American psychologist, one of the founders of applied psychology, particularly educational psychology, economic psychology, and forensic psychology.

Ovsyanniko-Kulikovskii, Dmitrii Nikolaevich (1853-1920), Russian literary critic and linguist. He was one of the first to study Sanscrit and Vedic mythology and philosophy in Russia, and was also the author of studies on the syntax of Russian. Following Potebnya, he claimed that language possesses a capacity for primordial representation, and developed the concept of an analogy between the word and a work of art, as well as pointing out the resemblance of scientific and artistic creativity. The psychology of creativity constituted the core of his work.

Pavlov, Ivan Petrovich (1849-1936), Russian and Soviet physiologist.

Pestalozzi, Johann Heinrich (1746-1827), Swiss educational reformer who saw the need for the education of intellectual, physical, and moral capacities, and the use of spontaneous events and planned work in the classroom. He opposed the use of rote learning, and suggested that students should understand each step or principle in a lesson before more complex material is presented. See, in English translation, *Pestalozzi's Educational Writings*, 1912.

Potebnya, Aleksandr Afanas'evich (1835-1891), Ukrainian and Russian linguist in literature, folklore, ethnology, as well as general linguistics and follower of Alexander von Humboldt. He viewed the "thought-speech act" as a creative mental event, and language, interpreted as a social element, as "objectified thought".

Rossolimo, Grigorii Ivanovich (1860-1928), Soviet psychoneurologist specializing in the anatomy and physiology of the nervous system, and numerous inventor of medical instruments. He constructed a battery of experimental tests to establish the state of mental functions in persons affected by different types of brain lesions, attempting to correlate psychological profiles with pathological state.

Rubinshtein, Sergei Leonidovich (1889-1960), Soviet psychologist who emphasized the close relationship between consciousness and praxis, as embodied in four principles, that mind was a function of material reality, that the psyche was a result of evolution and amenable to further change, that consciousness and praxis exist in a unity, and that theory and praxis also exist in a unity.

Sechenov, Ivan Mikhaelovich (1829-1905), founder of Russian physiology and a psychologist. Discovered how spinal reflexes are modified and inhibited by the central nervous system, specifically by cerebral effects. He also studied the feedback control of movement. For Sechenov, not only behavior, but consciousness as well, is composed of reflexes as its elemental constituent, and that the central issues of psychology could be resolved by means of the objective and natural scientific methods of physiology, rather than by philosophy. See, in English translation, *Selected Works*, Moscow, 1835.

Sherrington, Charles Scott (1857-1952), English physiologist in the area of sensory psychology, particularly tactual and muscular senses, conceived the notion of proprioceptor exterioceptor, and interioceptor. He introduced the concept of the integrative action of the nervous system based on a view of the reflex act as an integral process serving the function of adaptation, and discovered the phenomenon of reciprocal innervation as an element of the integration of neural activity, Sherrington saw the mind as a special essence not reducible to the functioning of the brain. His work served as a basis for Pavlov's study of conditional reflexes.

Shestov, Lev, pseud. (Schwarzmann, Lev Isaakovich) (1866-1938), Russian existentialist philosopher and author of studies of literary criticism on Shakespeare, Tolstoy, Dostoyevsky and Pascal.   In these studies Shestov illustrated particular themes in philosophy by reference to particular literary characters, in a "philosophy of tragedy," or "philosophy of the commonplace," that shifted the point of view of philosophical discourse from the universe to the individual. Shestov was also the author of major studies on Kierhegaard and on existentialist philosophy. His works display a mastery of paradox and aphorism.

Simon, Theodore (1873-1961), French psychiatrist, author of study of the correlation of physical development in children and intellectual capacity. He investigated children with disabilities in a laboratory of physiological psychology, which he invited Alfred Binet to join. Simon collaborated with Binet in the development of intelligence tests.

Sologub, Fedor pseud. (Fedor Kuz'mich Teternikov) (1863-1927). Soviet literary critic. See essay on Sologub by Yevgeny Zamyatin in *A Soviet Heretic: Essays by Yevgeny Zamyatin*, edited and translated by Mirra Ginsburg, University of Chicago Press, 1970, pp. 217-223.

Spinoza (Spinoza d'Espinosa), Baruch (Benedict) (1632-1677), Dutch-Jewish materialist philosopher ostracized by the Jewish community for his rationalist views and kept from assuming a teaching position at the university by the secular authorities. He viewed human beings as reflecting the same psychophysical parallelism that pervades the universe, believing that the two aspects of mind and body are basically one. He believed in natural causes for human actions, and that knowledge liberates the individual from external nature, enabling him to act in the light of necessity.

Steinach, E., author of articles on studies on mechanical stimulation of reflex in the frog which showed that the threshold value of the stimulation was less when the stimulus was applied to skin instead of to a cutaneous afferent nerve [cited by Sherrington].

Stern, William Lewis (1871-1938), German philosopher and psychologist in the area of child psychology and differential psychology. He attempted a synthesis, or reconciliation, between the scientific and philosophical approaches to human beings that would lead to a science of the total human individual in which the person would be viewed as a unique being. Stern also devised the notion of "intelligence quotient" from Binet's concept of mental age by dividing the latter by the child's chronological age.

Thorndike, Edward Lee (1874-1949), American psychologist in the area of animal intelligence and learning in children, developed the theory of connectionism, holding that there were connections between situations and responses, rather than associations between ideas. He discovered the law of effect (similar to Pavlov's law of reinforcement), according to which a response tendency could be stamped in or out, based on rewards or punishments.

Titchener, Edward Bradford (1867-1927), English and American psychologist who emphasized the human mind in general as the subject of psychology, as opposed to individual minds, and eschewed applications, whether of treatment or improvement. His method of study was that of introspection. He viewed consciousness as consisting in the states of sensation and imagery, and of effective states, and subsequently investigated dimensional attributes (quality, intensity, etc.), of mental life, as opposed to specific elements.

Ukhtomskii, (Prince) Aleksei Alekseevich (1884-1941), Russian and Soviet physiologist. Developed the concept of dominant as a special functional system, or constellation of processes in the nervous system, viewing it as the physiological mechanism of the organization and regulation of behavior. His study of the dominant and of learned rhythm (that the functioning of an organ recalls the rhythm of external stimuli) led him to a novel conception of the nature of fatigue. In physiology, he worked on the concept of a functional system and of the history of a system around the same time as Vygotsky.

Vagner [Wagner], Vladimir Aleksandrovich (1849-1934), biologist and psychologist, founder of animal psychology and comparative psychology in Russia, radical Social Darwinist. Vagner studied instincts in animals from an objective approach and showed that the mental regulation of behavior manifests itself in distinctive fashion. He criticized both anthropomorphist approaches to the study of animal instinct, and purely physiological interpretations that ignored psychological factors. He also suggested classifying patterns of behavior on a scale of evolutionary emergence.

Wundt, Wilhelm (1832-1920), German physiologist, founder of structuralism, a school of psychology that employed introspection as a means of analyzing conscious processes into basic elements, which he called sensations, which he then classified by modality, intensity and duration, and feelings, and then placed along three continua, that of pleasure-displeasure, that of tension-relaxation, and that of excitement-depression, and synthesized in creative fashion, through what he turned apperception, into a new unit, or psychic resultant.

Zalkind, Aron Borisovich (1888-1936), Soviet educator and psychiatrist working in mental health and early advocate of Freudian theory who spoke of the need for Party activists to pursue a psychologically healthy work routine. Author of a monograph on the culture of revolutionary epochs.

Zavadovskii, Boris Mikhaelovich (1895-1951), Soviet biologist specializing in the study of natural selection, the methodology of biology, and the endocrine system.

Note: These notes are drawn from, in order of frequency of use, *Great Soviet Encyclopedia*, 1970; Corsini, *Oxford Companion to Mind*; *French Biographical Dictionary*; *Dictionary of Scientific Biography*, Joravsky, *Vygotskii, Collected Works*.

BIBLIOGRAPHY

The following bibliography has been reconstructed from the few references in the text to specific works; from works quoted in the text by reference to their authors without, however, the page numbers, and sometimes even the titles, being given, but for which passages corresponding to the translation into Russian were located; and works which can be reasonably assumed to be the source of quotations given in the text, or of discussion with reference to a particular author, but for which the corresponding passage in the original could not be found. (In the present text, these "quotations" are given in translation from the Russian without bibliographic information.) Dates of publication into Russian are given for non-Russian texts that were translated prior to publication of the original text (1926), and English translations (generally the most recent one) are given where they exist.

Andreev, Leonid Nikolaevich. *"Darkness,"* translated by (originally published 1907).

Bekhterev, Vladimir Mikhaelovich. *General Principles of Human Reflexology*, London, 1933.

-----*Voprosy izuchenii trude (Questions in the Study of Labor*. St. Petersburg, 1922.

Binet, Alfred and Simon, Theodore. *The Development of Intelligence in Children*, New York, Armo, 1973 (Russian translation ,1911).

Blonskii, Pavel Petrovich. *Trudovaya Shkola (The Work Study School)*. 1919.

-----*Ocherki nauchnoi psikhologii (Outline of Scientific Psychology)*. 1921.

-----*Pedalogiya (Child Psychology)*. Moscow, 1925.

Buhler, Karl. *The Mental Development of the Child*, translated by Oscar Oesner. London, Routledge & Kegan Paul, 1930.

Chekhov, Anton Pavlovich. "Exclamation Point," "A Horsey Tale," "The House" in: Chukovskii, Kornei. *Crocodile*, translated by Richard Coe, London, Faber and Faber, 1964.

Dostoyevskii, Fedor Mikhaelovich. *The Idiot*, translated by Davi Magarshack. New York, Penguin, 1955.

-----*Crime and Punishment*, translated by Jessie Coulson. New York, Norton, 1964.

-----*House of the Dead*, translated by David McDuff. London, Penguin, 1985.

Ebbinghaus, Hermann. *Memory*, translated by Henry A. Ruger and Clara E. Bussenius. New York, Teacher's College, Columbia University, 1913.

Freud, Sigmund. *Psychopathology of Everyday Life*, translated by Alan Tyson. New York, Norton, 1966.

Frank, Semyon Lyudvigovich. *Dusha cheloveka (The Soul of Man)* Moscow, 1917.

Froebel, Friedrich. *A Selection from his Writings,* translated by Irene Lilley. London, Cambridge University Press, 1967.

Gaupp, Robert. *Psychologie des kindes (Psychology of Children)*. Leipzig, 1908 (Russian translation 1909).

Gessen, Sergei Iosifovich. *Osnovy pedagogiki (Foundations of Pedagogics)*. Berlin, 1923.

Gogol, Nikolai Vasilevich, *Dead Souls*, translated by George Reavey. New York, Norton, 1985.

-----*The Government Inspector*, translated by Constance Garnett. New York, Knopf, 1927.

Griboedov, Aleksandr Sergeevich. *The Misfortune of Being Clever*, translated by S. W. Pring. London, 1914, (also translated as Wit Works Woe , 1933.)

Groos, Karl. *The Play of Man*, translated into English by Elizabeth Baldwin. New York, Appleton, 1901.

Haeckel, Ernst Heinrich. *The Riddle of the Universe*, translated by Joseph McCabe. New York, 1900.

Herbart, Johann Friedrich. *Outline of Educational Doctrine*, translated by Alexis F. Lange. Folcroft, PA, Folcroft, 1977.(1898).

Ivanov-Razumnik pseud. (Ivanov, R. Vasil'evich). *History of Russian Social Thought (Istoriya russkoi obshchestvennoi)*. St. Petersburgi, M. M. Stasiulevich, 1907.

James, William. "What is an Emotion," Mind, 9, 1884, pp. 188-205; *Principles of Psychology*. Cambridge, Harvard University Press, 1890 (Russian translation 1902); *Talks to Teachers on Psychology and to Students on Some of Life's Ideals*. Cambridge, Harvard University Press, 1899, 1983

Jefferson, Joseph. *Rip Van Winkle as Played by Joseph Jefferson*. Toronto, George N. Morang, 1899.

Kerschensteiner, Georg. *The Idea of the Industrial School*, translated by Rudolf Pinter. New York, The Macmillan Company, 1913 (Russian translation 1918).

Key, Ellen. *The Century of the Child*, translated by, Francis Maro. New York, G.P. Putnam, 1909 (sections reprinted separately as The Education of the Child with introduction by Edward Bok, 1910).

Kohler, Wolfgang. *The Mentality of Apes*, translated by Ella Winter. New York, Vintage, 1917, 1959 (Russian translation 1930).

Kornilov, Konstantin Nikolaevich. *Ocherk psikhologii rebenka doshkolnogo vozrasta (Outline of the Psychology of the Pre-school Child*. Moscow, 1922.

Korolenko, Vladimir Galaktionovich. *The Blind Musician*, translated by Aline Delano. Boston, Little, Brown, 1890 (Westport, Conn., Greenwood, 1970).

Kretschmer, Ernst. *Physique and Character*, translated by W. J. H. Sprott. London, Routledge & Kegan Paul Ltd., 1925.

Krylov, Ivan Andreevich, "The Dragon Fly and the Ant," "The Wolf Against the Hunter," "The Fox and the Raven," in :*Krilof and His Fables*, translated by W.R.S. Ralston. London, Strahan & Co., 1869, 1920. Fables by M.J. Krylov. Translated into French from Complete Edition of 1825, 1828.

Lange, Carl Georg. *The Emotions*, translated from the authorized German translation by Dr. H. Karella of the Danish original by Istar A. Haupt. New York, Hafner, 1967 (originally published 1885).

Lange, Nikolai Nikolaevich. *Psychological Studies (Psikhologicheskie issledovaniya)*. Odessa 1893.

Lazarev, Petr Petrovich. *Soch., vols. 1-3*. Moscow-Leningrad, 1950-57.

Marshall, H. R.. *Pain, Pleasure, and Aesthetics*. New York, 1894.

Marx, Karl. *Capital*, translated by S. Moore, E. Aveling, and E. Untermann. Chicago, C.H. Kerr & Company, 1908-1909.

Meumann, Ernst. *Vorlesungen zur einführung in die experimentelle Pedagogik und ihre psychologische Grundlagen, (Projects at Experimental Pedagogics and their psychological Basis)*. Leipzig, W. Engelmann, 1907. (Russian translation 1914, 1917).

-----*Intelligenz und Wille, (Intelligence and Will)*.Leipzig, Quelle & Meyer, 1908 (Russian translation 1917).

Münsterberg, Hugo. *Psychology and the Teacher*. New York, D.Appleton, 1909 (Russian translation 1911).

Natorp, Paul. *Sozialpaedogogik (Public Education)*. Stuttgart, F. Frommann (E. Hauff), 1899. (Russian translation 1911).

Ovsyanniko-Kulikovskii, Dmitrii. *History of the Russian Intelligentsia (Istoriya russkoi intelligentsii)*. 1906-11.

Pavlov, Ivan. *The scientific investigation of the psychical faculties or processes in higher animals: the Huxley lecture on recent advances in science and their bearing on science and surgery.*

.Pushkin, Aleksandr Sergeevich. *Eugene Onegin,* translated by Charles Johnston. New York, Viking, 1978; *The Avaricious Knight,* Cambridge University Press, 1933.

Rousseau, Jean-Jacques. *Emile,* translated by Eleanor Worthington. Boston, Heath, 1906.

Rubinshtein, M. M. *Ocherk pedagogicheshkoi psikhologii v svyazi obshchem pedagogike (Outline of Pedagogical Psychology in Relation to General Pedagogics).* Moscow, 1916.

-----*Esteticheskoe vospitanie (Esthetic Education).* Moscow, [before 1923].

Sechenov, Ivan Mikhaelovich, *Selected Physiological and Psychological Works,* translated by S. Belsky. Moscow, Foreign Languages Publishing, 1965.

Shcherbina, A. M.. *Slepoi muzykant Korolenko (Korolenko's Blind Musician).* Moscow, 1916.

Sherrington, Charles Scott. *Integrative Action of the Nervous System.* New Haven, Yale University Press, 1947 (originally published in 1906).

Sologub, Fedor pseud. (Fedor Kuz'mich Teternikov). *The Petty Demon,* translated by S. D. Cioran. Ann Arbor, Ardis, 1983.

Stowe, Harriet Beecher. *Uncle Tom's Cabin.* Crowell, 1890.

Tagore, Rabindranath. *Personality.* New York, Macmillan, 1917. (Russian translation 1922).

Thorndike, Edward Lee. *Educational Psychology,* New York, Teacher's College. Columbia University, 1913-14.

Vygotsky, L. S. "Biogeneticheskii zakon" ("The Biogenetic Law"). Bol'shaya Sovetsk. Ents., Vol. VI (1927), pp. 275-279.

-----*Psychology of Art,* (originally completed 1925)

-----and Luria, Aleksandr Romanovich. *Etyudy po istorii povedeniya: obeq'yan, primitiv, rebenok (Studies on the History of Behavior: Ape, Primitive Man, Child).* Moscow, 1930.

Zalkind, Aron Borisovich. "Freidizm i marksizm" ("Freudian Theories and Marxism"). *Krasnaya Nov'*, No. 4, 1924.

INDEX